# Outcome Assessment in
# Advanced Practice Nursing

**Ruth M. Kleinpell**, PhD, RN-CS, FAAN, FAANP, FCCM, is currently the director of the Center for Clinical Research and Scholarship at Rush University Medical Center and a professor at Rush University College of Nursing in Chicago, Illinois. In addition, she is a nurse practitioner at Mercy Hospital and Medical Center in Chicago, Illinois. She received her diploma in nursing from Lutheran Medical Center School of Nursing, Cleveland, Ohio, and her baccalaureate, master's, and doctoral degrees in nursing from the University of Illinois College of Nursing, Chicago, Illinois. She received her Acute Care Nurse Practitioner certification at Rush University College of Nursing. Dr. Kleinpell is known for her work on outcomes research and has presented and published in the areas of assessing outcomes of advanced practice nursing, outcomes research, and other areas of nursing practice. She is a fellow of the American Academy of Nursing, the American Academy of Nurse Practitioners, the Institute of Medicine of Chicago, and the American College of Critical Care Medicine. Most recently, she received the 2012 Sigma Theta Tau International Nurse Researcher Hall of Fame Award.

# Outcome Assessment in Advanced Practice Nursing

## Third Edition

RUTH M. KLEINPELL, PHD, RN-CS, FAAN, FAANP, FCCM

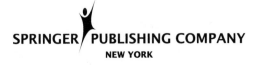

SPRINGER PUBLISHING COMPANY

NEW YORK

Springer Publishing Company, LLC
11 West 42nd Street
New York, NY 10036
www.springerpub.com

*Acquisitions Editor*: Margaret Zuccarini
*Production Editor*: Michael O'Connor
*Composition*: Newgen Imaging

*ISBN*: 978–0-8261–1047-3
*e-book ISBN*: 978–0-8261–1048-0

13 14 15 16 / 5 4 3 2 1

The author and the publisher of this Work have made every effort to use sources believed to be reliable to provide information that is accurate and compatible with the standards generally accepted at the time of publication. The author and publisher shall not be liable for any special, consequential, or exemplary damages resulting, in whole or in part, from the readers' use of, or reliance on, the information contained in this book. The publisher has no responsibility for the persistence or accuracy of URLs for external or third-party Internet websites referred to in this publication and does not guarantee that any content on such websites is, or will remain, accurate or appropriate.

Library of Congress Cataloging-in-Publication Data

Outcome assessment in advanced practice nursing / [edited by] Ruth M. Kleinpell. — 3rd ed.
    p. ; cm.
  Includes bibliographical references and index.
  ISBN 978-0-8261-1047-3 — ISBN 978-0-8261-1048-0 (e-ISBN)
  I. Kleinpell, Ruth M.
  [DNLM: 1. Advanced Practice Nursing—standards. 2. Outcome Assessment (Health Care)
3. Nurse Clinicians—standards. 4. Nurse Practitioners—standards.  WY 128]

  610.7306′92—dc23                                                                 2013000627

# Contents

# Contributors

**Anne W. Alexandrov, PhD, RN, CCRN, ANVP-BC, FAAN**
Assistant Dean and Professor
Doctor of Nursing Practice Program
  Director
Program Director, NET SMART
  Neurovascular APN Fellowship
  Program
University of Alabama at
  Birmingham
Birmingham, AL

**Rhonda Arthur, DNP, CNM, FNP, WHNP**
Director of Family Nursing
Frontier Nursing University
Hyden, KY

**Denise Bryant-Lukosius, RN, PhD**
Associate Professor
School of Nursing and Department of
  Oncology
McMaster University
Hamilton, ON
Canada

**Suzanne M. Burns, RN, MSN, RRT, ACNP, CCRN, FAAN, FCCM, FAANP**
Professor Emeritus
School of Nursing
University of Virginia
Consultant, Critical and Progressive
  Care Nursing and Clinical Nursing
  Research
Charlottesville, VA

**Margaret Faut Callahan, PhD, CRNA, FNAP, FAAN**
Professor and Dean
Marquette University College of
  Nursing
Milwaukee, WI

**Tamara Harrison Chaker, RN, MSN**
Acute Care Nurse Practitioner
David Geffen School of Medicine
University of California Los Angeles
  Medical Center
Ahmanson Cardiomyopathy Center
Los Angeles, CA

**Renée Charbonneau-Smith, RN, MScN**
Canadian Centre for Advanced Practice
   Nursing Research (CCAPNR)
McMaster University School of
   Nursing
Hamilton, ON
Canada

**Catherine C. Cohen, BSN, RN**
Columbia University School of Nursing
New York, NY

**Julie Creaser, RN, MN**
Clinical Nurse Specialist
David Geffen School of Medicine
University of California Los Angeles
   Medical Center
Ahmanson-UCLA Cardiomyopathy
   Center
Los Angeles, CA

**Judy E. Davidson, DNP RN CNS FCCM**
Director
Research Integration and Management
Clinical Research Services, Scripps
   Health
La Jolla, CA

**Alba DiCenso, RN, PhD**
Professor
School of Nursing and Department of
   Epidemiology and Biostatistics
McMaster University
Hamilton, ON
Canada

**Virginia Erickson, RN, PhD**
Coordinator, Staff Nurse
   Evidence-Based Practice
   Fellowship
Department of Nursing
Nursing Research and Education
Ronald Reagan UCLA Medical Center
Los Angeles, CA

**Kevin D. Frick, PhD**
Professor
Department of Health Policy and
   Management
Johns Hopkins Bloomberg School of
   Public Health
Baltimore, MD

**Anna Gawlinski, RN, DNSc, FAAN**
Adjunct Professor
UCLA School of Nursing
Department of Nursing
Nursing Research and Education
Ronald Reagan UCLA Medical Center
Los Angeles, CA

**Mary Jo Goolsby, EdD, MSN, NP-C, CAE, FAANP**
Vice President
Research, Education, and Professional
   Practice
American Association of Nurse
   Practitioners
Austin, TX

**Roger Green, DNP, FNP, FAANP**
Family Nurse Practitioner
Palm Springs, CA

**Saadia Israr, MMI**
Program Manager
Canadian Centre for Excellence
   in Oncology Advanced Practice
   Nursing
Juravinski Hospital and Cancer
   Centre
Hamilton, ON
Canada

**Melissa A. Johnson, MSN, RN, CNS, CNRN**
Clinical Nurse Specialist
Scripps Memorial Hospital
Encinitas, CA

**Ruth M. Kleinpell, PhD, RN-CS, FAAN, FAANP, FCCM**
Director
Center for Clinical Research and Scholarship
Rush University Medical Center
Professor
Rush University College of Nursing
Chicago, IL

**Michael J. Kremer, PhD, CRNA, FAAN**
Professor and Director
Nurse Anesthesia Program
Rush University
Chicago, IL

**Nancy Livingston, RN, MN**
Nurse Practitioner
David Geffen School of Medicine
University of California Los Angeles Medical Center
Ahmanson-UCLA Cardiomyopathy Center
Los Angeles, CA

**Kathy S. Magdic, DNP, RN, ACNP-BC, FAANP**
Assistant Professor and Coordinator
Acute Care Nurse Practitioner Program
University of Pittsburgh
Pittsburgh, PA

**Julie Marfell, DNP, FNP**
Chairperson
Department of Family Nursing
Frontier Nursing University
Hyden, KY

**Kathy McCloy, RN, MSN**
Acute Care Nurse Practitioner
UCLA Pulmonary Hypertension Program
David Geffen School of Medicine
Division of Pulmonary and Critical Care Medicine
University of California Los Angeles Medical Center
Los Angeles, CA

**Ann F. Minnick, PhD, RN, FAAN**
Senior Associate Dean for Research
Julia Eleanor Chenault Professor of Nursing
Vanderbilt University School of Nursing
Vanderbilt University
Nashville, TN

**Marguerite J. Murphy, DNP, RN**
Director, DNP Program
College of Nursing
Georgia Health Sciences University
Augusta, GA

**Beth D. Quatrara, DNP, RN, CMSRN, ACNS-BC**
Advanced Practice Nurse 3–Clinical Nurse Specialist
Director of PNSO Nursing Research Program
University of Virginia Health System
Charlottesville, VA

**Darlene Rourke, RN, MSN, CHFN**
Clinical Nurse Specialist
David Geffen School of Medicine
University of California Los Angeles Medical Center
Ahmanson-UCLA Cardiomyopathy Center
Los Angeles, CA

**Marilyn Wolf Schwartz, MLS**
Retired Medical Library Director
Naval Medical Center, San Diego, CA
Rocky Mountain University of Health Professions
Provo, UT

**Patricia W. Stone, PhD, RN, FAAN**
Centennial Professor in Health Policy
Columbia University School of Nursing
New York, NY

**Suzan Ulrich, DrPh, CNM, FACNM**
Associate Dean for Midwifery and
    Women's Health
Frontier Nursing University
Hyden, KY

**Elizabeth Vandenbogaart, RN, MSN**
Acute Care Nurse Practitioner
David Geffen School of Medicine
University of California Los Angeles
    Medical Center
Ahmanson-UCLA Cardiomyopathy
    Center
Los Angeles, CA

# Foreword

The ability to demonstrate the value that advanced practice nurses (APNs) bring to their patients' health and to the effective operation of health care systems in which they work is even more important today than 10 years ago. Outcomes are the data used today to quantify, evaluate, and validate the impact of all health care services. Outcomes are used to judge the safety, effectiveness, and overall quality of care. Patient, provider, and system outcomes data are used by governmental agencies (e.g., Medicare), health care organizations (e.g., hospitals, group practices), and payers to determine whether performance meets expectations. External audiences also use outcomes data, and publicly posted "provider report cards" featuring care outcomes are used by individual consumers as well as businesses to make health care choices. Additionally, policy makers use the data to determine who provides services and how they are paid. Clearly, outcomes data are critical to APN practice.

APNs serve at the front lines of health care and will make even greater contributions in the future to improve our health care system. This is in part because APNs have developed a reputation for providing accessible, high-quality, cost-effective care. The foundation for this reputation and for recent expansions of practice authority is based on published data demonstrating excellent APN care outcomes. As coinvestigator and coauthor of the recently published synthesis review of the literature on outcomes of APN care published from 1990 to 2008 (Newhouse et al., 2011), I continue to be impressed with the number of studies identifying the impact of APN care. However, the need for additional work to delineate APN outcomes continues.

So what do APNs need to do and how will this book help? All APNs must appreciate the critical importance of outcomes data in evaluating, improving, and changing practice. Armed with this knowledge, individual APNs must take the next step to incorporate outcomes assessment as a routine component of their day-to-day practice. They need to compare their outcome data to benchmarks and use the data to refine their practice and enhance the profession. APNs need to be able to discuss outcomes data from their practice and how they were achieved. Outcomes, which characterize their patients' health status, are particularly important for nurse midwives, nurse anesthetists, and nurse practitioners. In addition, for clinical nurse specialists who spend much of their time behind the scenes ensuring safe and high-quality care delivery, systems-related variables are critical to survival in these complex care systems.

This text provides APN students and educators, practicing APNs, and the administrators with whom they work with up-to-date information on APN outcomes assessment, the "who, what, when, where, how, and why." It includes critical perspectives on not only the health effects of APN practice, but also the economic impact of their practice. Chapters that synthesize current data on each APN role will guide practice innovations and enhance practice authority. Identified gaps in data will help to prioritize future research and develop new APN care models, which might lead to improvements in health and health care delivery. The authors of this work provide the essential information to accomplish all of these important objectives.

*Julie Stanik-Hutt, PhD, CRNP, CCNS, FAAN*
Associate Professor, Johns Hopkins University, School of Nursing
and Progressive Cardiac Care/Cardiology Nurse Practitioner Service,
Johns Hopkins Hospital

## REFERENCE

Newhouse, R., Stanik-Hutt, J., White, K., Johantgen, M., Bass, E., Zangaro, G.,...L. Weiner, J. (2011). Advanced practice registered nurse outcomes 1990–2008: A systematic review. *Nursing Economics, 29,* 230–250.

# *Preface*

Assessing outcomes of advanced practice nursing care is an important aspect of bringing recognition to the multifaceted roles of advanced practice nurses (APNs) and of their impact on outcomes. Since 2001, when the first edition of this book was published, the field of outcomes research has further grown and developed. This third edition of *Outcome Assessment in Advanced Practice Nursing* has been written to provide APNs with updated resources and information on measuring outcomes of practice. The chapters within this book focus on presenting an overview of advanced practice nursing outcomes research and discussing outcomes measurement in all areas of advanced practice nursing, including clinical nurse specialist, nurse practitioner, certified registered nurse anesthetist, and certified nurse midwife. Examples of outcome studies are presented from actual research in APN practice. Additional chapters focus on a discussion of outcomes assessment in specialty APN practice, community and ambulatory settings, information on locating instruments and measures for APN outcomes assessment, and information on an international initiative focused on the development of an APN research data collection toolkit. New to this edition is a chapter focusing on outcomes of APN care that are specifically related to the doctorate of nursing practice (DNP).

The contributors to this third edition are recognized expert practitioners, educators, and researchers, and collectively they offer invaluable insights into the process of conducting outcomes assessments in APN practice. The ever-expanding field of outcomes measurement can make conducting an outcomes assessment complex. *Outcome Assessment in Advanced Practice Nursing* provides APNs with up-to-date resources and examples of outcome measures, tools, and methods that can be used by APNs in their quest to measure outcomes of care. This third edition of the book was written to serve as a resource for assessing outcomes for APNs, regardless of specialty area of practice or practice setting. Having knowledge of the APN outcomes literature as well as the process of assessing outcomes of practice is important for all APNs. The true impact of APN care can only be established through continued focus on outcomes assessment and evaluation—something that this book encourages readers to actively pursue.

Ruth M. Kleinpell

*Outcome Assessment in*
*Advanced Practice Nursing*

# Chapter 1: Measuring Outcomes in Advanced Practice Nursing

RUTH M. KLEINPELL

The measurement of outcomes has been identified as one of the most important activities in assessing the effectiveness of an intervention, in identifying effective practices, and in identifying practices that need improvement (U.S. Department of Health and Human Services, Administration for Children and Families, 2010). In the broadest sense, outcomes in health care are the result of interventions based on the use of clinical judgment, scientific knowledge, skills, and experience (Doran, 2011; Kleinpell & Gawlinski, 2005; O'Grady, 2008). An increased focus on assessing the outcomes of advanced practice nursing (APN) has resulted from the growing emphasis on outcomes that has become a recognized component of the majority of health care initiatives. The demands for measuring outcomes of care have been emphasized by federal and state regulatory agencies, practice guidelines, employers, and consumer groups. Health care organizations are now actively monitoring patient outcomes as a means of evaluation as well as for requirements for accreditation and certification.

Contributing to the increased focus on improving outcomes are entities such as The Joint Commission, the National Quality Forum, and the Agency for Healthcare Research and Quality. Mandatory state reporting of hospital quality measures and other initiatives for improving health care quality have also prompted greater focus on outcomes measurement (Kapu & Kleinpell, 2012). As APNs assume an increasing role in providing care to patients in a growing number of settings, measuring the impact of their care on patient outcomes and quality-of-care measures becomes a necessary component of performance evaluation.

Additionally, health care restructuring continues to change the way in which care is delivered, and as APNs' roles change, the measurement of outcomes is an important parameter by which APN care can be evaluated. Moreover, as APNs are involved in providing care to a variety of patient groups and in various settings, they are often the most familiar with the clinical problems that need to be studied and are therefore the ideal practitioners to participate in the development of outcome-based initiatives (Resnick, 2006). Knowledge of the process of outcomes measurement and of available resources is essential for all APNs regardless of practice specialty or setting. This chapter reviews important issues in measuring outcomes in APN including a discussion of the state of the science on APN outcomes research.

## FOCUSING ON OUTCOMES OF APN

Although the measurement of APN outcomes is important, it is not a standard part of institutional or clinical practice. In a recent survey conducted by the University Health System Consortium, a large national group formed from the association of 103 academic medical centers, 25 organizations were surveyed on their use of APNs (Moote, Krsek, Kleinpell, & Todd, 2011). Survey responses indicated that productivity was measured with a variety of metrics, including patient encounters, number of procedures, gross charges, collections of professional fees, number of shared visits (Medicare), number of indirect billing visits (Blue Cross), and number of visits billed under the practitioner provider number. Few organizations had defined productivity targets, and most reported that they did not measure the impact of APN-led interventions, citing difficulties with linking providers to patients or difficulties with quantifying outcomes. Although a few organizations reported tracking outcomes, often overall by service, none had developed a focused plan for outcomes assessment. Those who did report tracking outcomes identified that they were monitoring length of stay (LOS; 15%); readmission rates (12%); family and patient satisfaction (12%); and specific clinical outcomes, such as ventilator days (8%), urinary tract infection (UTI) rates (4%), ventilator-associated pneumonia rates (4%), skin breakdown rates (4%), venous thromboembolism prophylaxis rates (4%), and catheter-related bloodstream infection rates (4%; Moote et al., 2011). The results of the study revealed that even in institutions that employ large numbers of APNs (i.e., 200 or more), no focused effort to assess outcomes had been implemented. Assessing the outcomes of APNs and their contributions to care is an essential component of their utilization. Yet, it can be challenging to develop focused processes to capture APNs' contributions to care.

## OUTCOMES MEASUREMENT IN APN PRACTICE

Measuring outcomes of APN practice involves identifying and choosing indicators to be monitored and choosing a methodology to conduct the outcomes assessment. The process of monitoring outcomes of APN practice can be complex, as time needs to be allocated to the planning and conduct of the outcomes assessment. The chapters in this book outline several examples of practice-based outcome assessments related to APN practice, including indicators monitored and how an outcomes assessment was conducted as well as sources for identifying outcome-related tools.

## OUTCOMES OF APN PRACTICE: WHAT EVIDENCE IS IN THE LITERATURE?

A review of the literature on outcomes measurement in advanced practice nursing published since 2000 provides specific examples of outcome parameters influenced by APN care (Exhibit 1.1). Several recent synthesis reviews highlight that a number of studies have been conducted that have focused on the evaluation of APN roles and on outcomes of APN care (Hatem, Sandall, Devane, Soltani, & Gates, 2009; Newhouse et al., 2011; Laurant et al., 2004). These systematic reviews have focused on all APN roles including nurse practitioner (NP), clinical nurse specialist (CNS), certified registered nurse anesthetist (CRNA), and certified nurse midwife (CNM) and have included two Cochrane Database systematic reviews on the impact of primary care NPs (Laurant et al., 2004) and CNM care (Hatem et al., 2009). A systematic review by Newhouse et al. (2011) reviewed the published literature on APN outcomes between 1990 and 2008 and found that care provided by APNs was similar and in some ways better than care provided by physicians alone. APN care was found to reduce LOS and costs of care for hospitalized patients and improve functional status; improve specific illness-related measures such as glucose control, lipid control, blood pressure, or duration of ventilation; reduce length of hospitalization, rehospitalizations, and emergency department (ED) or

**Exhibit 1.1** *Examples of Outcome Measures for APNs*

| |
|---|
| Blood glucose control |
| Symptom management |
| Patient lengths of stay |
| Costs of care |
| Smoking cessation |
| Adverse events (e.g., accidental extubation) |
| Patient and family knowledge |
| Patient self-efficacy |
| Urinary incontinence rates |
| Lipid management |
| Blood pressure control |
| Fall rates |
| Staff nurse knowledge |
| Staff nurse retention rates |
| Nosocomial infection rates |
| Readmission rates |
| Nutritional intake |
| Skin breakdown rates |
| Restraint use |
| Hand hygiene compliance |
| Patient and family satisfaction rates |
| Nurse satisfaction rates |
| Caregiver knowledge, satisfaction |
| Rates of adherence to best practices |

urgent care visits; and result in high patient satisfaction ratings, among other outcomes (Newhouse et al., 2011).

Several additional reviews have focused on NP effectiveness (Bourbonniere & Evans, 2002; Cunningham, 2004) or a comparison of NP and MD practice (Horrocks, Anderson, & Salisbury, 2002). Other explorations have included integrative reviews on the impact of APN care (Ingersoll, 2008) and in specialty areas of practice such as heart failure management (Brandon, Schuessler, Ellison, & Lazenby, 2009; Dickerson, Wu, & Kennedy, 2006; Kutzleb & Reiner, 2006; Lowery et al., 2011; Osevala, 2005), chronic kidney disease care (Bissonnette, 2011; Hamilton & Hawley, 2006), osteoporosis management (Greene & Dell, 2010), cystic fibrosis care (Rideout, 2007), and diabetes care management (Boville et al., 2007; Jessee & Rutledge, 2012).

Early studies assessing the outcomes of APN care explored the impact of APN practice and examined process and client outcome variables including client management, activities, cost of care, problem identification, physician acceptance, and disease- or condition-specific outcomes. Other studies measuring outcomes of APN care have explored a variety of factors including the impact of APN care on patients, patient satisfaction with care, quality of care provided by APNs as compared to physicians, and outcomes of care of APNs in comparison to other practitioners, including physician assistants, medical residents, and physicians (Scherr, Wilson, Wagner, & Haughian, 2012; Schuttelaar, Vermeulen, & Coenraads, 2011; Seale, Anderson, & Kinnersley, 2006; Sears, Wickizer, Franklin, Cheadle, & Berkowitz, 2007; Sears, Wickizer, Franklin, Cheadle, & Berkowitz, 2008; Sidani et al., 2006a). Additional studies have explored characteristics of APNs that impact outcomes, such as provider proficiency, complication rates, clinical competency, and personal activities (Bevis et al., 2008; Dierick-van Daele, Metsemakers, Derckx, Spreeuwenberg, & Vrijhoef, 2009; Gershengorn et al., 2011; Johantgen et al., 2012).

Identifying outcome measures that are "nurse-sensitive" has been identified as a way of linking nursing roles to specific health care outcomes. A number of nurse-sensitive outcome measures have been proposed including clinical outcomes such as symptom control and health status indicators; prevention of complications such as infection and complications of immobility; knowledge of disease and its treatment including patient knowledge of the illness process and knowledge of medications; and functional health outcomes including physical and social functioning (Doran, 2011). Specific nurse-sensitive outcomes of APN have also been identified (Exhibit 1.2; Ingersoll, McIntosh, & Williams, 2000).

Studies focusing on APN care in specialty areas of practice such as acute care have examined several aspects of patient care outcomes including rates of UTI and skin breakdown (Elpern et al., 2009; Russell, VorderBruegge, & Burns, 2002), use of laboratory tests (Gawlinski & McCloy, 2001), LOS (Burns et al., 2003; Gershengorn et al., 2011; Meyer & Miers, 2005; Miller, Burns et al., 2002), readmission rates and ED

Exhibit 1.2 *Nurse-Sensitive Outcomes of APN*

| |
|---|
| Patient satisfaction |
| Symptom resolution or reduction |
| Compliance/adherence |
| Patient/family knowledge |
| Collaboration among care providers |
| Functional status |
| Patient self-esteem |
| Knowledge and skill of other care providers |
| Length of time in hospital |
| Staff satisfaction with work |
| Costs of care |
| Patient preparedness for interventions |

Adapted from Ingersoll, McIntosh, and Williams (2000).

visits (Bissonnette, 2011; Brandon et al., 2009; Lowery et al., 2011; Paul, 2000), mortality (Burns et al., 2003; Gershengorn et al., 2011), costs of care (Burns & Earven, 2002; Burns et al., 2003; Dierick-van Daele et al., 2009; Meyer & Miers, 2005; Paul, 2000; Schuttelaar et al., 2011), discharge instructions (Kleinpell & Gawlinski, 2005), smoking cessation (Kleinpell & Gawlinski, 2005), use of angiotensin-converting enzyme-I, β-blockers and anticoagulation for cardiac patients (Kleinpell & Gawlinski, 2005), thoracostomy tube performance (Bevis et al., 2008), or ventilatory weaning (Burns & Earven, 2002; Burns et al., 2003; Hoffman, Miller, Zullo, & Donahoe, 2006). It is evident that a number of studies have evaluated APN outcomes; yet, as APN roles are diverse, information on APN outcomes remains needed, especially for new and evolving APN roles.

## CLASSIFYING APN OUTCOME STUDIES

Organizing studies related to APN outcomes according to categories can facilitate discussion and evaluation. A classic outcome categorization schema outlines outcomes based on care-, patient-, and performance-related measures (Jennings Staggers, & Brosch, 1999). Although not mutually exclusive, using these groupings to examine outcome studies of APN care can aid in summarizing important findings and in highlighting areas needing further study. Exhibit 1.3 outlines outcome measures used in advanced practice nursing effectiveness research grouped according to these areas.

**Exhibit 1.3** *Examples of Outcome Measures Used in APN Effectiveness Research*

| Care-Related | Patient-Related | Performance-Related |
|---|---|---|
| Costs of care | Patient satisfaction | Quality of care |
| Length of stay | Patient access to care | Interpersonal skills |
| In-hospital mortality | Patient compliance | Technical quality |
| Morbidity | Symptom resolution or reduction | Adherence to best practice guidelines |
| Readmission rates | Health maintenance | Completeness of documentation |
| Occurrence of drug reactions | Return to work | Time spent in role components |
| Procedure success rate/ complications | Stress levels | APN job satisfaction |
| Clinic wait time | Knowledge | Clinical competence |
| Time spent with patients | Blood pressure control | Performance ratings |
| Number of visits per patient | Diet and weight control | Collaboration |
| Number of patient hospitalizations | Blood glucose levels | Procedure complication rates |
| Use/ordering of lab tests | Clinic wait time | Revenue generation |
| Rate of drug prescription | Emergency department wait time | Physician recruitment and retention |
| Management of common medical problems | Patient self-esteem | Consultations |
| Number of consultations | Depressive symptoms | Time savings for house staff MDs |
| Infant immunizations | Patient/family knowledge | Resuscitation outcomes |
| Diagnoses made | Functional status | Clinical examination |
| Diagnostic screening tests ordered | Quality of life | Comprehensiveness |
| Acute care home visits | Caregiver knowledge, satisfaction | Relative value units (RVUs) |

*(continued)*

**Exhibit 1.3** *Examples of Outcome Measures Used in APN Effectiveness Research* *(continued)*

| Care-Related | Patient-Related | Performance-Related |
|---|---|---|
| Intravenous fluid volume | Patient well-being | |
| Total parenteral nutrition use | | |
| Number of blood transfusions | | |
| Prenatal/postpartum visits | | |
| Low birthweight rates | | |
| Rates of cesarean section | | |
| Number of induced labors | | |
| Analgesia/anesthesia used | | |
| Quality of life | | |
| Time to readmission | | |
| Length of time between discharge and readmission | | |
| Urinary incontinence | | |
| ED visits | | |
| Ventilator duration | | |
| Rates of UTI | | |
| Side rail use and fall rates | | |

## Care-Related Outcomes of APN

Care-related outcomes are those outcomes that result from APN involvement in care, or an APN intervention. Studies assessing the impact of APN care have ranged from studies exploring the impact on quantitative indices such as lab values, physiological values such as weight gain, clinical symptoms such as dyspnea or pain, and aspects of health such as physical function and mobility (Albers-Heitner et al., 2012; Bissonnette, 2011; Brandon et al., 2009; Lowery et al., 2011; Newhouse et al., 2011). Other studies in this category have measured the effect of APN care on length of patient hospitalization, hospital readmission rates, costs, appropriateness of prescribing decisions, timeliness of consultations, mortality, and morbidity rates (Boville et al., 2007; Brandon et al., 2009; Burns et al., 2003; Cowan et al., 2006; Delgado-Passler & McCaffery, 2006;

Dellasega & Zerbe, 2002; Ettner et al., 2006; Gawlinski et al., 2001; Lindberg et al., 2002; Litaker et al., 2003; Lowery et al., 2011; McCauley, Bixby, & Naylor, 2006; Meyer & Miers, 2005; Neff, Madigan, & Narsavage, 2003; Rideout, 2007; Russell et al., 2002; Vanhook, 2000). These studies have concluded that APNs perform a comprehensive range of activities that include both expanded nursing practice activities and collaborative physician-related activities (physical assessment and diagnosis, ordering diagnostic tests, prescribing treatments, seeking and giving consultations, case management). In general, these studies have found a variety of results related to APN care, ranging from no impact to significant impact on outcomes. Studies reporting significant results of APN care have cited such parameters as decreased length of hospitalization stay, annual cost savings, time savings per day for house staff, and decreased outpatient clinic waiting times (Albers-Heitner et al., 2012; Bissonnette, 2011; Burns et al., 2003; Cowan et al., 2006; Lowery et al., 2011; McCauley et al., 2006; Meyer & Miers, 2005; Morse, Warshawsky, Moore, & Pecora, 2006; Paul, 2000; Rideout, 2007; Russell et al., 2002; Wit, Bos-Schaap, Hautvast, Heestermans, & Umans, 2012). Table 1.1 outlines selected studies in this category of APN outcomes, including outcome measures explored.

Table 1.1  *Studies Assessing Care-Related Outcomes of Advanced Practice Nursing*

| Study | APN role | Outcome indicators | Findings |
|---|---|---|---|
| Wit et al. (2012); observation study of impact of NP led clinic for postoperative heart surgery patients | NP | Patient hospital length of stay, transfer time, postoperative complications | An NP-led clinic registered 1,967 patients over 10 years and was evaluated to be feasible and effective for postop care |
| Albers-Heitner et al. (2012); impact of NP care in primary care for adult patients with urinary incontinence | NP | Urinary incontinence quality of life, costs | One hundred eighty-six patients managed by NPs had significant changes in urinary incontinence and quality of life and less costs of care compared to 198 patients receiving usual care |
| Lowery et al. (2011); impact of NP disease management model for patients with chronic heart failure | NP | Congestive heart failure (CHF) readmissions, mortality rates | Patients managed by NPs ($n = 458$) had significantly fewer CHF and all-cause admissions at 1 year and lower mortality at both 1- and 2-year follow-up compared to 511 control patients |

*(continued)*

Table 1.1 *Studies Assessing Care-Related Outcomes of Advanced Practice Nursing* (continued)

| Study | APN role | Outcome indicators | Findings |
|-------|----------|--------------------|----------|
| Cibulka et al. (2011); NP directed oral care program for low-income pregnant women | NP | Oral care practice and dental exams | Patients ($n$ = 170) randomized to intervention had higher rates of toothbrushing and flossing and dental checkups and less intake of high-sugar drinks compared to controls |
| Coddington et al. (2011); impact of pediatric NP care at a nurse managed center on quality of care measures | NP | Pediatric health care effectiveness and data information set (HEDIS) quality indicators | NP care met or exceeded national HEDIS benchmark standards of care and targets for immunizations, treatment of upper respiratory infection, and access to care measures |
| Cheung et al. (2011); certified nurse midwife-led normal birth unit in China | CNM | Characteristics of deliveries | Two hundred twenty-six women managed by the CNM had significant differences in deliveries, rates of episiotomies, amniotomies (all decreased) and increased post delivery mobility compared to a matched retrospective cohort |
| Bissonnette (2011); impact of APN led chronic care model for kidney transplant patients | APN | Hospital admissions, emergency department (ED) visits, clinical practice guideline-based treatment | Compared to 119 control patients, 61 patients managed by APNs had fewer hospital readmissions and ED visits and higher percent of clinical practice guideline treatments |
| Greene and Dell (2010); impact of NP disease management program for patients with osteoporosis | NP | Number of patients treated for osteoporosis, hip fractures | Over a 6-year period there was a 263% increase in the number of DXA scans done each year, 153% increase in patients on anti-osteoporosis medications, and a 38.1% decrease in hip fractures |
| Begley et al. (2010); clinical and economic impact of nurse specialist and advanced practitioner care | APN | Focus group and Delphi study on patient/client outcomes | APN care improves patient/client outcomes including symptom management and appropriateness of medication regime, promotes self management and patient and family information and education, reduces exacerbations of conditions, prevents complications, and improves adherence to treatment |

*(continued)*

## Table 1.1  *continued*

| | | | |
|---|---|---|---|
| Brandon et al. (2009); impact of APN led telephone follow-up program for heart failure patients | APN | Rehospitalizations rates; self care behaviors, quality of life | Patients receiving the APN-led intervention had reduced rehospitalizations rates, improved patient self-care behaviors, and improved quality of life |
| Capezuti et al. (2007); impact of APN consultation and educational services on side rail use in nursing homes | APN | Side rail use and fall rates | APN led intervention resulted in significantly decreased side rail use and decreased falls |
| Rideout (2007); evaluation of a pediatric NP care coordinator model for hospitalized children, adolescents, and young adults with cystic fibrosis | NP | Timelines of inpatient consultations; weight gain, length of stay (LOS), patient/family satisfaction, change in forced expiratory volume in first second ($FEV^1$) | In 21 patients, there was a significant decrease in time to complete consultations, a decrease in LOS by 1.35 days ($p = .06$). Patient/parent satisfaction was high |
| Boville et al. (2007); impact of NP care in chronic disease management care of 110 patients with diabetes | NP | Glycemic control, lipid management, blood pressure control | NP care with the use of clinical algorithms for medication intensification resulted in improved glycemic control, lipid management, and control of hypertension |
| Krichbaum (2007); impact of NP led care model for elderly patients with hip fractures | NP | Health and functional status; return home outcomes | Six-month intervention for 30 patients demonstrated better function at 12 months with activities of daily living |
| Hamilton and Hawley (2006); impact of CNS care for patients with chronic renal failure in an outpatient anemia management program | CNS | Quality of life | CNS-managed patients had a statistically significant increase in quality of life indicators |
| Morse et al. (2006); assessment of an NP-led rapid response team (RRT) | NP | Codes outside the ICU, staff in-hospital mortality rates | An NP-led RRT resulted in decreased perceptions of the RRT, decreased in-hospital mortality rates and high satisfaction ratings from staff |
| Cowan et al. (2006); analysis of impact of acute care NP care for medical inpatients co-managed with MD compared to hospitalist-managed care | NP | LOS, hospital costs, readmission rates 4 month after discharge ($p < .001$) | Average LOS was lower in NP/MD co-managed patients (5 vs. 6 days) |

*(continued)*

**Table 1.1**  *Studies Assessing Care-Related Outcomes of Advanced Practice Nursing  (continued)*

| Study | APN role | Outcome indicators | Findings |
|---|---|---|---|
| Cragin et al. (2006); impact of nurse midwife care on patient outcomes | CNM | Perinatal outcomes | Midwifery patients had more optimal care processes with no differences in neonatal outcomes |
| Ettner et al. (2006); impact of NP on costs of care for medical inpatients | NP | Costs of care | The addition of a NP to general medicine teams was cost effective; NP care reinforced medical compliance, follow-up plans, and symptom management |
| McCauley et al. (2006); impact of APN care on elderly patients with heart failure | APN | Length of time between hospital discharge and readmission, hospital readmission LOS, costs | APN care resulted in reduced hospital readmission, reduced LOS of readmissions, and decreased overall health care costs |
| Shebasta et al. (2006); impact of pediatric NP on staff nurse satisfaction | NP | Staff nurse satisfaction | Involvement of a pediatric NP in patient care resulted in higher staff nurse satisfaction |
| Reigle et al. (2006); impact of acute care NP on cardiology patients | NP | LOS, prescription of appropriate discharge medications, documentation of patient education | NP-managed patients undergoing cardiac catheterization or percutaneous coronary intervention resulted in decreased LOS, more prescription of indicated medications, and more documentation of patient status and patient education |
| Stolee et al. (2006); impact of NP role for long-term care residents | NP | Ratings of effectiveness and satisfaction of NP role | NP care significantly impacted the primary care of residents in long-term care |
| Kutzleb and Reiner (2006); prospective quasi-experimental study assessing the impact of NP care on patients with heart failure | NP | Quality of life, functional status | NP-directed care resulted in increased patient quality of life and health and functioning ($p = .0003$) over a 12-month period |
| Forster et al. (2005); impact of CNS care on medical patients | CNS | Readmission, risk of adverse event, mortality, quality of care | CNS-managed patients had higher overall quality of care; no differences were observed in readmission rates, adverse events, or mortality rates compared to usual care managed patients |
| Meyer and Miers (2005); acute care NP and cardiovascular (CV) surgery | NP | LOS, costs of care | Care given by ACNPs on the CV team resulted in decreased LOS by 1.91 days and decreased cost of team care by $5,038.91 per patient |

*(continued)*

## Table 1.1 *continued*

| | | | |
|---|---|---|---|
| Ahrens et al. (2003); impact of CNS-led communication intervention with families of ICU patients | CNS | ICU LOS, hospital LOS, hospital costs | A structured CNS communication initiative resulted in shorter ICU LOS and lower costs of care |
| Neff et al. (2003); impact of APN care for home-care patients with COPD | APN | Dyspnea, activities of daily living, rehospitalizations ED visits | APN-directed pulmonary disease management resulted in shorter rehospitalization, LOS, and less rehospitalizations; a significantly higher number of patients in the APN group were discharged and remained at home compared to the control group ($p < .05$) |
| Burns et al. (2003); for mechanically ventilated patients in the ICU | NP | Ventilator duration, ICU LOS, mortality, costs of care | An outcomes-management model of ACNP care resulted in decreased ventilator duration ($p = .0001$), decreased ICU LOS ($p = .0008$), decreased hospital LOS ($p = .0001$), decreased mortality rates ($p = .02$), and more than $3,000,000 cost savings |
| Litaker et al. (2003); impact of NP-physician team in managing patients with chronic disease | NP | Glycosylated hemoglobin, HDL-C, satisfaction with care, health-related quality of life | Patients randomized to the NP-MD team care experienced significant improvements in mean $HbA_{1c}$ and HDL-C, and satisfaction with care |
| Tijhuis et al. (2002); impact of CNS care for patients with rheumatoid arthritis | CNS | Functional status, quality of life, disease activity, health utility, satisfaction with care | CNS-managed patients had a significant improvement ($p < .05$) in functional status, quality of life, health utility, and patient satisfaction |
| Russell et al. (2002); ACNP care neuroscience ICU patients | NP | LOS, rates of UTI, skin breakdown, foley catheter time, mobilization out of bed | Patients managed by ACNPs had shorter LOS ($p = .03$), shorter ICU neuroscience LOS ($p < .001$), lower rates of UTI and skin breakdown ($p < .05$), and shorter time to discontinuation of foley catheter and mobilization out of bed |
| Lindberg et al. (2002); impact of asthma NP care for 347 patients | NP | Asthma symptoms, quality of documentation, patient self-management | NP managed patients reported fewer asthma symptoms and more self-management; documentation quality of NP care was high |

*(continued)*

**Table 1.1**  *Studies Assessing Care-Related Outcomes of Advanced Practice Nursing  (continued)*

| Study | APN role | Outcome indicators | Findings |
|---|---|---|---|
| Dellasega and Zerbe (2002); impact of APN intervention on caregivers of frail rural older adults | APN | Caregiver physical health, well-being, and perceived stress | Caregivers who received APN intervention had higher self-rated emotional health scores, fewer depressive symptoms, and lower stress scores |
| Ley (2001); impact of CNS care for cardiac surgery patients | CNS | Cardiac surgical bleeding | A quality improvement initiative resulted in decreased preoperative exposure to clopidogrel and decreased postoperative bleeding |
| Larsen et al. (2001); impact of CNS care for adult sickle cell patients | CNS | Pain consultations, patient-controlled analgesia use, patient education | Implementation of a clinical pathway resulted increased pain consultations and patient-controlled analgesia use, and increased patient education |
| Gawlinski et al. (2001); ACNP care for cardiac ICU patients using extubation protocols | NP | Mechanical ventilation time, reintubation events, LOS | Decreased mean time to extubation, decreased rates of ventilator associated pneumonia, shorter LOS, decreased use of arterial blood gases |
| Brooten et al. (2001); impact of CNS care for women with high-risk pregnancies | CNS | Preterm infant, prenatal hospitalizations, infant rehospitalizations, costs of care, LOS, mortality | CNS managed patients had fewer preterm infants, fewer infant deaths, fewer prenatal hospitalizations, decreased LOS |
| Carroll et al. (2001); impact of APN care for unpartnered elders following acute myocardial infarction | APN | Patient education, self-efficacy, functional status | APN-led intervention resulted in increased self-efficacy and improved function |
| Dobscha et al. (2001); effectiveness of a CNS-led intervention to improve primary care provider recognition of depression | CNS | Recognition and management of depression | A CNS-led intervention resulted in improved recognition and initial management of depression in a VA primary care setting |
| Barnason et al. (2000); impact of CNS led recovery program for cardiac surgery patients | CNS | Factors facilitating and inhibiting adherence to cardiac therapy program | CNS-managed patients required less oxygen use on day 2 |

*(continued)*

## Table 1.1 *continued*

| | | | |
|---|---|---|---|
| Vanhook (2000); analysis of effect of the implementation of acute stroke team facilitated by NP | NP | Mortality rate, length of stay, hospital charges, time to arrival after symptom, onset | Mortality rated dropped from 5.7% to 3.8%, LOS dropped from 10 days in 1995 to 3.2 days in 1998, hospital charges were decreased 50%, time to arrival after symptom onset decreased from 22 to 7 hours |
| Paul (2000); retrospective review of impact of NP-managed heart failure clinic for 15 patients with congestive heart failure | NP | Hospital readmissions, emergency department visits, length of stay, charges reimbursement | Six months after implementation of heart failure clinic, hospital admissions decreased (from 151 hospital days to 22); mean length of stay decreased (from 4.3 days to 3.8 days), and mean inpatient hospital charged decreased from $40,624 per patient admission to $5,893; percent of recovered charges from reimbursement increased from 73% to 87% |

Table reviews studies published from 2000 to present. The prior edition of this book reported on studies published beginning in the 1960s and 1970s through 2009 (Kleinpell, 2009).

### *Patient-Related Outcomes of APN Care*

Patient-related outcomes of care are those outcomes that impact patient perceptions, preferences, or knowledge. Studies in this category have measured the effect of APN care on patient satisfaction, quality of life, patient access to care, health service utilization, patient compliance, patient complaints, patient knowledge, symptom management, social function, and psychological function. Findings from these studies have revealed that APN care results in increased patient satisfaction, patient compliance with treatment plans, cost savings in terms of annual costs and hospital charges, decreased lengths of hospital stay, decreased readmission rates, changes in patient clinical parameters such as lipid levels (Andrus & Donaldson, 2006; Hogan, Seifert, Moore, & Simonson, 2010; Paez & Allen, 2006), symptom management (McCorkle et al., 2009), patient self-efficacy (Jessee & Rutledge, 2012; Wand, White, Patching, Dixon, & Green, 2012), quality of life (Hanrahan, Wu, Kelly, Aiken, & Blank, 2011; McCorkle, Siefert, Dowd, Robinson, & Pickett, 2007), caregiver knowledge (Bradway et al., 2012), blood pressure control (Benkert et al., 2001), improvement in patient care practices such as pneumococcal vaccine administration (Mackey, Cole, & Lindenberg, 2005), cervical cancer screening (Kelley, Daly, Anthony, Zauszniewski, & Stange, 2002), and increased patient education, among others (Blue et al., 2001; Bryant & Graham, 2002; Cooper, Lindsay, Kinn, & Swann,

2002; Gracias et al., 2003; Sears et al., 2007; Sole, Hunkar-Huie, Schiller, & Cheatham, 2001). Table 1.2 outlines studies in this category of APN outcomes, including outcome measures explored.

Table 1.2  *Studies Assessing Patient Related Outcomes of APN Care*

| Study | APN role | Outcome indicators | Findings |
|---|---|---|---|
| Wand et al. (2012); impact of emergency department- (ED) based mental health NP | NP | Patient satisfaction, self efficacy, and psychological distress | An ED NP outpatient service decreased psychological distress, increased self-efficacy, and was rated with high patient satisfaction |
| Jessee and Rutledge (2012); impact of NP group visits to medically underserved patients with diabetes in family practice clinic | NP | Patient health, knowledge, and self-efficacy | NP intervention resulted in better clinical outcomes (A1C), greater patient knowledge and better self-efficacy than usual care groups |
| Bradway et al. (2012); impact of transitional care model for cognitively impaired older adults and their caregivers | APN | Care coordination, patient and care giver information and knowledge, experience | APN transitional care improved care coordination, caregiver information and knowledge, and the caregiver experience |
| Sung et al. (2011); NPs as coordinators of acute stroke team | NP | Time to CT scan, time to neurology evaluation, and time to initiate thrombolytic therapy | All significantly improved; time of patient arrival to patient treatment was also diminished |
| Hanrahan et al. (2011); impact of APN model of care management for community dwelling persons with HIV and serious mental illness | APN | Health-related quality of life, depression | In a 4-year randomized trial, control patients (n = 110) were compared to intervention patients (n = 128) who received the 12-month intervention and demonstrated significant improvement in depression and QOL |
| Hogan et al. (2010); cost effectiveness of certified registered nurse anesthetist care | CRNA | Cost of care | CRNAs are less costly to train than anesthesiologists and have the potential for providing anesthesia care efficiently |

*(continued)*

## Table 1.2 *continued*

| | | | |
|---|---|---|---|
| Hatem et al. (2009); comparison of nurse midwife care to other models of care | CNM | Childbirth complications | A review of 11 trials (12,276 women) indicated that midwife-led models of care were less likely to experience antenatal hospitalization, the use of regional analgesia, episiotomy, and instrumental delivery, and more likely to experience spontaneous vaginal birth and initiate breastfeeding |
| McCorkle et al. (2009); postsurgical care for women undergoing gynecological cancer surgery | APN | Functional status, symptom distress | Women receiving the 6-month APN intervention had improved functional status, less symptom distress, and less uncertainty compared to controls |
| Sears et al. (2007); impact of 3-year pilot program to expand NP care in state workers' compensation system | NP | Medical costs and disability outcomes | Likelihood of work time loss was less for NP claims; duration of lost work time and medical costs did not differ with MDs |
| McCorkle et al. (2007); randomized clinical trial of an APN intervention for patients with a radical prostatectomy | APN | Quality of life depressive symptoms | Patients experienced more moral distress related to sexual functioning while spouses experienced marital interaction distress; both patients and spouses reported decreased depression |
| Paez and Allen (2006); NP management of hypercholesterolemia following coronary revascularization | NP | Low density lipoprotein (LDL) cholesterol change | Case management by an NP resulted in significant reduction in LDL cholesterol levels |
| McCabe (2005); impact of CNS care for patients with atrial fibrillation | CNS | Patient self-care management, complications of treatment, care fragmentation | CNS care resulted in improved patient functioning and self-care management, reduced complications of treatment, and decreased fragmentation of care |
| Tsay et al. (2005); impact of CNS care for patients with end-stage renal disease | CNS | Perceived stress, depression, quality of life | CNS managed patients had less perceived stress ($p = .0005$), depression ($p = .001$), and improved quality of life ($p = .02$) |
| Krein et al. (2004); randomized clinical trial of NP care for patients with diabetes | NP | Glycemic control, patient satisfaction | There were no differences in glycemic control; patients managed by NPs had higher satisfaction |

*(continued)*

**Table 1.2  *Studies Assessing Patient Related Outcomes of APN Care  (continued)***

| Study | APN role | Outcome indicators | Findings |
|---|---|---|---|
| Gracias et al. (2003); NP care in surgical ICU for 900 patient days | NP | Influence on compliance with clinical practice guideline use for DVT/PE, stress ulcer, and anemia | Compliance was significantly higher for NP team for all 3 clinical practice guidelines (DVT/PE $p < .001$, stress ulcer $p < .001$, and anemia $p < .02$) |
| Cooper et al. (2002); NP care in ER for 199 patients | NP | Patient care, patient satisfaction, clinical documentation | Patients reported higher levels of satisfaction with NP care compared to MD care ($p < .001$), and NP clinical documentation was rated of higher quality ($p < .001$). There were no differences in level of symptoms, recovery times, or unplanned follow up between the groups |
| Corner et al. (2003); longitudinal study assessing impact of palliative care APN on cancer patients over 28 days | APN | Quality of life, anxiety scores | Significant improvements were found in emotional ($p = .03$) and cognitive functioning ($p = .03$) and a decrease in anxiety scores ($p = .003$) |
| Kelley et al. (2002); impact of NP preventive care for cervical cancer screening | NP | Cervical cancer screening | NP preventive care for cervical cancer resulted in a significant increase in documentation of cervical cancer screening (from 2% to 69%) |
| Bryant and Graham (2002); client satisfaction of 506 patients who received care by 36 APNs at 26 different practice sites | APN | Client satisfaction scores | Client satisfaction scores were high indicating they were very satisfied with APN care |
| Dellasega et al. (2002); impact of APN intervention for caregivers of frail rural older adults | APN | Caregiver physical health and well-being, stress, burden | Caregivers in the APN-managed group experienced more positive physical and emotional health outcomes and fewer depressive symptoms |
| Moore et al. (2002); randomized clinical trial of APN care for patients with lung cancer | APN | Quality of life, patient satisfaction, resource use, costs of care | APN-managed patients reported less dyspnea at 3 months ($p = .03$), better care for emotional functioning ($p = .03$), and higher quality of life ($p = .01$) |

*(continued)*

### Table 1.2 *continued*

| | | | |
|---|---|---|---|
| Rantz et al. (2001); CNS care for nursing home patients | CNS | Resident assessment measures, falls, activity behavior, pressure ulcers | CNS care resulted in improvement in quality measures including falls, behavior symptoms, activity, and pressure ulcers |
| Sole et al. (2001); NP care on trauma service during a 6-month period | NP | Types of patients cared for, diagnoses, orders, patient disposition | NPs identified new diagnoses in 53% of patients; they were also more likely to order rehabilitation and discharge planning, bowel management, and nutrition-based orders |
| Willoughby and Burroughs (2001); descriptive study of impact of CNS care for skin care for diabetic patients | CNS | Foot care practices | CNS managed patients were more likely to use appropriate foot-care practices |
| Benkert et al. (2001); assessment of blood pressure control for patients with hypertension in a nurse-managed center | NP | Blood pressure control | Insured and uninsured patients managed by NPs had comparable blood pressure control; uninsured patients averaged 3.2 more visits per year |
| Blue et al. (2001); randomized control trial of NP care for 165 heart failure patients | NP | Readmission, lengths of stay (LOS) | Compared with usual care, patients in NP group had fewer readmissions for heart failure ($p = .018$) and spent fewer days in hospital for heart failure ($p = .0051$) |
| Diesch et al. (2000); impact of CNS-guided imagery intervention for coronary artery bypass surgery patients | CNS | Pain, fatigue, anxiety, narcotic use, LOS, patient satisfaction | CNS guided imagery intervention resulted in decreased pain, fatigue, anxiety, narcotic use, and LOS, and increased patient satisfaction |
| Lacko et al. (2000); quasi-experimental study assessing impact of APN-education intervention for staff nurses | APN | Delirium-screening abilities of staff nurses | An APN educational intervention resulted in improved delirium-screening abilities of staff nurses |
| Wheeler (2000); quasi-experimental comparative study of CNS managed care for patients with total knee replacement | CNS | LOS, complications | CNS-managed patients received more nursing care interventions, had decreased LOS, and fewer complications |

*(continued)*

Table 1.2  *Studies Assessing Patient Related Outcomes
of APN Care  (continued)*

| Study | APN role | Outcome indicators | Findings |
|---|---|---|---|
| Ryden et al. (2000); randomized control trial of APN intervention for long-term care residents | APN | Incontinence, pressure ulcers, aggressive behavior | APN-managed patients experienced greater improvement or less decline in incontinence, pressure ulcers, and aggressive behavior |
| Ritz et al. (2000); randomized clinical trial of APN intervention for newly diagnosed patients with breast cancer | APN | Well-being, mood states, uncertainty, costs of care | Uncertainty decreased significantly in the intervention group at 1, 3, and 6 months with the strongest effect on subscales of complexity, inconsistency, and unpredictability There were no differences in costs. |

Table reviews studies published from 2000 to present. The prior edition of this book reported on studies published beginning in the 1960s and 1970s through 2009 (Kleinpell, 2009).

### Performance-Related Outcomes of APN Care

Performance-related outcomes include those outcomes that reflect the quality of care provided by APNs. Studies in this category have compared APN care with care provided by other midlevel providers, such as physician assistants, or other health care providers, such as medical residents and physicians. Studies in this category have also measured the effect of APN care on quality of care, interpersonal skills, technical quality, completeness of documentation, time spent in role components, patient perceptions of care, and clinical examination comprehensiveness (Aubrey & Yoxall, 2001; Bevis et al., 2008; Considine, Martin, Smit, Winter, & Jenkins, 2006; Hoffman et al., 2006; Kirkwood, Pesudovs, Loh, & Coster, 2005; Lambing, Adams, Fox, & Divine, 2004; Lenz, Mundinger, Hopkins, Lin, & Smolowitz, 2002; Mundinger et al., 2000; Pioro et al., 2001; Seale et al., 2006; Sidani et al., 2006b; Sullivan-Marx & Maislin, 2000; Vazirani, Hays, Shapiro, & Cowan, 2005; Woods, 2006). Specialty care comparisons of APN care and physician care have included detection rates of recurrent or metastatic disease (McFarlane et al., 2012), quality of fundus photography (Lamirel et al., 2012), and cardiac arrest and mortality resulting from rapid response team calls (Scherr et al., 2012), among others. Clinical outcomes, processes of care, utilization, and cost effectiveness have been found to be equivalent or superior to physician, physician assistant, and medical resident care (Dierick-van Daele et al., 2009; Gershengorn et al., 2011; Johantgen et al., 2012; Sullivan-Marx & Maislin, 2000).

Table 1.3 outlines studies in this category of APN outcomes, including outcome measures explored. Of those studies conducted

## Table 1.3 *Studies Assessing Performance-Related Outcomes of APN Care*

| Study | APN role | Outcome indicators | Findings |
|---|---|---|---|
| Scherr et al. (2012); comparison of NP-led program for rapid response teams compared to MD care | NP | Cardiac arrests, mortality rates | No differences in number of cardiac arrests or mortality rates for 255 patients; nurses reported confidence in knowledge of NP team |
| Schuttelaar et al. (2012); comparison of NP care and dermatologist care for children with eczema | NP | Costs of care, quality of life, patient satisfaction | NP care compared to dermatologist care was found to be cost effective and to result in improved quality of life and patient satisfaction |
| McFarlane et al. (2012); comparison of APN and physician consultant follow up of patients after colorectal surgery | APN | Detection rates of recurrent or metastatic disease | APN-led clinic for colorectal cancer follow up can achieve satisfactory results with detection rates of recurrent or metastatic disease comparable to MD consultant care |
| Lamirel et al. (2012); quality of NP-directed ophthalmoscopy for emergency department (ED) patients | NP | Quality of nonmydriatic fundus photography performed by NPs | Exams for 350 patients by NPs were evaluated as comparable for quality by 2 neuro-ophthalmologist raters |
| Johantgen et al. (2012); comparison of nurse midwife and physician labor and delivery care | CNM | Processes of care and infant outcomes | CNM care was found to have lower use of epidurals, episiotomies, and labor induction and perineal lacerations; no differences were found for Apgar scores, birth weight, or NICU admission compared to MD |
| Gershengorn et al. (2011); comparison of NP care and medical resident care for MICU patients | NP | Hospital mortality, length of stay, discharge disposition | No difference in hospital mortality, length of stay (ICU, hospital), or posthospital discharge disposition for NP compared to MD care |
| Dierick-van Daele et al. (2009); comparison of NP and general medical practitioner care in primary care | NP | Costs of care, follow up consultations | 12 NPs were compared to 50 GPs working in 15 general primary care practices. Direct costs were lower for NP care. Practices did not differ for direct costs plus costs from a societal perspective for patients aged less than 65 years. Cost differences were attributed to differences in salary |
| Bevis et al. (2008); comparison of outcomes of thoracostomies performed by NPs versus MDs | NP | Insertion complications, lengths of stay (LOS), morbidity | No differences in insertion complications, LOS, or morbidity |

*(continued)*

**Table 1.3  *Studies Assessing Performance-Related Outcomes of APN Care  (continued)***

| Study | APN role | Outcome indicators | Findings |
|---|---|---|---|
| Considine et al. (2006); comparison of NP care with ED MD care for patients with hand/wrist wounds, hand/wrist fractures, and cast removal | NP | ED wait times, treatment time, ED LOS | There were no differences in median LOS |
| Hoffman et al. (2006); comparison of NP and critical care fellow care for 192 ICU mechanically ventilated patients | NP | LOS, days of mechanical ventilation, readmissions, mortality | There were no differences in LOS, days of mechanical ventilation, readmissions, weaning status, or mortality |
| Seale, Anderson, and Kinnersley (2006); comparison of treatment advice of primary care NP versus general MD practitioners | NP | Treatment advice during same day appointments | A statistically significant greater proportion of NPs talk concerned treatments, with discussion of how to use treatments and of side effects |
| Sidani et al. (2006); comparison of processes of care (roles and coordination of services) of acute care NPs and physician residents | NP | Patient perceptions of care | NPs engaged in management and informal coordination activities more than MDs while MDs engaged in more formal coordination activities. NPs encouraged more patient participation in care and provided more patient education |
| Woods (2006); comparison of neonatal NP and MD care for neonates | NP | Assessment and clinical examination comprehensiveness, completeness of management plan, procedures performed, medications ordered, quality of record keeping | Management and care were found to be similar; there were no statistically significant differences in the standard and quality of care; however, NPs did not perform as well as MDs in terms of overall completeness or comprehensiveness of care |
| Vazirani et al. (2005); 2-year review of NP care for inpatients | NP | Perceptions of NP role by 156 MDs and 123 staff nurses | Physicians reported greater collaboration ($p < .001$) and better communication ($p = .006$); nurses reported better communication with NPs than with MDs ($p < .001$) |
| Hoffman et al. (2005); comparison of acute care NP care with critical care fellows care for 526 ICU patients | NP | Readmission, duration of mechanical ventilation, LOS | There were no differences in readmission, mortality, duration of mechanical ventilation, LOS, or disposition |

*(continued)*

## Table 1.3 *continued*

| | | | |
|---|---|---|---|
| Kleinpell (2005); 5-year longitudinal study of 437 acute NPs | NP | Role and role components | ACNPs reported spending a majority of time in direct patient care management (85% to 88%). Other care aspects of the role include teaching, research, program development, quality assurance, and administrative components |
| Krichbaum et al. (2005); impact of APN intervention to reinforce protocols for care for long-term care residents | APN | Urinary incontinence, pressure ulcers, depression, aggression | An APN-directed intervention resulted in improved resident outcomes for urinary incontinence pressure ulcers, depression, and aggression |
| Seale et al. (2006); comparison of NP and MD care for geriatric inpatients | NP | Time spent in activities including patient care, documentation, care, readmission, and mortality rates | Readmission and mortality rates were similar. NPs spent more time planning; MDs spent more time on literature reviews. Charges per length of stay were lower for MDs |
| Aigner et al. (2004); comparison of NP and MD care for nursing home residents | NP | ED visits, hospitalizations, LOS, costs, annual history and physical exams | No differences were found between the groups for outcomes; NP-managed patients were seen more often, reflecting increased patient access to care |
| Lenz et al. (2004); comparison of NP and MD care for primary care patients | NP | Health status, disease-specific physiologic measures, ED visits satisfaction | No differences were found between the groups in any measure |
| Scisney-Matlock et al. (2004); comparison of hypertension care by physicians versus physician-APN care | NP | Blood pressure control, patient knowledge of hypertension | NP-MD-managed patients had lower BP readings and higher scores for discussion of BP readings |
| Hoffman et al. (2003); ACNP care in comparison to pulmonary critical care fellows in ICU | NP | Activities and roles in the ICU | ACNPs and fellows spent a similar proportion of time performing required tasks. Physicians spent more time in nonunit activities such as education while ACNPs spent more time interacting with patients and patients' families and collaborating with health care team |
| Lenz et al. (2002); comparison of NP and MD care for adults with type 2 diabetes | NP | Processes of care, hemoglobin AIC testing, documentation | NPs were more likely than MDs to document HgA1C levels, general education, patient height, urinalysis results, education about nutrition, weight, exercise, and medications |

*(continued)*

**Table 1.3** *Studies Assessing Performance-Related Outcomes of APN Care  (continued)*

| Study | APN role | Outcome indicators | Findings |
|---|---|---|---|
| Aubrey and Yoxall (2001); neonatal NPs provided the same comparison of neonatal NP versus MD care in resuscitation of 245 preterm infants at birth | NP | Resuscitation outcomes | Resuscitation teams led by NPs had the same number of interventions as those led by MDs. Babies resuscitated by NPs were intubated more quickly and received surfactant sooner ($p = .0001$) and were less likely to be hypothermic on admission to the ICU ($p = .013$) |
| Pioro et al. (2001); comparison of NP and MD care for 381 general medical patients | NP | LOS, costs, consultations, complications, transfers to ICU | There were no significant differences between NP and MD care |
| Sullivan-Marx and Maislin (2000); exploratory comparison study of NP ($n = 43$) and family MD ($n = 46$) relative work values in the Medicare fee schedule for 3 office visit codes | NP | Relative work values and intensity for 3 current procedural terminology (CPT) codes for office visits: 99203-office visit for new patient, 99213-office visit for established patient with low complexity medical decisions, and 99215-office or outpatient visit of established patient with high complexity medical decisions | No significant differences between NPs and MDs were found in the 3 CPT codes for relative work values and intensity. NPs estimated higher intraservice (face-to-face) time with patients ($p < .01$) and MDs higher pre-service time ($p < .05$) (reviewing health records, lab data) and post coordination of care, contact with family and insurer) |
| Mundinger et al. (2000); randomized trial of NP and MD care in primary care in 4 community-based and 1 hospital-based clinic. Care delivered to 806 NP patients was compared to care given to 510 physician patients | NP | Patient satisfaction health status physiologic test results 1 year service utilization | No significant differences found in patients' health status at 6 months; no differences in health service use at 6 months or 1 year; no differences in initial appointment; satisfaction with provider attributes was higher for physician at 6 months; for patients with hypertension, diastolic value was lower |
| Karlowicz and McMurray (2000); comparison of neonatal NP and pediatric residents' care of 201 low-birth-weight infants | NP | LOS, survival to discharge, costs | There were no significant differences between NP and MD care |

Table reviews studies published from 2000 to present. The prior edition of this book reported on studies published beginning in the 1960s and 1970s through 2009 (Kleinpell, 2009).

and published in the literature, those categorized as assessing performance-related outcomes of APN practice represent the largest number of studies.

Although categorization of APN studies facilitates analysis and critique, the categories are not mutually exclusive. Several studies combined measures of care-, patient-, and performance-related outcome measures.

## SOURCES FOR IDENTIFYING OUTCOME MEASURES AND OUTCOME INSTRUMENTS

Sources for identifying outcome measures include the literature on outcomes, outcomes measurement manuals, regulatory and accrediting agencies, governmental sources, and clinical practice guidelines. A number of data-gathering tools can be used to collect outcome data including flow charts, check sheets, protocols, guideline-based performance measures, critical pathways, and instruments. A growing number of instruments that have established reliability and validity are available for use in outcomes measurement studies. Sources for finding outcomes measurement tools include the literature, specialty organizations and institutes, software programs, and Internet sources.

Other sources of outcome and performance measures include textbooks, journal supplements, software, and Internet sources devoted to maintaining collections of instruments, tests, rating scales, and other tools that can be used for outcomes research. Issues to consider in choosing tools and instruments for outcomes measurement studies include instrument purpose and intended study population, length and completion time, degree and type of reliability, and validity testing conducted with the instrument, administration and scoring aspects, and associated fees for use and/or scoring. The use of objective documentation tools can also help to evaluate APN work activities and measure performance and outcomes (Whitcomb, Craig, & Welker, 2000). Such tools, like a customized APN productivity tool, can be used to track outcomes of APN care based on daily role components (Steuer & Kopan, 2011). The chapter by Schwartz et al. in this book further reviews sources of outcome instruments including Internet resources.

## HIGHLIGHTING THE IMPACT OF APN CARE NATIONALLY AND INTERNATIONALLY

The contributions of APN care are demonstrated not only in an impressive number of published studies but also in authoritative resources.

A recent scientific statement from the American Heart Association related to cardiology care and emerging training models identified that APNs with expertise in cardiac care contribute to cost-effective care, improved staffing, and continuity of care (Morrow et al., 2012). Similarly, the Society of Critical Care Medicine highlights the role of NPs in critical care and the impact on patient care in acute care and intensive care unit settings (Kleinpell, Buchman, & Boyle, 2012). An Agency for Healthcare Research and Quality review on the impact of APNs focused on the outcomes of APN care and APN-led initiatives on patient safety and quality of care (O'Grady, 2008). Additionally, a growing number of international studies and initiatives have also identified the increasing role that APNs play in providing patient- and family-centered care and in impacting quality of care (Albers-Heitner et al., 2012; Ball, Walton, & Hawes, 2007; Begley et al., 2010; Cheng, 2012; Cheung et al., 2011; Fagerström & Glasberg, 2011; Partiprajak, 2012; Schuttelaar et al., 2011). A country review of the APN role in Ireland, commissioned by the National Council for the Professional Development of Nursing and Nurse Midwifery, assessed the clinical and economic impact of the roles (Begley et al., 2010). Using a variety of data collection tools and Delphi methodology, the study demonstrated that care provided by clinical specialist and advanced practitioners improves patient/client outcomes, is safe, acceptable, and cost neutral. APN care was found to improve symptom management, appropriateness of medication regime, self-management, patient and family education, and reduce exacerbations of conditions, prevent complications, and improve adherence to treatment plans (Begley et al., 2010).

Other reviews of APN roles in Canada (DiCenso et al., 2010), Scotland (National Health Services, 2012), Australia (Chang, Gardner, Duffield, & Ramis, 2010; Jennings et al., 2008), Ireland (Meskell, 2012), the Netherlands (Dierick-van Daele et al., 2010), and Finland (Fagerström & Glasberg, 2011) highlight the importance of assessing outcomes to ensure continued role development.

## SUMMARY

Studies measuring the impact of APN care have found that APNs improve access to care, competently manage care for patients in a variety of health care settings, are accepted by patients, and provide high-quality care. Several studies additionally identified that the APN-led approach to care improves both the processes and outcomes of care, highlighting specific aspects such as increased use of clinical practice guidelines (Begly et al., 2010; Bissonnette, 2011; Gracias et al., 2008;

Russell et al., 2002). Additional research on APNs has further explored the impact of APN care on care-, patient-, and performance-related outcomes. Identifying domains of APN practice may help in categorizing role functions that are unique to APN practice and that can be examined in terms of their effect on patient outcomes. Beal (2000) examined the practice of NPs working in a neonatal intensive care unit and identified nine domains of NP practice including (1) diagnostic/patient monitoring, (2) management of patient health/illness, (3) administering/monitoring therapeutic interventions and regimens, (4) monitoring/ensuring quality of health care practices, (5) organization and work role, (6) helping role, (7) teaching/coaching role, (8) management of rapidly changing situations, and (9) consulting role. In evaluating what a particular APN role encompasses in terms of role functions, outcomes that are impacted by APN care can be more readily identified. Developing APN-specific metrics that reflect the direct-care role components can also help to facilitate the tracking of outcomes (Kapu, Thomson-Smith, & Jones, 2012).

A predominant number of studies have focused solely on comparing APN care to other health care providers. Although it is important to establish that APN care is not different (or better) than that of other health care providers, research on the unique contributions and outcomes of APN care is needed. Several synthesis reviews on the impact of APNs on patient outcomes have confirmed that additional studies are needed to demonstrate APN importance to cost and quality outcomes in a variety of populations (Hatem et al., 2009; Newhouse et al., 2011; Laurant et al., 2004).

The current emphasis on quality of care and care effectiveness mandates that APNs demonstrate their impact on patient care, health care outcomes, and systems of care. Assessing the outcomes of APN care has become a necessary rather than an optional component of performance evaluation. It is only through demonstrating the outcomes of APN care for patients, providers, and health care systems that the value of this care can be defined. Additionally, as the APN role is expanding to a variety of unique practice settings including in patient hospital settings, subacute care, urgent care, home care, long-term care, as well as traditional primary care settings, the impact of the APN in these settings needs to be further explicated.

## RECOMMENDATIONS FOR APN OUTCOME STUDIES

The Institute of Medicine report on the future of nursing highlighted the importance of promoting the ability of APNs to practice to the full extent of their education and training and to further identify nurses' contributions to delivering high quality care (Institute of Medicine of the National Academies, 2010). Inherent in this focus is the need to demonstrate the outcomes of APN care.

The use of practice-level outcome studies has been proposed as a way to practically measure the effect of APN care (Buppert, 2000). As randomized clinical trials are often not feasible in clinical practice settings, the use of practice-level outcome studies can enable measurement of an APN intervention by comparing the patient's improvement with the patient's baseline measurements (Buppert, 2000). Other study designs such as quasi-experimental, qualitative or descriptive, or the use of case studies can also be employed in assessing APN outcomes. Additionally, APNs and researchers who have conducted outcomes research on the impact of the APN role need to be encouraged to disseminate the results through publications and presentations.

Use of nationally recognized outcome measures and instruments rather than self-developed tools should be incorporated into APN outcomes research. The use of outcome measures that have an impact on health policy (such as costs, access to care, and quality of life) should also be adopted. Additionally, research with the use of randomization and experimental designs that incorporate multiple sites and/or large patient populations are also needed in APN outcomes research. Finally, successful methods and processes used to conduct outcomes research need to be shared to facilitate replication and to disseminate knowledge. The need for outcomes research on the APN role continues to exist. Measuring outcomes of advanced practice nursing is needed to establish the continued impact of APN care and highlight the effectiveness of APNs, as well as to identify the unique contributions that APNs bring to patient care in the evolving health care arena.

## REFERENCES

Ahrens, T., Yancey, V., & Kollef, M. (2003). Improving family communications at the end of life: Implications for length of stay in the intensive care unit and resource use. *American Journal of Critical Care, 12*(4), 317–23; discussion 324.

Aigner, M. J., Drew, S., & Phipps, J. (2004). A comparative study of nursing home resident outcomes between care provided by nurse practitioners/physicians versus physicians only. *Journal of the American Medical Directors Association, 5*(1), 16–23.

Albers-Heitner, C. P., Joore, M. A., Winkens, R. A., Lagro-Janssen, A. L., Severens, J. L., & Berghmans, L. C. (2012). Cost-effectiveness of involving nurse specialists for adult patients with urinary incontinence in primary care compared to care-as-usual: An economic evaluation alongside a pragmatic randomized controlled trial. *Neurourology and Urodynamics, 31*(4), 526–534.

Albers-Heitner, C. P., Lagro-Janssen, T. A., Joore, M. M., Berghmans, B. L., Nieman, F. F., Venema, P. P.,...Winkens, R. R. (2011). Effectiveness of involving a nurse specialist for patients with urinary incontinence in primary care: Results of a pragmatic multicentre randomised controlled trial. *International Journal of Clinical Practice, 65*(6), 705–712.

Albers-Heitner, P., Berghmans, B., Joore, M., Lagro-Janssen, T., Severens, J., Nieman, F., & Winkens, R. (2008). The effects of involving a nurse practitioner in primary care for adult patients with urinary incontinence: The PromoCon study (Promoting Continence). *BMC Health Services Research, 8*, 84.

Andrus, M. R., & Donaldson, A. R. (2006). Outcomes of a lipid management program in a rural nurse practitioner clinic. *The Annals of Pharmacotherapy, 40*(4), 782.

Anetzberger, G. J., Stricklin, M. L., Gauntner, D., Banozic, R., & Laurie, R. (2006). VNA HouseCalls of greater Cleveland, Ohio: Development and pilot evaluation of a program for high-risk older adults offering primary medical care in the home. *Home Health Care Services Quarterly, 25*(3–4), 155–166.

Aubrey, W. R., & Yoxall, C. W. (2001). Evaluation of the role of the neonatal nurse practitioner in resuscitation of preterm infants at birth. *Archives of Disease in Childhood: Fetal and Neonatal Edition, 85*(2), F96–F99.

Badger, M. J., Lookinland, S., Tiedeman, M., Anderson, V., & Eggett, D. (2002). Nurse practitioners' treatment of febrile infants in Utah: Comparison to physician practice nationally. *Journal of the American Academy of Nurse Practitioners, 14*(12), 540–553.

Ball, C., & Cox, C. L. (2003). Part one: Restoring patients to health outcomes and indicators of advanced nursing practice in adult critical care. *International Journal of Nursing Practice, 9*(6), 356–367.

Ball, S. T., Walton, K., & Hawes, S. (2007). Do emergency department physiotherapy practitioner's, emergency nurse practitioners and doctors investigate, treat and refer patients with closed musculoskeletal injuries differently? *Emergency medicine Journal, 24*(3), 185–188.

Barnason, S., & Rasmussen, D. (2000). Comparison of clinical practice changes in a rapid recovery program for coronary artery bypass graft patients. *The Nursing Clinics of North America, 35*(2), 395–403.

Baxter, J., & Leary, A. (2011). Productivity gains by specialist nurses. *Nursing Times, 107*(30–31), 15–17.

Beal, J. A., & Quinn, M. (2002). The nurse practitioner role in the NICU as perceived by parents. *MCN, The American Journal of Maternal/Child Nursing, 27*, 183–188.

Becker, D., Kaplow, R., Muenzen, P. M., & Hartigan, C. (2006). Activities performed by acute and critical care advanced practice nurses: American Association of Critical-Care Nurses Study of Practice. *American Journal of Critical Care, 15*(2), 130–148.

Begley, C., Murphy, K., Higgins, A., Elliot, J., et al. (2010). Evaluation of *clinical nurse and midwife practitioner roles in Ireland (SCAPE): Final Report*. Dublin, National Council for the Professional Development of Nursing and Midwifery in Ireland. http://www.tcd.ie/Nursing_Midwifery/assets/research/pdf/SCAPE_Final_Report_13th_May.pdf Accessed August 10 2012.

Benatar, D., Bondmass, M., Ghitelman, J., & Avitall, B. (2003). Outcomes of chronic heart failure. *Archives of Internal Medicine, 163*(3), 347–352.

Benkert, R., Buchholz, S., & Poole, M. (2001). Hypertension outcomes in an urban nurse-managed center. *Journal of the American Academy of Nurse Practitioners, 13*(2), 84–89.

Bevis, L. C., Berg-Copas, G. M., Thomas, B. W., Vasquez, D. G., Wetta-Hall, R., Brake, D.,...Harrison, P. (2008). Outcomes of tube thoracostomies performed by advanced practice providers vs trauma surgeons. *American Journal of Critical Care, 17*(4), 357–363.

Bissonnette, J. (2011). Evaluation of an advanced practice nurse led interprofessional collaborative chronic care approach for kidney transplant patients: The TARGET study. Retrieved from http://www.ruor.uottawa.ca/en/handle/10393/19975.

Blue, L., Lang, E., McMurray, J. J., Davie, A. P., McDonagh, T. A., Murdoch, D. R.,...Morrison, C. E. (2001). Randomised controlled trial of specialist nurse intervention in heart failure. *BMJ, 323*(7315), 715–718.

Borgmeyer, A., Gyr, P. M., Jamerson, P. A., & Henry, L. D. (2008). Evaluation of the role of the pediatric nurse practitioner in an inpatient asthma program. *Journal of Pediatric Health Care, 22*(5), 273–281.

Bourbonniere, M., & Evans, L. K. (2002). Advanced practice nursing in the care of frail older adults. *Journal of the American Geriatrics Society, 50*(12), 2062–2076.

Boville, D., Saran, M., Salem, J. K., Clough, L., Jones, R. R., Radwany, S. M., & Sweet, D. B. (2007). An innovative role for nurse practitioners in managing chronic disease. *Nursing Economics, 25*(6), 359–364.

Bradway, C., Trotta, R., Bixby, M. B., McPartland, E., Wollman, M. C., Kapustka, H.,...Naylor, M. D. (2012). A qualitative analysis of an advanced practice nurse-directed transitional care model intervention. *The Gerontologist, 52*(3), 394–407.

Brandon, A. F., Schuessler, J. B., Ellison, K. J., & Lazenby, R. B. (2009). The effects of an advanced practice nurse led telephone intervention on outcomes of patients with heart failure. *Applied Nursing Research, 22*(4), e1–e7.

Brooten, D., Youngblut, J. M., Brown, L., Finkler, S. A., Neff, D. F., & Madigan, E. (2001). A randomized trial of nurse specialist home care for women with high-risk pregnancies: Outcomes and costs. *The American Journal of Managed Care, 7*(8), 793–803.

Bryant, R., & Graham, M. C. (2002). Advanced practice nurses: A study of client satisfaction. *Journal of the American Academy of Nurse Practitioners, 14*(2), 88–92.

Bryant-Lukosius, D., & DiCenso, A. (2004). A framework for the introduction and evaluation of advanced practice nursing roles. *Journal of Advanced Nursing, 48*(5), 530–540.

Bryant-Lukosius, D., DiCenso, A., Browne, G., & Pinelli, J. (2004). Advanced practice nursing roles: Development, implementation and evaluation. *Journal of Advanced Nursing, 48*(5), 519–529.

Buchholz, S. W., & Purath, J. (2007). Physical activity and physical fitness counseling patterns of adult nurse practitioners. *Journal of the American Academy of Nurse Practitioners, 19*(2), 86–92.

Buppert, C. (2000). Measuring outcomes in primary care practice. *Nurse Practitioner, 25(1),* 88–98.

Burns, S. M., & Earven, S. (2002). Improving outcomes for mechanically ventilated medical intensive care unit patients using advanced practice nurses: A 6-year experience. *Critical Care Nursing Clinics of North America, 14*(3), 231–243.

Burns, S. M., Earven, S., Fisher, C., Lewis, R., Merrell, P., Schubart, J. R.,...Bleck, T. P. (2003). Implementation of an institutional program to improve clinical and financial outcomes of mechanically ventilated patients: One-year outcomes and lessons learned. *Critical Care Medicine, 31*(12), 2752–2763.

Callahan, C. M., Boustani, M. A., Unverzagt, F. W., Austrom, M. G., Damush, T. M., Perkins, A. J.,...Hendrie, H. C. (2006). Effectiveness of collaborative care for older adults with Alzheimer disease in primary care: A randomized controlled trial. *The Journal of the American Medical Association, 295*(18), 2148–2157.

Capezuti, E., Wagner, L. M., Brush, B. L., Boltz, M., Renz, S., & Talerico, K. A. (2007). Consequences of an intervention to reduce restrictive side rail use in nursing homes. *Journal of the American Geriatrics Society, 55*(3), 334–341.

Carroll, D. L., Robinson, E., Buselli, E., Berry, D., & Rankin, S. H. (2001). Activities of the APN to enhance unpartnered elders self-efficacy after myocardial infarction. *Clinical Nurse Specialist, 15*(2), 60–66.

Case, R., Haynes, D., Holaday, B., & Parker, V. G. (2010). Evidence-based nursing: The role of the advanced practice registered nurse in the management of heart failure patients in the outpatient setting. *Dimensions of Critical Care Nursing, 29*(2), 57–62; quiz 63.

Chang, A. M., Gardner, G. E., Duffield, C., & Ramis, M. A. (2010). A Delphi study to validate an advanced practice nursing tool. *Journal of Advanced Nursing, 66*(10), 2320–2330.

Chen, D. Y., Jing, J., Schneider, P. F., & Chen, T. H. (2009). Comparison of the long-term efficacy of low dose 131I versus antithyroid drugs in the treatment of hyperthyroidism. *Nuclear Medicine Communications, 30*(2), 160–168.

Cheng, C. (2012). The impact of an APN-led clinic on patients with psychosis. In Seventh Annual International Nurse Practitioner/Advanced Practice Nursing Network Conference, London, England, UK, August 20–22, 2012, 19–20.

Cheung, N. F., Mander, R., Wang, X., Fu, W., Zhou, H., & Zhang, L. (2011). Clinical outcomes of the first midwife-led normal birth unit in China: A retrospective cohort study. *Midwifery, 27*(5), 582–587.

Cibulka, N. J., Forney, S., Goodwin, K., Lazaroff, P., & Sarabia, R. (2011). Improving oral health in low-income pregnant women with a nurse practitioner-directed oral care program. *Journal of the American Academy of Nurse Practitioners, 23*(5), 249–257.

Coddington, J., Sands, L., Edwards, N., Kirkpatrick, J., & Chen, S. (2011). Quality of health care provided at a pediatric nurse-managed clinic. *Journal of the American Academy of Nurse Practitioners, 23*(12), 674–680.

Considine, J., Martin, R., Smit, D., Winter, C., & Jenkins, J. (2006). Emergency nurse practitioner care and emergency department patient flow: Case-control study. *Emergency Medicine Australasia, 18*(4), 385–390.

Corner, J., Halliday, D., Haviland, J., Douglas, H. R., Bath, P., Clark, D., ... Webb, T. (2003). Exploring nursing outcomes for patients with advanced cancer following intervention by Macmillan specialist palliative care nurses. *Journal of Advanced Nursing, 41*(6), 561–574.

Cooper, M. A., Lindsay, G. M., Kinn, S., & Swann, I. J. (2002). Evaluating Emergency Nurse Practitioner services: A randomized controlled trial. *Journal of Advanced Nursing, 40*(6), 721–730.

Cooper, J. M., Loeb, S. J., & Smith, C. A. (2010). The primary care nurse practitioner and cancer survivorship care. *Journal of the American Academy of Nurse Practitioners, 22*(8), 394–402.

Counsell, S. R., Callahan, C. M., Clark, D. O., Tu, W., Buttar, A. B., Stump, T. E., & Ricketts, G. D. (2007). Geriatric care management for low-income seniors: A randomized controlled trial. *The Journal of the American Medical Association, 298*(22), 2623–2633.

Cowan, M. J., Shapiro, M., Hays, R. D., Afifi, A., Vazirani, S., Ward, C. R., & Ettner, S. L. (2006). The effect of a multidisciplinary hospitalist/physician and advanced practice nurse collaboration on hospital costs. *The Journal of Nursing Administration, 36*(2), 79–85.

Cragin, L., & Kennedy, H. P. (2006). Linking obstetric and midwifery practice with optimal outcomes. *Journal of Obstetric, Gynecologic, and Neonatal Nursing, 35*(6), 779–785.

Cunningham, R. S. (2004). Advanced practice nursing outcomes: A review of selected empirical literature. *Oncology Nursing Forum, 31*(2), 219–232.

Curran, C. R., & Roberts, W. D. (2002). Columbia University's competency and evidence-based Acute Care Nurse Practitioner Program. *Nursing Outlook, 50*(6), 232–237.

Dahl, J., & Penque, S. (2001). The effects of an advanced practice nurse-directed heart failure program. *Dimensions of Critical Care Nursing, 20*(5), 20–28.

DeJong, S. R., & Veltman, R. H. (2004). The effectiveness of a CNS-led community-based COPD screening and intervention program. *Clinical Nurse Specialist, 18*(2), 72–79.

Delgado-Passler, P., & McCaffrey, R. (2006). The influences of postdischarge management by nurse practitioners on hospital readmission for heart failure. *Journal of the American Academy of Nurse Practitioners, 18*(4), 154–160.

Dellasega, C., & Zerbe, T. M. (2002). Caregivers of frail rural older adults. Effects of an advanced practice nursing intervention. *Journal of Gerontological Nursing, 28*(10), 40–49.

DiCenso, A., Bryant-Lukosius, D., Martin-Misener, R., Donald, F., Abelson, J., Bourgeault, I., ... Harbman, P. (2010). Factors enabling advanced practice nursing role integration in Canada. *Nursing Leadership, 23 Spec No 2010*, 211–238.

Dick, K., & Frazier, S. C. (2006). An exploration of nurse practitioner care to homebound frail elders. *Journal of the American Academy of Nurse Practitioners, 18*(7), 325–334.

Dickerson, S. S., Wu, Y. W., & Kennedy, M. C. (2006). A CNS-facilitated ICD support group: A clinical project evaluation. *Clinical Nurse Specialist, 20*(3), 146–153.

Dierick-van Daele, A. T., Metsemakers, J. F. M., Derckx, E. W., Spreeuwenberg, C., & Vrijhoef, H. J. (2009). Nurse practitioners substituting for general practitioners: Randomized control trial. *Journal of Advanced Nursing, 65,* 391–401.

Dierick-van Daele, A. T., Spreeuwenberg, C., Derckx, E. W., van Leeuwen, Y., Toemen, T., Legius, M.,... Vrijhoef, H. J. (2010). The value of nurse practitioners in Dutch general practices. *Quality in Primary Care, 18*(4), 231–241.

Diesch, P., Soukup, M., Adams, P. C., & Wild, M. (2000). Guided imagery replication study using coronary artery bypass graft patients. *Nursing Clinics of North America, 25,* 417–425.

Doran, D., Mildon, B., & Clarke, S. (2011). Towards a national report card in nursing: A knowledge synthesis. *Nursing Leadership, 24*(2), 38–57.

Dulisse, B., & Cromwell, J. (2010). No harm found when nurse anesthetists work without supervision by physicians. *Health Affairs, 29*(8), 1469–1475.

Elpern, E. H., Killeen, K., Ketchem, A., Wiley, A., Patel, G., & Lateef, O. (2009). Reducing use of indwelling urinary catheters and associated urinary tract infections. *American Journal of Critical Care, 18*(6), 535–41; quiz 542.

Esperat, M. C., Hanson-Turton, T., Richardson, M., Tyree Debisette, A., & Rupinta, C. (2012). Nurse-managed health centers: Safety-net care through advanced nursing practice. *Journal of the American Academy of Nurse Practitioners, 24*(1), 24–31.

Ettner, S. L., Kotlerman, J., Afifi, A., Vazirani, S., Hays, R. D., Shapiro, M., & Cowan, M. (2006). An alternative approach to reducing the costs of patient care? A controlled trial of the multi-disciplinary doctor-nurse practitioner (MDNP) model. *Medical Decision Making, 26*(1), 9–17.

Fanta, K., Cook, B., Falcone, R. A., Rickets, C., Schweer, L., Brown, R. L., & Garcia, V. F. (2006). Pediatric trauma nurse practitioners provide excellent care with superior patient satisfaction for injured children. *Journal of Pediatric Surgery, 41*(1), 277–281.

Fagerström, L., & Glasberg, A. L. (2011). The first evaluation of the advanced practice nurse role in Finland - the perspective of nurse leaders. *Journal of Nursing Management, 19*(7), 925–932.

Forster, A. J., Clark, H. D., Menard, A., Dupuis, N., Chernish, R., Chandok, N.,... van Walraven, C. (2005). Effect of a nurse team coordinator on outcomes for hospitalized medicine patients. *The American Journal of Medicine, 118*(10), 1148–1153.

Fry, M. (2011). Literature review of the impact of nurse practitioners in critical care services. *Nursing in Critical Care, 16*(2), 58–66.

Fulton, J. (2012). *Validation of clinical nurse specialist core practice outcomes.* In Seventh Annual International Nurse Practitioner/Advanced Practice

Nursing Network Conference, London, England, UK, August 20–22, 2012, 37.

Fulton, J. S., & Baldwin, K. (2004). An annotated bibliography reflecting CNS practice and outcomes. *Clinical Nurse Specialist, 18*(1), 21–39.

Gawlinski, A., & McCloy, K. (2001). Measuring outcomes in cardiovascular advanced practice nursing. In R. Kleinpell (Ed.), *Assessing outcomes in advanced practice nursing*. New York, NY: Springer Publishing.

Gershengorn, H. B., Wunsch, H., Wahab, R., Leaf, D. E., Leaf, D., Brodie, D., ...Factor, P. (2011). Impact of nonphysician staffing on outcomes in a medical ICU. *Chest, 139*(6), 1347–1353.

Gracias, V. H., Sicoutris, C. P., Meredith, D. M., Haut, E., et al. (2003). Critical care nurse practitioners improve compliance with clinical practice guidelines in the surgical intensive care unit. *Critical Care Medicine, 31*(12), A93.

Gracias, V. H., Sicoutris, C. P., Stawicki, S. P., Meredith, D. M., Horan, A. D., Gupta, R., & Schwab, C. W. (2008). Critical care nurse practitioners improve compliance with clinical practice guidelines in "semiclosed" surgical intensive care unit. *Journal of Nursing Care Quality, 23*(4), 338–344.

Green, A., & Davis, S. (2005). Toward a predictive model of patient satisfaction with nurse practitioner care. *Journal of the American Academy of Nurse Practitioners, 17*(4), 139–148.

Greene, D., & Dell, R. M. (2010). Outcomes of an osteoporosis disease-management program managed by nurse practitioners. *Journal of the American Academy of Nurse Practitioners, 22*(6), 326–329.

Gross, P. A., Aho, L., Ashtyani, H., Levine, J., McGee, M., Moran, S., ...Skurnick, J. (2004). Extending the nurse practitioner concurrent intervention model to community-acquired pneumonia and chronic obstructive pulmonary disease. *Joint Commission Journal on Quality and Safety, 30*(7), 377–386.

Gross, P. A., Patriaco, D., McGuire, K., Skurnick, J., & Teichholz, L. E. (2002). A nurse practitioner intervention model to maximize efficient use of telemetry resources. *The Joint Commission Journal on Quality Improvement, 28*(10), 566–573.

Grumbach, K., & Grundy, P. (2010). *Outcomes of implementing patient centered medical home interventions: A review of the evidence from prospective evaluation studies in the United States.* Retrieved September 10, 2012 from http://www.pcpcc.net/files/evidence_outcomes_in_pcmh.pdf

Hamilton, R., & Hawley, S. (2006). Quality of life outcomes related to anemia management of patients with chronic renal failure. *Clinical Nurse Specialist, 20*(3), 139–43; quiz 144.

Hanrahan, N. P., Wu, E., Kelly, D., Aiken, L. H., & Blank, M. B. (2011). Randomized Clinical Trial of the Effectiveness of a Home-Based Advanced Practice Psychiatric Nurse Intervention: Outcomes for Individuals with Serious Mental Illness and HIV. *Nursing Research and Practice, 2011*(</Is>), 840248.

Hardie, H., & Leary, A. (2010). Value to patients of a breast cancer clinical nurse specialist. *Nursing Standard, 24*(34), 42–47.

Hatem, M., Sandall, J., Devane, D., Soltani, H., & Gates, S. (2009). Midwife-led versus other models of care for childbearing women. *Cochrane Database of Systematic Reviews, 4*, CD004667.

Hoffman, L., Tasota, F., Scharfenberg, C., Zullo, T., & Donahoe, M. (2002). Management of ventilator dependent patients: 5-Month comparison of an acute care nurse practitioner versus physicians-in-training. *American Journal of Respiratory and Critical Care Medicine, 165*, A388.

Hoffman, L. A., Tasota, F. J., Zullo, T. G., Scharfenberg, C., & Donahoe, M. P. (2005). Outcomes of care managed by an acute care nurse practitioner/attending physician team in a subacute medical intensive care unit. *American Journal of Critical Care, 14*(2), 121–30; quiz 131.

Hoffman, L. A., Miller, T. H., Zullo, T. G., & Donahoe, M. P. (2006). Comparison of 2 models for managing tracheotomized patients in a subacute medical intensive care unit. *Respiratory Care, 51*(11), 1230–1236.

Hogan, P. F., Seifert, R. F., Moore, C. S., & Simonson, B. E. (2010). Cost effectiveness analysis of anesthesia providers. *Nursing Economics, 28*(3), 159–169.

Horrocks, S., Anderson, E., & Salisbury, C. (2002). Systematic review of whether nurse practitioners working in primary care can provide equivalent care to doctors. *BMJ, 324*(7341), 819–823.

Ingersoll, G. L. (2008). Outcomes evaluation and performance improvement: An integrative review of research on advanced practice nursing. In A. B. Hamric, J. A. Spross, & C. M. Hanson, (Eds). *Advanced practice nursing: An integrative approach*. Philadelphia, PA: Saunders Elsevier.

Ingersoll, G. L., McIntosh, E., & Williams, M. (2000). Nurse-sensitive outcomes of advanced practice. *Journal of Advanced Nursing, 32*(5), 1272–1281.

Institute of Medicine of the National Academies. (2010). *The future of nursing. Leading change, advancing health*. Washington, DC: National Academy of Sciences.

Jackson, D. J., Lang, J. M., Ecker, J., Swartz, W. H., & Heeren, T. (2003). Impact of collaborative management and early admission in labor on method of delivery. *Journal of Obstetric, Gynecologic, and Neonatal Nursing, 32*(2), 147–57; discussion 158.

Jackson, D. J., Lang, J. M., Swartz, W. H., Ganiats, T. G., Fullerton, J., Ecker, J., & Nguyen, U. (2003). Outcomes, safety, and resource utilization in a collaborative care birth center program compared with traditional physician-based perinatal care. *American Journal of Public Health, 93*(6), 999–1006.

Jackson, P. L., Kennedy, C., Sadler, L. S., Kenney, K. M., Lindeke, L. L., Sperhac, A. M., & Hawkins-Walsh, E. (2001). Professional practice of pediatric nurse practitioners: Implications for education and training of PNPs. *Journal of Pediatric Health Care, 15*(6), 291–298.

Jennings, B. M., Staggers, N., & Brosch, L. R. (1999). A classification scheme for outcome indicators. *Image – The Journal of Nursing Scholarship, 31*(4), 381–388.

Jennings, N., O'Reilly, G., Lee, G., Cameron, P., Free, B., & Bailey, M. (2008). Evaluating outcomes of the emergency nurse practitioner role in a major urban emergency department, Melbourne, Australia. *Journal of Clinical Nursing, 17*(8), 1044–1050.

Jessee, B. T., & Rutledge, C. M. (2012). Effectiveness of nurse practitioner coordinated team group visits for type 2 diabetes in medically underserved

Appalachia. *Journal of the American Academy of Nurse Practitioners, 24*(12), 735–743. doi:10.1111/j.1745-7599.2012.00764.x

Johantgen, M., Fountain, L., Zangaro, G., Newhouse, R., Stanik-Hutt, J., & White, K. (2012). Comparison of labor and delivery care provided by certified nurse-midwives and physicians: A systematic review, 1990 to 2008. *Women's Health Issues, 22*(1), e73–e81.

Johnson, K. C., & Daviss, B. A. (2005). Outcomes of planned home births with certified professional midwives: Large prospective study in North America. *BMJ, 330*(7505), 1416.

Kane, R. L., Flood, S., Keckhafer, G., & Rockwood, T. (2001). How EverCare nurse practitioners spend their time. *Journal of the American Geriatrics Society, 49*(11), 1530–1534.

Kannusamy, P. (2006). A longitudinal study of advanced practice nursing in Singapore. *Critical Care Nursing Clinics of North America, 18*(4), 545–551.

Kapu, A. N., & Kleinpell, R. (2012). Developing nurse practitioner associated metrics for outcome assessment [online ahead of print]. *Journal of the American Academy of Nurse Practitioner,* 1–8. doi:10.1111/1745-7599/12001

Kapu, A. N., Thomson-Smith, C., & Jones, P. (2012). NPs in the ICU: The Vanderbilt initiative. *The Nurse Practitioner, 37*(8), 46–52.

Karlowicz, M. G., & McMurray, J. L. (2000). Comparison of neonatal nurse practitioners' and pediatric residents' care of extremely low-birth-weight infants. *Archives of Pediatrics & Adolescent Medicine, 154*(11), 1123–1126.

Kelley, C. G., Daly, B. J., Anthony, M. K., Zauszniewski, J. A., & Stange, K. C. (2002). Nurse practitioners and preventive screening in the hospital. *Clinical Nursing Research, 11*(4), 433–449.

Kirkwood, B. J., Pesudovs, K., Loh, R. S., & Coster, D. J. (2005). Implementation and evaluation of an ophthalmic nurse practitioner emergency eye clinic. *Clinical & Experimental Ophthalmology, 33*(6), 593–597.

Kirton, O. C., Folcik, M. A., Ivy, M. E., Calabrese, R., Dobkin, E., Pepe, J., ... Palter, M. (2007). Midlevel practitioner workforce analysis at a university-affiliated teaching hospital. *Archives of Surgery, 142*(4), 336–341.

Kleinpell, R. M. (2012). Assessing outcomes of nurse practitioners and physicians assistants in the ICU. In R. M. Kleinpell, T. Buchman, & W. A. Boyle. (Eds.), Integrating nurse practitioners and physician assistants in the ICU: Strategies for optimizing contributions to care. *Society of Critical Care Medicine,* 73–86.

Kleinpell, R. M., Ely, E. W., & Grabenkort, R. (2008). Nurse practitioners and physician assistants in the intensive care unit: An evidence-based review. *Critical Care Medicine, 36*(10), 2888–2897.

Kleinpell, R. M., & Gawlinski, A. (2005). Assessing outcomes in advanced practice nursing practice: The use of quality indicators and evidence-based practice. *AACN Clinical Issues, 16*(1), 43–57.

Krichbaum, K. (2007). GAPN postacute care coordination improves hip fracture outcomes. *Western Journal of Nursing Research, 29*(5), 523–544.

Krichbaum, K., Pearson, V., Savik, K., & Mueller, C. (2005). Improving resident outcomes with GAPN organization level interventions. *Western Journal of Nursing Research, 27*(3), 322–337.

Krein, S. L., Klamerus, M. L., Vijan, S., Lee, J. L., Fitzgerald, J. T., Pawlow, A., Reeves,...Hayward, R. A. (2004). Case management for patients with poorly controlled diabetes: A randomized trial. *The American Journal of Medicine, 116*(11), 732–739.

Kutzleb, J., & Reiner, D. (2006). The impact of nurse-directed patient education on quality of life and functional capacity in people with heart failure. *Journal of the American Academy of Nurse Practitioners, 18*(3), 116–123.

Lacko, L. A., Dellasega, C., Salerno, F. A., Singer, H., DeLucca, J., & Rothenberger, C. (2000). The role of the advanced practice nurse in facilitating a clinical research study. Screening for delirium. *Clinical Nurse Specialist, 14*(3), 110–5; quiz 116.

Lambing, A. Y., Adams, D. L., Fox, D. H., & Divine, G. (2004). Nurse practitioners' and physicians' care activities and clinical outcomes with an inpatient geriatric population. *Journal of the American Academy of Nurse Practitioners, 16*(8), 343–352.

Lamirel, C., Bruce, B. B., Wright, D. W., Delaney, K. P., Newman, N. J., & Biousse, V. (2012). Quality of nonmydriatic digital fundus photography obtained by nurse practitioners in the emergency department: The FOTO-ED study. *Ophthalmology, 119*(3), 617–624.

Laurant, M., Reeves, D., Hermens, R., Braspenning, J., Grol, R., & Sibbald, B. (2004). Substitution of doctors by nurses in primary care. *Cochrane Database of Systematic Reviews,* 2004(4), Article CD001271. doi: 10.1002/14651858. CD001271.pub2.

Lenz, E. R., Mundinger, M. O., Hopkins, S. C., Lin, S. X., & Smolowitz, J. L. (2002). Diabetes care processes and outcomes in patients treated by nurse practitioners or physicians. *The Diabetes Educator, 28*(4), 590–598.

Lenz, E. R., Mundinger, M. O., Kane, R. L., Hopkins, S. C., & Lin, S. X. (2004). Primary care outcomes in patients treated by nurse practitioners or physicians: Two-year follow-up. *Medical Care Research and Review, 61*(3), 332–351.

Ley, S. J. (2001). Quality care outcomes in cardiac surgery: The role of evidence-based practice. *AACN Clinical Issues, 12*(4), 606–17; quiz 633.

Lin, S. X., Gebbie, K. M., Fullilove, R. E., & Arons, R. R. (2004). Do nurse practitioners make a difference in provision of health counseling in hospital outpatient departments? *Journal of the American Academy of Nurse Practitioners, 16*(10), 462–466.

Litaker, D., Mion, L., Planavsky, L., Kippes, C., Mehta, N., & Frolkis, J. (2003). Physician - nurse practitioner teams in chronic disease management: The impact on costs, clinical effectiveness, and patients' perception of care. *Journal of Interprofessional Care, 17*(3), 223–237.

Lowery, J., Hopp, F., Subramanian, U., Wiitala, W., Welsh, D. E., Larkin, A.,...Vaitkevicius, P. (2012). Evaluation of a nurse practitioner disease management model for chronic heart failure: A multi-site implementation study. *Congestive Heart Failure, 18*(1), 64–71.

McFarlane, K., Dixon, L., Wakeman, C. J., Robertson, G. M., Eglinton, T. W., & Frizelle, F. A. (2012). The process and outcomes of a nurse-led colorectal cancer follow-up clinic. *Colorectal Disease, 14*(5), e245–e249.

Malloy, M. H. (2010). Infant outcomes of certified nurse midwife attended home births: United States 2000 to 2004. *Journal of Perinatology, 30*(9), 622–627.

Mackey, T. A., Cole, F. L., & Lindenberg, J. (2005). Quality improvement and changes in diabetic patient outcomes in an academic nurse practitioner primary care practice. *Journal of the American Academy of Nurse Practitioners, 17*(12), 547–553.

McCabe, P. J. (2005). Spheres of clinical nurse specialist practice influence evidence-based care for patients with atrial fibrillation. *Clinical Nurse Specialist, 19*(6), 308–17; quiz 318.

McCauley, K. M., Bixby, M. B., & Naylor, M. D. (2006). Advanced practice nurse strategies to improve outcomes and reduce cost in elders with heart failure. *Disease Management, 9*(5), 302–310.

McCorkle, R., Dowd, M., Ercolano, E., Schulman-Green, D., Williams, A. L., Siefert, M. L.,...Schwartz, P. (2009). Effects of a nursing intervention on quality of life outcomes in post-surgical women with gynecological cancers. *Psycho-Oncology, 18*(1), 62–70.

McCorkle, R., Siefert, M. L., Dowd, M. F., Robinson, J. P., & Pickett, M. (2007). Effects of advanced practice nursing on patient and spouse depressive symptoms, sexual function, and marital interaction after radical prostatectomy. *Urologic Nursing, 27*(1), 65–77; discussion 78.

Meskell, P. (2012). Evaluation of an advanced nurse practitioner (emergency care)—An Irish perspective. *The Journal for Nurse Practitioners, 8*(3), 200–205.

Meyer, S. C., & Miers, L. J. (2005). Cardiovascular surgeon and acute care nurse practitioner: Collaboration on postoperative outcomes. *AACN Clinical Issues, 16*(2), 149–158.

Moore, S., Corner, J., Haviland, J., Wells, M., Salmon, E., Normand, C.,...Smith, I. (2002). Nurse led follow up and conventional medical follow up in management of patients with lung cancer: Randomised trial. *BMJ, 325*(7373), 1145.

Moote, M., Krsek, C., Kleinpell, R., & Todd, B. (2011). Physician assistant and nurse practitioner utilization in academic medical centers. *American Journal of Medical Quality, 26*(6), 452–460.

Morrow, D. A., Fang, J. C., Fintel, D. J., Granger, C. G., Katz, J. N., Kushner, F. G. et al. (2012). Scientific statement from the American Heart Association care unit and the emerging need for new medical staffing and training models: A evolution of critical care cardiology: Transformation of the cardiovascular intensive. *Circulation.* doi:10.1161/CIR.0b013e31826890b0

Morse, K. J., Warshawsky, D., Moore, J. M., & Pecora, D. C. (2006). A new role for the ACNP: The rapid response team leader. *Critical Care Nursing Quarterly, 29*(2), 137–146.

Mundinger, M. O., Kane, R. L., Lenz, E. R., Totten, A. M., Tsai, W. Y., Cleary, P. D., Friedewald, W. T.,...Shelanski, M. L. (2000). Primary care outcomes in patients treated by nurse practitioners or physicians: A randomized trial. *The Journal of the American Medical Association, 283*(1), 59–68.

National Health Services, Scotland, United Kingdom. (2012). *Advanced practice nursing toolkit*. Retrieved August 21, 2012 from http://www.advanced practice.scot.nhs.uk/.

Naylor, M. D., Bowles, K. H., McCauley, K. M., Maccoy, M. C., Maislin, G., Pauly, M. V., & Krakauer, R. (2011). High-value transitional care: Translation of research into practice [online ahead of print]. *Journal of Evaluation in Clinical Practice*, doi: 10.1111/j.1365-2753.2011.01659.x.

Naylor, M. D., Brooten, D. A., Campbell, R. L., Maislin, G., McCauley, K. M., & Schwartz, J. S. (2004). Transitional care of older adults hospitalized with heart failure: A randomized, controlled trial [online ahead of print]. *Journal of the American Geriatrics Society, 52*(5), 675–684.

Naylor, M. D., & Kurtzman, E. T. (2010). The role of nurse practitioners in reinventing primary care. *Health Affairs, 29*(5), 893–899.

Neff, D. F., Madigan, E., & Narsavage, G. (2003). APN-directed transitional home care model: Achieving positive outcomes for patients with COPD. *Home Healthcare Nurse, 21*(8), 543–550.

Newhouse, R. P., Stanik-Hutt, J., White, K. M., Johantgen, M., Bass, E. B., Zangaro, G., ... Weiner, J. P. (2011). Advanced practice nurse outcomes 1990–2008: A systematic review. *Nursing Economics, 29*(5), 230–50; quiz 251.

O'Grady, E. (2008). Advanced practice registered nurses: The impact on patient safety and quality. In *Patient safety and quality: An evidence based handbook for nurses*. Agency for Healthcare Research and Quality. Retrieved September 20 2012 from http://www.ahrq.gov/qual/nurseshdbk/docs/O'GradyE_ APRN.pdf.

Oliver, S., & Leary, A. (2010). Return on investment: Workload, complexity and value of the CNS. *British Journal of Nursing, 21*(1), 32, 34–37.

Oliveria, S. A., Altman, J. F., Christos, P. J., & Halpern, A. C. (2002). Use of non-physician health care providers for skin cancer screening in the primary care setting. *Preventive Medicine, 34*(3), 374–379.

Osevala, M. L. (2005). Advance-practice nursing in heart-failure management: An integrative review. *The Journal of Cardiovascular Management, 16*(3), 19–23.

Paez, K. A., & Allen, J. K. (2006). Cost-effectiveness of nurse practitioner management of hypercholesterolemia following coronary revascularization. *Journal of the American Academy of Nurse Practitioners, 18*(9), 436–444.

Partiprajak, S. (2012). Outcomes of advanced practice nurse led type 2 diabetes support group. *7th Annual International Nurse Practitioner/Advanced Practice Nursing Network Conference*, August 20–22, 2012, London, England, United Kingdom.

Pine, M., Holt, K. D., & Lou, Y. B. (2003). Surgical mortality and type of anesthesia provider. *AANA Journal, 71*(2), 109–116.

Paul, S. (2000). Impact of a nurse-managed heart failure clinic: A pilot study. *American Journal of Critical Care, 9*(2), 140–146.

Pohl, J. M., Tanner, C., Pilon, B., & Benkert, R. (2011). Comparison of nurse managed health centers with federally qualified health centers as safety net providers. *Policy, Politics & Nursing Practice, 12*(2), 90–99.

Pioro, M. H., Landefeld, C. S., Brennan, P. F., Daly, B., Fortinsky, R. H., Kim, U., & Rosenthal, G. E. (2001). Outcomes-based trial of an inpatient nurse practitioner service for general medical patients. *Journal of Evaluation in Clinical Practice, 7*(1), 21–33.

Rantz, M. J., Popejoy, L., Petroski, G. F., Madsen, R. W., Mehr, D. R., Zwygart-Stauffacher, M.,…Maas, M. (2001). Randomized clinical trial of a quality improvement intervention in nursing homes. *The Gerontologist, 41*(4), 525–538.

Reavis, C. (2004). Nurse practitioner-delivered primary health care in urban ambulatory care settings. *American Journal for Nurse Practitioners, 8*(5), 41–49.

Reigle, J., Molnar, H. M., Howell, C., & Dumont, C. (2006). Evaluation of inpatient interventional cardiology. *Critical Care Nursing Clinics of North America, 18*(4), 523–529.

Resnick, B. (2006). Outcomes research: You do have the time! *Journal of the American Academy of Nurse Practitioners, 18*(11), 505–509.

Rideout, K. (2007). Evaluation of a PNP care coordinator model for hospitalized children, adolescents, and young adults with cystic fibrosis. *Pediatric Nursing, 33*(1), 29–35; quiz 35.

Roblin, D. W., Becker, E. R., Adams, E. K., Howard, D. H., & Roberts, M. H. (2004a). Patient satisfaction with primary care: Does type of practitioner matter? *Medical Care, 42*(6), 579–590.

Roblin, D. W., Howard, D. H., Becker, E. R., Kathleen Adams, E., & Roberts, M. H. (2004b). Use of midlevel practitioners to achieve labor cost savings in the primary care practice of an MCO. *Health Services Research, 39*(3), 607–626.

Rosenfeld, P., McEvoy, M. D., & Glassman, K. (2003). Measuring practice patterns among acute care nurse practitioners. *The Journal of Nursing Administration, 33*(3), 159–165.

Ruiz, R. J., Brown, C. E., Peters, M. T., & Johnston, A. B. (2001). Specialized care for twin gestations: Improving newborn outcomes and reducing costs. *Journal of Obstetric, Gynecologic, and Neonatal Nursing, 30*(1), 52–60.

Russell, D., VorderBruegge, M., & Burns, S. M. (2002). Effect of an outcomes-managed approach to care of neuroscience patients by acute care nurse practitioners. *American Journal of Critical Care, 11*(4), 353–362.

Ryden, M. B., Snyder, M., Gross, C. R., Savik, K., Pearson, V., Krichbaum, K., & Mueller, C. (2000). Value-added outcomes: The use of advanced practice nurses in long-term care facilities. *The Gerontologist, 40*(6), 654–662.

Scherr, K., Wilson, D. M., Wagner, J., & Haughian, M. (2012). Evaluating a new rapid response team: NP-led versus intensivist-led comparisons. *AACN Advanced Critical Care, 23*(1), 32–42.

Schuttelaar, M. L., Vermeulen, K. M., & Coenraads, P. J. (2011). Costs and cost-effectiveness analysis of treatment in children with eczema by nurse practitioner vs. dermatologist: Results of a randomized, controlled trial and a review of international costs. *The British Journal of Dermatology, 165*(3), 600–611.

Scisney-Matlock, M., Makos, G., Saunders, T., Jackson, F., & Steigerwalt, S. (2004). Comparison of quality-of-hypertension-care indicators for groups treated by physician versus groups treated by physician-nurse team. *Journal of the American Academy of Nurse Practitioners, 16*(1), 17–23.

Seale, C., Anderson, E., & Kinnersley, P. (2005). Comparison of GP and nurse practitioner consultations: An observational study. *The British Journal of General Practice, 55*(521), 938–943.

Seale, C., Anderson, E., & Kinnersley, P. (2006). Treatment advice in primary care: A comparative study of nurse practitioners and general practitioners. *Journal of Advanced Nursing, 54*(5), 534–541.

Sears, J. M., Wickizer, T. M., Franklin, G. M., Cheadle, A. D., & Berkowitz, B. (2007). Nurse practitioners as attending providers for workers with uncomplicated back injuries: Using administrative data to evaluate quality and process of care. *Journal of Occupational and Environmental Medicine, 49*(8), 900–908.

Sears, J. M., Wickizer, T. M., Franklin, G. M., Cheadle, A. D., & Berkowitz, B. (2008). Expanding the role of nurse practitioners: Effects on rural access to care for injured workers. *The Journal of Rural Health, 24*(2), 171–178.

Shebesta, K. F., Cook, B., Rickets, C., Schweer, L., Brown, R. L., Garcia, V. F., & Falcone, R. A. (2006). Pediatric trauma nurse practitioners increase bedside nurses' satisfaction with pediatric trauma patient care. *Journal of Trauma Nursing, 13*(2), 66–69.

Sidani, S., Doran, D., Porter, H., LeFort, S., O'Brien-Pallas, L. L., Zahn, C., et al. (2006a). Outcomes of nurse practitioners in acute care. *Internet Journal of Advanced Nursing Practice, 8*(1).

Sidani, S., Doran, D., Porter, H., LeFort, S., O'Brien-Pallas, L. L., Zahn, C.,...Sarkissian, S. (2006b). Processes of care: Comparison between nurse practitioners and physician residents in acute care. *Nursing Leadership, 19*(1), 69–85.

Simonson, D. C., Ahern, M. M., & Hendryx, M. S. (2007). Anesthesia staffing and anesthetic complications during cesarean delivery: A retrospective analysis. *Nursing Research, 56*(1), 9–17.

Sole, M. L., Hunkar-Huie, A. M., Schiller, J. S., & Cheatham, M. L. (2001). Comprehensive trauma patient care by nonphysician providers. *AACN Clinical Issues, 2*, 438–446

Steuer, J., & Kopan, K. (2011). Productivity tool serves as outcome measurement for NPs in acute care practice. *The Nurse Practitioner, 36*(5), 6–7.

Stolee, P., Hillier, L. M., Esbaugh, J., Griffiths, N., & Borrie, M. J. (2006). Examining the nurse practitioner role in long-term care: Evaluation of a pilot project in Canada. *Journal of Gerontological Nursing, 32*(10), 28–36.

Sullivan-Marx, E. M., & Maislin, G. (2000). Comparison of nurse practitioner and family physician relative work values. *Journal of Nursing Scholarship, 32*(1), 71–76.

Sung, S. F., Huang, Y. C., Ong, C. T., & Chen, Y. W. (2011). A parallel thrombolysis protocol with nurse practitioners as coordinators minimized door-to-needle time for acute ischemic stroke. *Stroke Research and Treatment, 2011*, 198518.

Swindle, R. W., Rao, J. K., Helmy, A., Plue, L., Zhou, X. H., Eckert, G. J., & Weinberger, M. (2003). Integrating clinical nurse specialists into the treatment of primary care patients with depression. *International Journal of Psychiatry in Medicine, 33*(1), 17–37.

Sze, E. H., Ciarleglio, M., & Hobbs, G. (2008). Risk factors associated with anal sphincter tear difference among midwife, private obstetrician, and resident deliveries. *International Urogynecology Journal and Pelvic Floor Dysfunction, 19*(8), 1141–1144.

Tijhuis, G. J., Zwinderman, A. H., Hazes, J. M., Van Den Hout, W. B., Breedveld, F. C., & Vliet Vlieland, T. P. (2002). A randomized comparison of care provided by a clinical nurse specialist, an inpatient team, and a day patient team in rheumatoid arthritis. *Arthritis and Rheumatism, 47*(5), 525–531.

Tsay, S. L., Lee, Y. C., & Lee, Y. C. (2005). Effects of an adaptation training programme for patients with end-stage renal disease. *Journal of Advanced Nursing, 50*(1), 39–46.

United States Department of Health and Human Services, Administration for Children and Families. (2010). *Measuring outcomes guidebook*. Retrieved August 22, 2012 from http://www.acf.hhs.gov/programs/ocs/ccf/ccf_resources/measuring_outcomes.pdf

Urden, L., & Stacy, K. (2012). Clinical nurse specialist productivity and outcomes. In Seventh Annual International Nurse Practitioner/Advanced Practice Nursing Network Conference, London, England, UK, August 20–22, 2012, 31.

Vanhook, P. (2000, February 19). Presence of nurse practitioner on stroke team reduced morbidity, mortality. American Heart Association 25th International Stroke Conference Report. *Reuters Medical News.*

Varughese, A. M., Byczkowski, T. L., Wittkugel, E. P., Kotagal, U., & Dean Kurth, C. (2006). Impact of a nurse practitioner-assisted preoperative assessment program on quality. *Paediatric Anaesthesia, 16*(7), 723–733.

Vazirani, S., Hays, R. D., Shapiro, M. F., & Cowan, M. (2005). Effect of a multidisciplinary intervention on communication and collaboration among physicians and nurses. *American Journal of Critical Care, 14*(1), 71–77.

Wagner, L. M., Capezuti, E., Brush, B., Boltz, M., Renz, S., & Talerico, K. A. (2007). Description of an advanced practice nursing consultative model to reduce restrictive siderail use in nursing homes. *Research in Nursing & Health, 30*(2), 131–140.

Wand, T., White, K., Patching, J., Dixon, J., & Green, T. (2012). Outcomes from the evaluation of an emergency department-based mental health nurse practitioner outpatient service in Australia. *Journal of the American Academy of Nurse Practitioners, 24*(3), 149–159.

Wheeler, E. C. (2000). The CNS's impact on process and outcome of patients with total knee replacement. *Clinical Nurse Specialist, 14*(4), 159–69; quiz 170.

Whitcomb, R., Craig, R., & Welker, C. (2000). Measuring how acute care nurse practitioners affect outcomes. *Dimensions of Critical Care Nursing, 19*(6), 34–35.

Whitcomb, R., Wilson, S., Chang-Dawkins, S., Durand, J., Pitcher, D., Lauzon, C., & Aleman, D. (2002). Advanced practice nursing. Acute care model in progress. *The Journal of Nursing Administration, 32*(3), 123–125.

Willoughby, D., & Burroughs, D. (2001). A CNS-managed diabetes foot-care clinic: A descriptive survey of characteristics and foot-care behaviors of the patient population. *Clinical Nurse Specialist, 15*(2), 52–57.

Wit, M. A., Bos-Schaap, A. J., Hautvast, R. W., Heestermans, A. A., & Umans, V. A. (2012). Nursing role to improve care to infarct patients and patients undergoing heart surgery: 10 years' experience. *Netherlands Heart Journal, 20*(1), 5–11.

Wojner, A. W. (2001). *Outcomes management: Application to clinical practice.* St Louis, MO: Mosby.

Woods, L. (2006). Evaluating the clinical effectiveness of neonatal nurse practitioners: An exploratory study. *Journal of Clinical Nursing, 15*(1), 35–44.

# Chapter 2: Analyzing Economic Outcomes in Advanced Practice Nursing

KEVIN D. FRICK, CATHERINE C. COHEN, AND PATRICIA W. STONE

## Chapter Objectives

1. Present an overview of five different types of economic evaluations that an advanced practice nurse (APN) may encounter.
2. Contrast economic evaluation methodology with that of comparative-effectiveness studies.
3. Outline appropriate outcome measures for each type of analysis.
4. Summarize and critique published examples of each type of economic evaluation.
5. Discuss methodological issues of importance to economic evaluations.

## Chapter Discussion Questions

1. Compare and contrast comparative-effectiveness research with cost-effectiveness research.
2. Describe a scenario for study where a cost–utility methodology would be appropriate. Provide an example.

3. If studying three interventions with no single standard outcome measure (or validated means of clinical outcome aggregation), which methodology may be most appropriate?
4. What is a key assumption required for a successful cost–benefit analysis (CBA)? How are the outcomes of CBAs presented?
5. Use a "two-step" approach to determine cost of a new antibiotic formulation that requires 4 minutes of reconstitution preparation by the RN immediately prior to IV infusion.

Cost effectiveness of health care practice is an increasingly important topic in the delivery of care and consequently in nursing research. The growing proportion of older adults in the U.S. population, various improvements in healthcare technology, direct-to-consumer advertising for a long list of pharmaceuticals, increasing costs of doing business in other sectors besides health care, and international competitive pressures on wages and benefits have drawn greater attention to the costs of health care over time. The focus on cost is not the only factor raising the importance of studying and contemplating the cost effectiveness of health care in the United States. Other relevant factors include (1) the scientific recommendations related to the conduct of cost-effectiveness analyses that have been issued in the United States, (2) a format for formulary submissions offered by the Academy of Managed Care Pharmacy, (3) recognition by parties in the United States of other recommendations around the globe, (4) conferences related to cost effectiveness sponsored by the National Institute of Nursing Research, and (5) an increasing focus on comparative effectiveness more generally.

In 2010, U.S. health care spending increased 3.9% (greater than the rate of inflation) to a total of $2.6 trillion or 17.9% of the gross domestic product (Centers for Medicare & Medicaid Services, 2012). This increasing level of expenditure and the greater proportion of the gross domestic product being spent on health care forces policy makers to consider the costs as well as the effectiveness of new treatments, devices, or interventions. Health policy makers increasingly request analyses, including projected economic outcomes prior to the approval of funding for or reimbursement of these new activities.

In the current health care environment, advanced practice nurses (APNs) need to be knowledgeable about the interpretation of cost and effectiveness data in particular, when they are combined in a cost-effectiveness study.

The increased demand for economic information has resulted in a number of economic evaluations in the literature specific to nursing (e.g., Anderson, Walsh, Louey, Meade, & Fairbrother, 2002; Brooten et al., 2002; Crowther, 2003; Spetz, 2005) and a plethora of cost-effectiveness studies (Neumann, Greenberg, Olchanski, Stone, & Rosen, 2005). Not only are APNs and other clinicians now expected to review publications containing economic outcomes related to their services, but they must also participate in these analyses and interpret others for appropriateness of implementing findings into practice (e.g., Chiu & Newcomer, 2007; Chummun & Tiran, 2008; Lee, Chan, Chen, Gin, & Lau, 2007; Subramanian et al., 2007).

To accomplish these goals, APNs must understand how to distinguish comparative-effectiveness research from cost-effectiveness analysis (CEA) research. Comparative-effectiveness research has been defined as the conduct and synthesis of research comparing the benefits and harms of different interventions and strategies to prevent, diagnose, treat, and monitor health conditions in "real-world" settings; its purpose is to improve health outcomes by developing and disseminating evidence-based information about the everyday effectiveness of interventions (Federal Coordinating Council for Comparative Effectiveness Research U.S. President, U.S. Congress, & U.S. Department of Health and Human Services, 2009; Iglehart, 2009; Volpp & Das, 2009). This is in contrast to efficacy research, such as a randomized controlled trial, where the question is typically whether the treatment can work under a controlled environment. Because comparative-effectiveness research is aimed to inform actual patient situations, it is very much patient-centered and thus is also called patient-centered outcomes research. This methodology not only highlights the everyday needs of the patients, but it may also incorporate many different types of patient outcomes. Cost-effectiveness research is one type of patient-centered outcomes research that focuses on economic outcomes of two or more comparable health care interventions and is an important component of a comprehensive comparative-effectiveness assessment (Garber, 2011; Jacobson, 2007; Stone, 2001a, 2001b).

A number of different methods are employed to address economic outcomes of health care. The purposes of this chapter are (1) to present an overview of five different types of economic evaluations an APN may encounter, (2) discuss appropriate outcome measures for each type of analysis, (3) present and critique published examples of each type of economic evaluation, and (4) discuss methodological issues of importance to economic evaluations.

## TYPES OF ECONOMIC EVALUATIONS

Five different methods of economic evaluations are commonly used in assessing the economic impact of new health care interventions and technology. Table 2.1 presents a brief overview of these methods (Drummond, Sculpher, Torrance, O'Brien, & Stoddart, 2005). In all of these economic outcome evaluations, alternative strategies are compared and the incremental cost of the competing strategies is computed according to the following formula:

Incremental costs = $C1 - C2$

where $C1$ represents the cost of the new intervention and $C2$ represents the cost of the comparator (e.g., the next-best strategy). There is more variation between methods regarding how effectiveness is measured, although the focus remains on incremental changes in effectiveness (i.e., comparing the outcome of one intervention with that of another).

### Table 2.1  Types of Economic Evaluations

| Type of Study | Definition | Effect Measurement |
|---|---|---|
| Cost minimization analysis (CMA) | An analysis that computes the incremental costs of alternatives that achieve the same outcome | Not measured |
| Cost consequence analysis (CCA) | An analysis in which incremental costs and effects are computed, without any attempt to aggregate them | Natural occurring units* |
| Cost-effectiveness analysis (CEA) | An analysis in which incremental costs and effects are presented in a ratio | Natural occurring units |
| Cost-utility analysis | A special type of CEA, in which quality of life is considered | Quality-adjusted life years |
| Cost-benefit analysis (CBA) | An analysis in which incremental costs and effects are computed, and all benefits and costs are measured in dollars | Dollars |

*Examples of natural occurring units are life-years gained, disability-days saved, or cases avoided.

### Cost-Minimization Analysis

In a true cost-minimization analysis (CMA), only the costs are evaluated and the alternatives are assumed or have been found to offer equivalent outcomes. Many of these studies begin as cost-effectiveness studies (discussed in more detail below), in which the investigators expected one intervention to be both more effective and more expensive. As a result, in most published economic evaluations labeled as CMAs, some level of effectiveness of the strategies being compared is measured (e.g., Goodman et al., 2007; Patel, Duquaine, & McKinnon, 2007). In each study, clinical outcomes were measured prior to the study being published as a CMA. In the Goodman et al. (2007) study, the authors measured a number of outcomes of a fitness-for-life program and found no statistically significant differences between groups. In the Patel et al. (2007) study, outcomes associated with changes in the dosing of meropenem were found to be similar prior to the study being published as a cost-minimization study.

### Cost–Consequence Analysis

A cost–consequence analysis (CCA) is a study in which the costs and the consequences of two or more alternatives are measured, but costs and consequences are listed separately. This methodology is often chosen when there is no obvious summary measure for the outcomes applicable to the interventions being studied. In a CCA, the analyst expects the decision makers to form their own opinions about the relative importance of the findings. To facilitate decision making, the analysts provide an array of consequences applicable to each strategy. Two studies serve as examples of this methodology being used in the nursing literature. Sørensen and Frich (2008) analyzed the consequences of a nurse follow-up intervention for chronic nonmalignant pain patients and described outcomes in terms of the eight SF-36 subscales. Dawes et al. (2007) compared nurse-supported early discharge for women receiving major abdominal or pelvic surgery with those receiving usual care. In addition to studying costs, Dawes et al. examined results from the SF-36, complications, length of hospital stay, readmissions, and satisfaction.

### Cost-Effectiveness Analysis

CEA also measures incremental costs. In CEA, incremental consequences are measured in a single common natural unit, such as life-years gained or cases avoided. In addition, costs and effects are summarized in an incremental cost-effectiveness ratio, which is calculated using the following formula:

Cost-effectiveness ratio = $(C1 - C2)/(E1 - E2)$

where $C1$ equals the cost of the new intervention, $C2$ equals the cost of the comparator, $E1$ equals the effect of the new intervention, and $E2$ equals the effect of the comparator. For CEA, analysts often attach the resource utilization data-collection process to a randomized trial, usually powered on something other than the cost-effectiveness result (e.g., Paez & Allen [2006] examined nurse management of hypercholesterolemia patients), or employ a decision-analytic approach and model the problem through the use of a decision tree (e.g., Kang, Mandsager, Biddle, & Weber [2012] examined different methods of monitoring for methicillin-resistant *Staphylococcus aureus* in academic hospitals; Honkanen, Schackman, Mushlin, & Lachs [2005] modeled external hip protectors being used in nursing homes). A sample decision tree is diagrammed in Figure 2.1.

The decision is between choosing alternative 1 or alternative 2. Both alternatives have associated probabilities of good and bad outcomes. In addition, there are the associated costs of each strategy. The use of decision analysis and decision trees is a defined mathematical modeling technique. It is suggested that anyone interested in using this technique seek training opportunities. There are a number of highly readable texts available to the APN wishing to understand this approach better (Drummond et al., 2005; Haddix, Teutsch, & Corso, 2002; Muennig, 2008; Petitti, 2000).

A number of examples of CEA can be found in the recent nursing literature (Ganz, Simmons, & Schnelle, 2005; Honkanen et al., 2005; Kang et al., 2012; Paez & Allen, 2006; Rost, Pyne, Dickinson, & LoSasso,

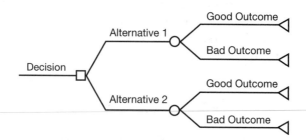

Figure 2.1 *Example of a Decision Tree*

2005). Paez and Allen (2006) provide an excellent example of deriving a CEA from a randomized trial. The study included 228 consecutive adults with hypercholesterolemia and chronic heart disease who were hospitalized. The intervention was follow-up care regarding lipid management, including lifestyle modification with services being provided by a nurse practitioner; this was compared with usual care enhanced with a small amount of extra information on lipids. The results were expressed as the extra dollars spent per unit change in low-density lipoprotein cholesterol (LDL-C) at 1 year and per percentage reduction in LDL-C at 1 year. Although this is an acceptable health outcome, it only facilitates comparison with other studies that are focusing on interventions for hypercholesterolemia. In contrast, Ganz et al. used a Markov simulation cohort (i.e., simulating what happens to a cohort of individuals over multiple periods through time) to estimate the cost effectiveness of having recommended staffing levels. This group used data from the literature, showed the sources very clearly, and expressed their results in dollars per quality-adjusted life year (QALY, discussed in more detail below).

The QALY is a common outcome unit at this point in time, as it has been recommended by a number of organizations around the world and facilitates comparisons among different studies. More generally, many economic analysts recommend using a standard outcome measure, such as dollars per life year ($/LY), because it is appropriate to different health care situations. Consequently, results can be compared across a variety of patient populations and settings. Although easy to understand, an outcome measure of $/LY considers only survival, not suboptimal health states and/or quality of life. This is a concern, as quality of life is often considered an important issue to individuals considering different health care treatments. This leads directly into the more detailed discussion of QALYs and their application, which follows.

### Cost–Utility Analysis

Cost–utility analysis (CUA) considers the effectiveness of the interventions on both the quantity and the quality of life in a single multidimensional measure, QALY. The QALY is a measure of the quantity of life gained weighted by the quality of that life. Quality of life is measured by a utility, which is a measure of preference for a given health state rated on a scale of 0 (death) to 1 (perfect health). Because dollars spent to gain a QALY are not disease specific, the measure is useful for informing health policy decisions and is recommended for such use by the U.S. Public Health Service's Panel on Cost-Effectiveness in Health and Medicine (Gold, Siegel, Russell, & Weinstein, 1996). However, variance in the interpretation of what QALYs are actually measuring ("Determinants of health economic decisions in actual practice: The role of behavioral economics," 2006) and lack of universal agreement as to what society should be willing to pay to gain a QALY persists (Donaldson et al., 2011; Hirth, Chernew, Miller, Fendrick, & Weissert, 2000; Ubel, Hirth, Chernew, & Fendrick, 2003). In fact, a 2009 meeting of the International Society of Pharmacoeconomics and Outcomes Research (ISPOR) devoted a development workshop to determining how to define and measure the value of QALY. Despite ongoing debate, the figure of $50,000/ QALY is still often cited in the United States (Braithwaite, Meltzer, King, Leslie, & Roberts, 2008).

One group of researchers considered a nursing intervention to increase adherence to antiretroviral therapy among HIV-infected patients (Freedberg et al., 2006). The design of this study illustrates how data from a randomized clinical trial can be combined with a computer-modeling exercise to conduct the CEA. The authors modeled the associated change in virologic suppression as well as changes in cost- and quality-adjusted survival. Comparing these results with the costs of the intervention and the therapy, the authors found the intervention to be highly cost effective, with a ratio of $14,100 per QALY gained compared with standard therapy.

### Cost–Benefit Analysis

CBA is a form of economic evaluation in which consequences are summarized in monetary units. In CBA, a single dollar figure representing costs minus benefits is calculated. As long as the decision maker agrees with the methods used to place a dollar value on outcomes, this provides the decision maker with a direct indication of whether the value of the benefits is greater than the cost. Simon et al. (2007) determined the net economic benefit of a nurse specialist-led program for patients with depression and diabetes. Their study used a randomized trial design and compared this program with "usual care" intervention. The care provided included psychotherapy and pharmaceutical treatment. A sufficient amount of other health services utilization was saved so that if a day without depression was counted as $10 (the type of assumption necessary for a CBA), the total positive economic benefit per patient was $952. The authors also conducted a statistical analysis to demonstrate that the 95% confidence

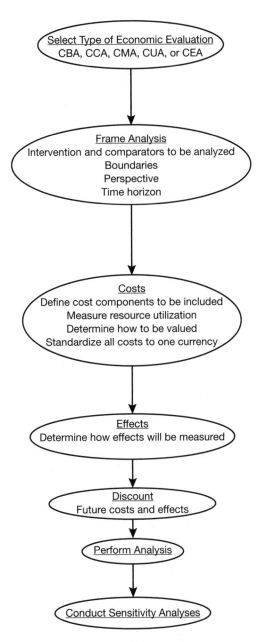

Figure 2.2 *Basic Steps in Economic Evaluations*

interval regarding the point estimate of economic net benefit did not include zero.

## COMMON ISSUES IN ALL ECONOMIC EVALUATIONS

The basic steps in conducting economic evaluations are illustrated in Figure 2.2. In addition, because this is essentially a new language to many APNs, Table 2.2 defines some of the concepts and common terminology used in these analyses.

### Selecting the Type of Economic Evaluation

The first step is to select the appropriate type of analysis to conduct. Considerations should include (1) the goal of the analysis (e.g., whether to compare only interventions affecting a single disease with a well-defined most important symptom or to compare interventions for different diseases or interventions for a condition with a complex set of symptoms), (2) whether the effectiveness of the interventions is equivalent (and, if so, this suggests a CMA), (3) the effectiveness measures available (e.g., can QALYs be generated), (4) the potential impact of the interventions on either quality or quantity of life (if both, then a CUA is most appropriate), (5) the availability of data, (6) the expertise available, and (7) ethical issues.

### Table 2.2  *Common Terminology in Economic Evaluations*

| Term | Definition |
|---|---|
| Boundaries of the study | The scope of the study |
| Comparator(s) | The alternative(s) to which the new intervention is compared |
| Consumer price index (CPI) | A measure of average change in price over time. This is used to adjust costs that are estimated in different years |
| Discounting | The process of converting future costs and effects to the present value |
| Incremental cost-effectiveness ratio | The ratio of the difference of the costs of two alternatives to the difference in effectiveness between the same two alternatives. Used in cost-effectiveness and cost–utility analyses |
| Perspective | The viewpoint from which the analysis is conducted |
| Sensitivity analysis | Calculations in which a parameter is varied and indicates the degree of influence it has on the analysis. Often used when a parameter is uncertain |
| Time horizon | The period of time for which the costs and effects are measured |

### Framing the Analysis

Once the economic method has been selected, the researcher frames the analysis. This includes selecting the appropriate comparator(s) to analyze. For example, when testing the cost effectiveness of a new educational program, the researcher might consider implementation in a hospital setting, initiation in an outpatient clinic, and a lack of teaching altogether as comparators given that outcomes may be different among them. At the least, the comparison of new interventions should be to the current practice, or status quo. Benchmarking to an established standard of care emphasizes the fact that analyses do not compare an intervention with "doing nothing." In addition, often more than one comparator is appropriate to include in the analysis. This is especially true when multiple alternatives have been found to offer similar clinical outcomes or if there are potentially multiple levels of intensity of the interventions (e.g., increasing home health visits from twice a week to daily).

Boundaries (i.e., the scope) of the study delimit the costs and effects that are included in the analysis. Many interventions have some spillover effects that must be considered. The question becomes how far to follow such effects to adequately assess the economic impact of the intervention. For example, if the aim of an educational program for mothers of infants admitted to a neonatal intensive care unit is to decrease the mothers' levels of anxiety and improve the physiologic outcomes of the infants, then it logically follows that the boundaries would include both the mothers and the infants. This intervention may affect the overall parenting skills of the mother, however, and may have additional positive effects on other children in the family. In theory, all these effects are relevant, but in framing the study it is important to draw practical and feasible limits around the analysis.

In all types of economic evaluations, the perspective or viewpoint taken in the analysis also drives the set of costs and benefits included. Studies may be motivated by policy decisions relevant to specific institutions or individuals. In this case, the perspective of primary interest may be that of a managed care organization, hospital, employer, state health department, or other party. An economic evaluation conducted from the perspective of the hospital (i.e., providing a result most relevant to a hospital decision maker) should not consider costs (or savings) associated with family caregiving in the home. If the goal of the analysis is to affect broad resource allocation and health policy issues, however, then the societal perspective is appropriate and recommended (Gold et al., 1996). This perspective incorporates all costs and all health effects regardless of who incurs them. This is advantageous because if a systematic analysis is performed to compare the results of multiple studies and all have used the societal perspective, it makes comparison easier. Gathering data for the societal perspective also allows any other perspective to be calculated as a subset of the societal perspective. A general rule is to take a societal perspective and then, if desired, present the same results from a different perspective.

The time horizon refers to the period of time for which the costs and benefits are measured in the analysis. The time horizon may vary from less than 1 year to the patient's entire life span. The appropriate time horizon to consider will depend on the probable length of effect of the interventions being compared. Once the framing of the analysis is complete, the analyst is ready to estimate costs. The distinction between the time of the intervention and the time horizon for the analysis must be kept in mind. An intervention that lasts less than 1 year (e.g., nurses providing counseling to adolescents on high-risk behaviors) may have effects that last a lifetime.

### Costs

Terminology pertaining to costs of resources has traditionally been divided into "direct" and "indirect" costs (Gold et al., 1996), with other labels like "friction costs" sometimes being applied to the cost of hiring a new employee and sometimes being applied to an entire method of valuing productivity (Brouwer & Koopmanschap, 2005; Gold et al., 1996). However, because economists and accountants do not use the same definitions and sometimes even economists have not been able to agree on a universal set of definitions, the terminology has become complicated. In health economics, direct costs have been defined as changes in resource use directly attributable to the provision of care, whereas indirect costs have referred to costs associated with the loss of productivity from morbidity and/or mortality (Liljas, 1998). Accountants, on the other hand, refer to direct costs as variable costs (e.g., supplies) and indirect costs as overhead costs (e.g., rent) (Anthony & Young, 1994). In light of these past inconsistencies in defining and measuring costs, the APN conducting an economic evaluation should be sure to clarify and clearly communicate how the cost terms are defined. The trend in the CEA literature is to avoid the term "indirect." Given this trend and the potential for confusion, we urge APNs to likewise avoid using this term.

Economists and analysts often use a "two-step" approach to determine the costs attributable to an intervention. The first step in the estimation is determining the amount of resources attributable or consumed. Once the attributable resources have been determined, the "money" valuation or costs of the resources may be estimated. Using a two-step approach increases the clarity and transparency of the analysis and allows readers of the analysis to understand how the costs of attributable resources may be similar or different in their own setting.

The resources and associated costs can be categorized as in Exhibit 2.1, which is an adaptation of a grouping that appeared earlier in the literature (Luce, Manning, Siegel, & Lipscomb, 1996). In CEA, financial health care costs are directly related to the intervention itself and associated costs or savings of future health care, which the intervention may impact. For example, financial health care costs associated with a hepatitis B virus (HBV) immunization program should include the costs of obtaining and administering the immunization. In addition, they should include "downstream" costs (as well as savings), such as hospitalizations, outpatient visits, and other treatment costs associated with the diagnosis of HBV itself. Financial costs associated with other related diseases, such as cirrhosis or cancer, should also be

**Exhibit 2.1  *Cost Components to Consider for Inclusion***

| |
|---|
| Direct health-care costs* |
|    Intervention |
|    Hospitalization |
|    Outpatient visits |
|    Long-term care |
|    Other health care |
|    Patient time receiving care |
| Direct non-health care |
| Transportation |
| Family/caregiver time |
|    Social services |
| Productivity costs* |
| Other |

*Not recommended for inclusion in cost-utility analyses by the United States Public Health Service's Panel on Cost-Effectiveness in Health and Medicine (Gold, Siegel, Russell & Weinstein, 1996).

included. Similarly, the value of the time a patient spends either seeking care or participating in an intervention constitutes a real use of resources for the individual and society. Thus, relevant patient–time costs may include both the time involved in receiving the treatment and the time spent waiting to receive care.

Consumption of resources other than those associated with the provision of health care also should be considered in economic evaluations conducted from the societal perspective. Financial non-health care costs may include, for example, child care costs for a parent attending a smoking cessation program, increase in a family's food expenditure as a result of a dietary prescription, the cost of transportation to and from a clinic, and the like.

Historically, patient time and other non-health care resources have not been consistently included in analyses (Jacobs & Fassbender, 1998; Stone, Chapman, Sandberg, Liljas, & Neumann, 2000). Nonetheless, if an analysis is conducted from the societal perspective, inclusion of such factors is recommended (Gold et al., 1996). In addition, because health care is becoming more community based, nursing interventions may directly influence these costs. For example, a home visit by an APN case manager may not only increase the ability of the APN to conduct a holistic assessment, but may also save resources related to patient time, transportation, and family caregiving. Bhandari (2011) included patient transportation costs of an iron supplementation therapy in a cost-minimization study and found that new iron preparations reduced these costs compared to standard of care.

Productivity costs are the costs associated with morbidity or mortality. Morbidity costs are those associated with lost or impaired ability to work or to engage in leisure activities (e.g., loss of income due to time for recuperation or convalescence after coronary bypass surgery). Mortality costs are related to loss of life and are usually measured according to what the individual would have been capable of earning. Two issues are important to note concerning productivity costs.

First, the U.S. Public Health Service's Panel on Cost-Effectiveness in Health and Medicine recommended that productivity costs be excluded from CUAs (Gold et al., 1996). The authors expressed concern that including both productivity costs and QALYs would represent a double counting because people may be considering productivity and earning potential when responding to tradeoffs involving health and quality of life. Thus, when QALYs are used, productivity is already included in the denominator of the cost-effectiveness ratio.

Second, the assumption that productivity costs should be excluded from CUAs is controversial and has been debated by experts in the field (Brouwer, Koopmanschap, & Rutten, 1997a, 1997b; Weinstein & Manning, 1997; Weinstein et al., 1997). In light of this controversy, some analysts have presented results both with and without the inclusion of productivity costs (Krahn, Guasparini, Sherman, & Detsky, 1998; Moradi-Lakeh, Shakerian, & Esteghamati, 2012). APNs conducting CUAs may also wish to present results both with and without the inclusion of productivity costs as well as continue to monitor recommendations made in the United States and elsewhere.

Some interventions (e.g., a successful smoking cessation program) extend life. Costs related to resource consumption in "added life years" are recommended for inclusion in economic evaluations. Added life-year costs are related to the consumption of health care resources (financial health care costs) and other types of consumption (all other cost categories). Because not all analyses increase life expectancy (e.g., use of cochlear implants or an educational intervention program aimed at decreasing parental anxiety), resource consumption in added life years is not always applicable. Sometimes, living longer and healthier can cost less annually but sum to more over a lifetime (van Baal et al., 2008).

Finally, income transfers such as Social Security payments are redistributions of money and are therefore not real costs to society. Consequently, although these "transfer costs" may be tracked and may be important for analyses from the government's perspective, they should not be included with other societal costs. What should be included in a societal cost analysis are the costs of administering an income transfer program.

When trying to determine which costs to include, the process should begin with an outline of the categories of costs included, using the list in Exhibit 2.1. Once this is complete, a researcher should consider the cost "ingredients" that the intervention impacts under each category (Drummond et al., 2005). After the ingredients are identified, discussions about which costs are most relevant and which are important to measure can take place. Moreover, the perspective of the analysis will drive the decisions about which cost component to include. The treatment of the cost component (e.g., productivity costs captured in quality of life adjustments) is determined by the specific economic analytic method chosen.

Once the consumption of resources has been estimated, the resource must be assigned a dollar value. Economists use the term "opportunity costs," which reflects the value of the next-best alternative use of the resources. Determining the actual opportunity cost of a resource is difficult. Following are some general guidelines for assigning a dollar value to a resource.

In many markets, market prices (or charges) equate to costs. This does not apply in health care as often as in other fields. This incongruence is particularly notable for charges associated with hospitalizations. Although health care institutions bill for standard amounts, some payers are able to successfully negotiate lower charges for care. However, payers who are willing to pay higher levels of reimbursement or unable to negotiate lower levels of reimbursement will ultimately pay more for the same care. The practice of obtaining higher payments from some patrons is termed "cost shifting." Therefore, for these institutional categories, an adjustment to prices is necessary to accurately represent exchange of funds, the cost. In fact, many customers, such as large insurance organizations, pay only a fraction of these charges. Large payers negotiate payment rates for services rendered based on the cost of the service and allowed profit margins (or excess revenues for not-for-profit institutions). Payers with the least market power (e.g., uninsured individuals) are the only ones who are likely to pay anything near the actual cost. If a hospital were just to break even based on the negotiated rates, then it is clear that the actual amount charged does not represent anything close to the actual cost.

Instead of using charges, a common source of valuation for hospital costs is the hospital's own cost-accounting system. For researchers internal to the institution, these will often be easy to access. These cost-accounting systems are developed by finance departments to help administrative decision making and are based on past accounting studies and algorithms. Although the market price of medical care often does not represent actual costs, the market prices of the goods in the cost-accounting system are expected to represent the relevant cost. If a cost-accounting system is available, the APN can usually determine the specific monetary health care cost components, such as variable costs (e.g., staffing and supplies) and fixed overhead costs (e.g., rent and percentage of administration costs).

Another alternative is to use hospital cost-to-charge ratios (CCRs), which are calculated by dividing the total costs in a cost center by the total charges for the same resource. CCRs are recognized as a gross adjustment to charges. This type of adjustment is better than using charges alone, but is not preferable to cost-accounting systems when they are available. Published sources also are often used as the source of valuation of the resource (Stone et al., 2000). Governmental fee schedules are also often used to represent costs of particular procedures (Armstrong, Malone, & Erder, 2008).

When cost estimations come from various sources, it is important to standardize all costs to the same currency and year. For example, non-

U.S. currency figures may be converted into U.S. dollars using the appropriate foreign exchange factor for that time period (Board of Governors of the Federal Reserve System, http://www.federalreserve.gov/releases/g5a/current/default.htm). A study of stoma therapy nurses demonstrates the concept of exchange rates (Becker, Schulten-Oberbörsch, Beck, & Vestweber, 1999). The concept of purchasing-power parity, which not only accounts for the exchange rate but also attempts to yield the capacity to purchase the same quantity of goods, is also commonly used (Urdahl, Knapp, Edgell, Ghandi, & Haro, 2003). In addition, because $1 in 1988 does not have the same purchasing power as $1 in the year 2008, the costs from different years must be adjusted into a standard year format by the use of the consumer price index (CPI), for which data are available from the Bureau of Labor Statistics (BLS) website (www.bls.gov), and a single year-to-year calculation can be done using the inflation calculator provided at that website (http://data.bls.gov/cgi-bin/cpicalc.pl). This inflation calculator is based on general market goods inflation. The BLS also calculates a medical inflation rate (http://www.bls.gov/spotlight/2009/health_care/). Because the costs of health care are rising more rapidly than costs in most other markets, analysts often use the medical inflation rate to inflate costs that pertain only to health care resources. A recent study of the costs of nurse turnover demonstrates inflation adjustment for calculations that could serve as an input to cost–benefit analyses related to retention efforts (Jones, 2008). Finally, there is discussion as to whether to use the consumer price index (CPI) or the producer price index for inflation adjustment in general. Again, this largely depends on perspective. True opportunity costs are likely to be reflected in the producer price index. However, if the perspective is a payer perspective, then the CPI is likely to be more appropriate.

### Discounting

Once all costs and benefits have been calculated, future costs and benefits are discounted to present value. Discounting reflects the principle that suggests people place greater value on something they have today than on something they will have in the future. Interest rates are an example of this principle. Future costs and benefits are discounted to present value using the following formula:

$$F/(1 + r)n$$

where $F$ is the future value (usually measured in dollars at today's value), $r$ is the discount rate, and $n$ is the number of years in the future

(Stone, 1998). Currently, in the United States, experts recommend using a 3% discount rate to discount both costs and effects (Gold et al., 1996). However, because prevention interventions are aimed at improving future health, by discounting future benefits, the intervention may not seem as beneficial. Therefore, some analysts are uncomfortable discounting future health benefits and only discount costs (Stone et al., 2000). Thus, to increase the comparability of analyses, APNs in the United States should discount both costs and effects at 3% and, if desired, the results without discounting may also be presented (Gold et al., 1996). Moreover, prior to the recommendations being issued by the U.S. Public Health Service's Panel on Cost-Effectiveness in Health and Medicine in 1996, many analysts used a 5% discount rate, so this was suggested as an additional discount rate to use for comparison (Gold et al., 1996).

### Analysis

In conducting economic evaluations, data gathered may include resource utilization, value of resources, effectiveness of treatment, and preferences regarding health outcomes. Based on the data gathered, the "base-case" analysis is computed. If the recommendations made by the U.S. Public Health Service's Panel on Cost-Effectiveness in Health and Medicine are followed, this initial analysis is labeled a "reference case" (Gold et al., 1996). A best practice when presenting results (whether they represent the reference case or not) is to include a table listing all parameters, the value assigned to each parameter, and the source of the value.

### Sensitivity Analysis

Many of the data points gathered include some assumptions or uncertainty in the parameter. For clarification, the analysis based only on the best point estimates is referred to as the "base case," regardless of whether the recommendations of the panel are followed. Thus, any CEA includes a base case, but not all base-case analyses are reference case analyses.

The assumptions that are made in the base case should be clearly stated before the results are presented to increase the transparency of the analysis. In addition, sensitivity analyses should be conducted to explore the implications of alternative assumptions. Sensitivity analysis is an important element of a sound economic evaluation (Drummond et al., 2005; Gold et al., 1996).

Sensitivity analyses are calculations in which a parameter is varied. These analyses indicate the degree of influence the particular value has on the analysis. The range used for a parameter should be specified along with the point estimate in Table 2.2.

A univariate sensitivity analysis examines the degree to which changing a single assumption changes the outcome of the entire analysis. By varying the value of the variable over a reasonable set of parameters, the investigator is able to determine how that variable may impact the results under different assumptions. The impact on the results has multiple interpretations. One is how the magnitude of the cost-effectiveness ratio changes; in other words, whether the ratio changes from spending $10,000/QALY gained to $30,000/QALY gained. However, a second level of interpretation is whether the decision to implement or not implement a new intervention changes. If a decision maker believes that any program costing less than $50,000 is a candidate for implementation, then the change from $10,000/QALY to $30,000/QALY will not change the decision about whether to consider a new intervention for implementation. Ganz et al. (2005) used a series of univariate sensitivity analyses to explore which parameter led to the greatest change in the incremental cost effectiveness of raising nurse staffing in skilled nursing facilities from the median level to the recommended level. The authors found that the parameter leading to the largest changes was the probability of admission to acute hospital from the nursing home. They also described the relationship between the incremental cost-effectiveness ratio and other variables.

Although univariate sensitivity analyses are insightful, looking at one source of uncertainty by itself is usually inadequate. The alternative is multivariate sensitivity analysis. A multivariate sensitivity analysis examines multiple sources of uncertainty at one time and may generate a more accurate understanding of the uncertainty of the cost-effectiveness results. This can be done by changing all parameters to their most or least favorable levels—but still working with predetermined levels of the values for each variable. A second approach makes use of the fact that variables can sometimes be expected to change together; in such cases, the analyst might explore how the cost-effectiveness ratio changes as the two variables are varied over their ranges. Finally, an analyst can conduct what is referred to as a probabilistic sensitivity analysis.

In this case, the analyst must define distributions from which the values for parameters may be drawn. A random draw is then taken from each distribution and the results of the analysis are calculated. The results of the first analysis are recorded and the process is repeated—at least thousands and sometimes tens of thousands of times. The analyst must then describe the range of results by describing the distribution of ratios. Honkanen et al. (2006) use this technique to describe the distribution of cost-effectiveness results in a study of hip protector use intended to prevent fractures in a community-dwelling geriatric population. One result this group found was that the incremental cost-effectiveness ratio was less than $50,000/QALY in 68% of repeated random results for women initiating hip protector use at age 75. A decision maker faced with this information would have to determine whether being 68% certain of a favorable economic result is sufficient to move forward with a policy change.

## CONCLUSIONS

The checklist in Exhibit 2.2 may be useful when reporting or reading a report of an economic evaluation. This checklist draws on criteria for high-quality cost-effectiveness studies and draws on a number of sets

### Exhibit 2.2 *CEA Checklist for Journal Report*

**1. Framework**

- Background of the problem
- General framing and design of the problem
- Target population for the intervention
- Other program descriptors
- Description of comparator programs
- Boundaries of the analysis
- Time horizon
- Statement of the perspective of the analysis

**2. Data and methods**

- Description of event pathway
- Identification of outcomes of interest in the analysis
- Description of model used
- Modeling assumptions
- Diagram of event pathway/model

*(continued)*

## Exhibit 2.2 *continued*

▩ Software used

▩ Complete information about the sources of effectiveness data, cost data, and preference weights

▩ Methods for obtaining estimates of effectiveness, costs, and preferences

▩ Critique of data quality

▩ Statement of year costs

▩ Statement of method used to adjust costs for inflation

▩ Statement of type of currency

▩ Sources and methods for obtaining expert judgment

▩ Statement of discount rates

### 3. Results

▩ Results of model validation

▩ Reference case results (discounted and undiscounted): total costs and effectiveness, incremental costs and effectiveness, and incremental cost-effectiveness ratios

▩ Results of sensitivity analyses

▩ Other estimates of uncertainty, if available

▩ Graphical representation of cost-effectiveness results

▩ Aggregate cost and effectiveness information

▩ Disaggregated results, as relevant

▩ Secondary analyses using 5% discount rate

▩ Other secondary analyses, as relevant

### 4. Discussion

▩ Summary of reference case results

▩ Summary of sensitivity analysis assumptions having important ethical implications

▩ Limitations of the study

▩ Relevance of the study results for specific policy questions or decisions

▩ Results of related CEAs

▩ Distributive implications of the intervention

### 5. Technical report available upon request

Adapted from Gold et al. (1996).

of criteria that have been specified in related literature (Drummond et al., 2005; Eldessouki & Smith, 2012; Gold et al., 1996).

With the continuing development of new treatments, technologies, and models of care delivery, health–economic evaluations have become increasingly important. The demand for economic outcome research is growing, as is the number of published analyses. In this chapter, we have introduced various methods used in economic evaluation and have described the concepts and terminology used in these analyses.

The quality of studies has been variable and not necessarily improving. As more studies are conducted and submitted for peer-reviewed publication, editors are not always able to find reviewers with the appropriate expertise; hence, studies that are poorly conducted in general or for which specific elements are poor can make their way into print. APNs who plan to read these analyses need to understand methodology enough to recognize what makes a good study and what makes a study that is barely acceptable or even fails the test of acceptability.

APNs interested in exploring this type of outcome evaluation are encouraged to seek additional training in these methods.

If APNs participate in and conduct economic evaluations concerning the care they provide, the cost effectiveness of APN care may be demonstrated. When the analysis uses a standard methodology and the assumptions are transparent, the results are more easily interpreted. If the outcome measure is a standard ratio, such as dollars per QALY gained, the results may furnish a strong argument to health policy decision makers concerning the funding and continued recognition of APNs as cost-effective health-care providers.

## Answers to Chapter Discussion Question

1. Both comparative effectiveness and cost-effectiveness are forms of research that determine relative effectiveness of an intervention, diagnostic procedure, or preventive strategy in a real-world environment. Cost-effectiveness methodology contrasts two or more interventions by including economic outcome(s). Comparative-effectiveness methodology compares a potentially broader range of benefit and harms in the everyday environment, but does not necessarily include economic outcomes or analysis.

2. CUA presents outcomes in terms of cost per QALY gained. Therefore, scenarios in which quality of life, mortality, as well as cost are of

interest would be appropriate. For example, Biesheuvel-Leliefeld et al. (2012) designed a cost–utility study to test the quality of life improvement of a nursing-led intervention for recurrent major depressive disorder, and reported in cost per QALY gained.

3. Cost–consequence methodology is intended for subjects with multiple relevant outcome measures, often when these outcomes cannot be summarized into a single measure. Cost and consequences are listed from each intervention of interest in the results and analysis.

4. CBA requires that the benefits of the tested interventions be monetized. Therefore, a researcher must assume a particular monetary value that accurately represents derived benefit or QALY gained, which may be controversial. The outcome measure for CBA is a dollar amount that is the sum of all costs minus the benefits. In this way, the costs and benefits are compared in the same units, which is particularly helpful if potential benefits include nonclinical parameters (Riegelman, 2005).

5. The first step is to identify all the factors that will influence the total cost of the therapy. These may include the price of the antibiotic itself, the nurse's time for preparation, the patient's time in the clinical setting, and any physical materials for preparation (i.e., needle, syringe, tubing) depending on the study perspective. Benefits may include shortened time in the hospital, reduced complications, and fewer rehospitalizations. The second step would be assigning a dollar value to each cost, as exemplified in Hamrick, Nye, and Gardner (2007).

## WEB LINKS

CEA Registry website—A database of medical publications containing CEA that have been audited by the Center for the Evaluation of Value and Risk in Health (CEVR), part of the Institute for Clinical Research and Health Policy Studies at Tufts Medical Center. All papers included are original analyses, written in English, and use QALY outcome measure(s). The website also includes a dictionary of relevant economic terms among other resources.
Website: https://research.tufts-nemc.org/cear4/

Board of Governors of the Federal Reserve System—On this website, the Federal Reserve offers exchange rates between the U. S. dollar and foreign currencies annually, monthly, and daily, recorded as far back as 1971. These data are useful if research analyses require converting

values to or from U. S. currency for the sake of comparison between or aggregation of costs in a common monetary unit.
Website: http://www.federalreserve.gov/releases/g5a/current/default. htm).

BLS—The BLS website (www.bls.gov) lists CPI, which allows comparison for the real value of money between time periods. The CPI calculator can determine conversion of the U. S. dollar's value between any years ranging from 1913 to present.
Website: http://data.bls.gov/cgi-bin/cpicalc.pl

Federal Reserve Bank of St. Louis Economic Data (FRED)—This website offers extensive economic indicators data useful for economic analyses. For example, these data include the U.S. inflation rate by day, month, or year.
Website: http://research.stlouisfed.org/

Health Economics Resource Center (HERC)—HERC is a resource for cost-effectiveness research that includes help identifying costs, definitions of economic concepts, and a bibliography of over 300 cost-effectiveness studies. This United States Department of Veterans Affairs website also contains actual VA health economic data with registration.
Website:    http://www.herc.research.va.gov/methods/methods_cost_ oc.asp

## REFERENCES

Anderson, P. J., Walsh, J. M., Louey, M. A., Meade, C., & Fairbrother, G. (2002). Comparing first and subsequent suprapubic catheter change: Complications and costs. *Urologic Nursing, 22*(5), 324–5, 328.

Anthony, R. N., & Young, D. W. (1994). *Management control in nonprofit organizations* (5th ed.). Boston, MA: Irwin McGraw-Hill.

Armstrong, E. P., Malone, D. C., & Erder, M. H. (2008). A Markov cost-utility analysis of escitalopram and duloxetine for the treatment of major depressive disorder. *Current Medical Research and Opinion, 24*(4), 1115–1121.

Becker, A., Schulten-Oberbörsch, G., Beck, U., & Vestweber, K. H. (1999). Stoma care nurses: Good value for money? *World Journal of Surgery, 23*(7), 638–42; discussion 642.

Bhandari, S. (2011). Update of a comparative analysis of cost minimization following the introduction of newly available intravenous iron therapies in hospital practice. *Therapeutics and Clinical Risk Management, 7,* 501–509.

Biesheuvel-Leliefeld, K. E., Kersten, S. M., van der Horst, H. E., van Schaik, A., Bockting, C. L., Bosmans, J. E., … van Marwijk, H. W. (2012). Cost-effectiveness of nurse-led self-help for recurrent depression in the primary care setting: Design of a pragmatic randomised controlled trial. *BMC Psychiatry, 12,* 59.

Braithwaite, R. S., Meltzer, D. O., King, J. T., Leslie, D., & Roberts, M. S. (2008). What does the value of modern medicine say about the $50,000 per quality-adjusted life-year decision rule? *Medical Care, 46*(4), 349–356.

Brooten, D., Naylor, M. D., York, R., Brown, L. P., Munro, B. H., Hollingsworth, A. O., … Youngblut, J. M. (2002). Lessons learned from testing the quality cost model of Advanced Practice Nursing (APN) transitional care. *Journal of Nursing Scholarship, 34*(4), 369–375.

Brouwer, W. B., & Koopmanschap, M. A. (2005). The friction-cost method: Replacement for nothing and leisure for free? *PharmacoEconomics, 23*(2), 105–111.

Brouwer, W. B., Koopmanschap, M. A., & Rutten, F. F. (1997a). Productivity costs measurement through quality of life? A response to the recommendation of the Washington Panel. *Health Economics, 6*(3), 253–259.

Brouwer, W. B., Koopmanschap, M. A., & Rutten, F. F. (1997b). Productivity costs in cost-effectiveness analysis: Numerator or denominator: A further discussion. *Health Economics, 6*(5), 511–514.

Centers for Medicare & Medicaid Services. (2012, April 11). *National healthcare expenditures data.* Retrieved from https://www.cms.gov/Research-Statistics-Data-and-Systems/Statistics-Trends-and-Reports/NationalHealthExpendData/NationalHealthAccountsHistorical.html

Chiu, W. K., & Newcomer, R. (2007). A systematic review of nurse-assisted case management to improve hospital discharge transition outcomes for the elderly. *Professional Case Management, 12*(6), 330–6; quiz 337.

Chummun, H., & Tiran, D. (2008). Increasing research evidence in practice: A possible role for the consultant nurse. *Journal of Nursing Management, 16*(3), 327–333.

Crowther, M. (2003). Optimal management of outpatients with heart failure using advanced practice nurses in a hospital-based heart failure center. *Journal of the American Academy of Nurse Practitioners, 15*(6), 260–265.

Dawes, H. A., Docherty, T., Traynor, I., Gilmore, D. H., Jardine, A. G., & Knill-Jones, R. (2007). Specialist nurse supported discharge in gynaecology: A randomised comparison and economic evaluation. *European Journal of Obstetrics, Gynecology, and Reproductive Biology, 130*(2), 262–270.

Determinants of health economic decisions in actual practice: The role of behavioral economics. (2006). [Summary of the presentation given by Professor Daniel Kahneman at the ISPOR Tenth Annual International Meeting First Plenary Session, May 16, 2005, Washington, DC, USA.]. *Value in Health, 9*(2), 65–67.

Donaldson, C., Baker, R., Mason, H., Jones-Lee, M., Lancsar, E., Wildman, J., … Smith, R. (2011). The social value of a QALY: Raising the bar or barring the raise? *BMC Health Services Research, 11,* 8.

Drummond, M., Sculpher, M. J., Torrance, G. W., O'Brien, B. J., & Stoddart, G. L. (2005). Methods for the economic evaluation of health care programmes (3rd ed.). New York, NY: Oxford University Press.

Eldessouki, R., & Smith, M. D. (2012). Health care system information sharing: A step toward better health globally. *Value Health Regional Issues, 1,* 118–129.

Federal Coordinating Council for Comparative Effectiveness Research (U.S.), United States. President., United States. Congress., & U.S. Department of Health and Human Services. (2009). *Report to the President and the Congress.* Washington, DC: U.S. Department of Health and Human Services.

Freedberg, K. A., Hirschhorn, L. R., Schackman, B. R., Wolf, L. L., Martin, L. A., Weinstein, M. C.,...Losina, E. (2006). Cost-effectiveness of an intervention to improve adherence to antiretroviral therapy in HIV-infected patients. *Journal of Acquired Immune Deficiency Syndromes, 43,* S113–S118.

Ganz, D. A., Simmons, S. F., & Schnelle, J. F. (2005). Cost-effectiveness of recommended nurse staffing levels for short-stay skilled nursing facility patients. *BMC Health Services Research, 5,* 35.

Garber, A. M. (2011). How the Patient-Centered Outcomes Research Institute can best influence real-world health care decision making. *Health Affairs, 30*(12), 2243–2251.

Gold, M. R., Siegel, J. E., Russell, L. B., & Weinstein, M. C. (1996). *Cost effectiveness in health and medicine.* New York, NY: Oxford University Press.

Goodman, H., Parsons, A., Davison, J., Preedy, M., Peters, E., Shuldham, C.,...Cowie, M. R. (2008). A randomised controlled trial to evaluate a nurse-led programme of support and lifestyle management for patients awaiting cardiac surgery 'Fit for surgery: Fit for life' study. *European Journal of Cardiovascular Nursing, 7*(3), 189–195.

Haddix, A. C., Teutsch, S. M., & Corso, P. S. (2002). *Prevention effectiveness: A guide to decision analysis and economic evaluation* (2nd ed.). New York, NY: Oxford University Press.

Hamrick, I., Nye, A. M., & Gardner, C. K. (2007). Nursing home medication administration cost minimization analysis. *Journal of the American Medical Directors Association, 8*(3), 173–177.

Hirth, R. A., Chernew, M. E., Miller, E., Fendrick, A. M., & Weissert, W. G. (2000). Willingness to pay for a quality-adjusted life year: In search of a standard. *Medical Decision Making, 20*(3), 332–342.

Honkanen, L. A., Mushlin, A. I., Lachs, M., & Schackman, B. R. (2006). Can hip protector use cost-effectively prevent fractures in community-dwelling geriatric populations? *Journal of the American Geriatrics Society, 54*(11), 1658–1665.

Honkanen, L. A., Schackman, B. R., Mushlin, A. I., & Lachs, M. S. (2005). A cost-benefit analysis of external hip protectors in the nursing home setting. *Journal of the American Geriatrics Society, 53*(2), 190–197.

Iglehart, J. K. (2009). Prioritizing comparative-effectiveness research–IOM recommendations. *The New England Journal of Medicine, 361*(4), 325–328. doi: NEJMp0904133 [pii] 10.1056/NEJMp0904133

Jacobs, P., & Fassbender, K. (1998). The measurement of indirect costs in the health economics evaluation literature. A review. *International Journal of Technology Assessment in Health Care, 14*(4), 799–808.

Jacobson, G. A. (2007). Comparative clinical effectiveness and cost-effectiveness research: Background, history and overview. (RL34208). Washington, DC: Congressional Research Service.

Jones, C. B. (2008). Revisiting nurse turnover costs: Adjusting for inflation. *The Journal of Nursing Administration, 38*(1), 11–18.

Kang, J., Mandsager, P., Biddle, A. K., & Weber, D. J. (2012). Cost-effectiveness analysis of active surveillance screening for methicillin-resistant Staphylococcus aureus in an academic hospital setting. *Infection Control and Hospital Epidemiology, 33*(5), 477–486.

Krahn, M., Guasparini, R., Sherman, M., & Detsky, A. S. (1998). Costs and cost-effectiveness of a universal, school-based hepatitis B vaccination program. *American Journal of Public Health, 88*(11), 1638–1644.

Lee, A., Chan, S., Chen, P. P., Gin, T., & Lau, A. S. (2007). Economic evaluations of acute pain service programs: A systematic review. *The Clinical Journal of Pain, 23*(8), 726–733.

Liljas, B. (1998). How to calculate indirect costs in economic evaluations. *PharmacoEconomics, 13*(1 Pt 1), 1–7.

Luce, B. R., Manning, W. G., Siegel, J. E., & Lipscomb, J. (1996). Estimating costs in cost-effectiveness analysis. In M. Gold, J. E. Siegel, L. Russell, & M. Weinstein (Eds.), *Cost-effectiveness in health and medicine* (pp. 176–213). New York, NY: Oxford University Press.

Moradi-Lakeh, M., Shakerian, S., & Esteghamati, A. (2012). Immunization against Haemophilus Influenzae Type b in Iran; Cost-utility and Cost-benefit Analyses. *International Journal of Preventive Medicine, 3*(5), 332–340.

Muennig, P. (2008). Health selection vs. causation in the income gradient: What can we learn from graphical trends? *Journal of Health Care for the Poor and Underserved, 19*(2), 574–579.

Neumann, P. J., Greenberg, D., Olchanski, N. V., Stone, P. W., & Rosen, A. B. (2005). Growth and quality of the cost-utility literature, 1976–2001. *Value in Health, 8*(1), 3–9.

Paez, K. A., & Allen, J. K. (2006). Cost-effectiveness of nurse practitioner management of hypercholesterolemia following coronary revascularization. *Journal of the American Academy of Nurse Practitioners, 18*(9), 436–444.

Patel, G. W., Duquaine, S. M., & McKinnon, P. S. (2007). Clinical outcomes and cost minimization with an alternative dosing regimen for meropenem in a community hospital. *Pharmacotherapy, 27*(12), 1637–1643.

Petitti, D. B. (2000). *Meta-analysis, decision analysis, and cost-effectiveness analysis: Methods for quantitative synthesis in medicine* (2nd ed.). New York, NY: Oxford University Press.

Riegelman, R. K. (2005). Studying a study & testing a test (5th ed.). Philadelphia, PA: Lippincott Williams & Wilkins.

Rost, K., Pyne, J. M., Dickinson, L. M., & LoSasso, A. T. (2005). Cost-effectiveness of enhancing primary care depression management on an ongoing basis. *Annals of Family Medicine, 3*(1), 7–14.

Simon, G. E., Katon, W. J., Lin, E. H., Rutter, C., Manning, W. G., Von Korff, M., ... Young, B. A. (2007). Cost-effectiveness of systematic depression treatment among people with diabetes mellitus. *Archives of General Psychiatry, 64*(1), 65–72.

Sørensen, J., & Frich, L. (2008). Home visits by specially trained nurses after discharge from multi-disciplinary pain care: A cost consequence analysis based on a randomised controlled trial. *European Journal Of Pain, 12*(2), 164–171.

Spetz, J. (2005). The cost and cost-effectiveness of nursing services in health care. *Nursing Outlook, 53*(6), 305–309.

Stone, P. W. (1998). Methods for conducting and reporting cost-effectiveness analysis in nursing. *Image, 30*(3), 229–234.

Stone, P. W. (2001a). Dollars and sense: A primer for the novice in economic analyses (Part I). *Applied Nursing Research, 14*(1), 54–55.

Stone, P. W. (2001b). Dollars and sense: A primer for the novice in economic analyses (Part II). *Applied Nursing Research, 14*(2), 110–112.

Stone, P. W., Chapman, R. H., Sandberg, E. A., Liljas, B., & Neumann, P. J. (2000). Measuring costs in cost-utility analyses. Variations in the literature. *International Journal of Technology Assessment in Health Care, 16*(1), 111–124.

Subramanian, S., Hoover, S., Gilman, B., Field, T. S., Mutter, R., & Gurwitz, J. H. (2007). Computerized physician order entry with clinical decision support in long-term care facilities: Costs and benefits to stakeholders. *Journal of the American Geriatrics Society, 55*(9), 1451–1457.

Ubel, P. A., Hirth, R. A., Chernew, M. E., & Fendrick, A. M. (2003). What is the price of life and why doesn't it increase at the rate of inflation? *Archives of Internal Medicine, 163*(14), 1637–1641.

Urdahl, H., Knapp, M., Edgell, E. T., Ghandi, G., & Haro, J. M. (2003). Unit costs in international economic evaluations: Resource costing of the Schizophrenia Outpatient Health Outcomes Study. *Acta Psychiatrica Scandinavica Supplementum, 107*(Supp. 416), 41–47.

van Baal, P. H., Polder, J. J., de Wit, G. A., Hoogenveen, R. T., Feenstra, T. L., Boshuizen, H. C., ... Brouwer, W. B. (2008). Lifetime medical costs of obesity: Prevention no cure for increasing health expenditure. *PLoS Medicine, 5*(2), e29.

Volpp, K. G., & Das, A. (2009). Comparative effectiveness–thinking beyond medication A versus medication B. *The New England Journal of Medicine, 361*(4), 331–333.

Weinstein, M. C., & Manning, W. G. (1997). Theoretical issues in cost-effectiveness analysis. *Journal of Health Economics, 16*(1), 121–128.

Weinstein, M. C., Siegel, J. E., Garber, A. M., Lipscomb, J., Luce, B. R., Manning, W. G., & Torrance, G. W. (1997). Productivity costs, time costs and health-related quality of life: A response to the Erasmus Group. *Health Economics, 6*(5), 505–510.

# Chapter 3: Selecting Advanced Practice Nurse Outcome Measures

SUZANNE M. BURNS AND BETH QUATRARA

## Chapter Objectives

1. Discuss reasons why measuring outcomes of advanced practice nurses (APNs) is essential to the role of the APN.
2. Identify at least three nurse-sensitive outcome measure categories.
3. Discuss the benefits and pitfalls of using benchmark/aggregate data to measure APN outcomes.
4. Describe methods to measure and monitor APN outcome data.

## Chapter Discussion Questions

1. Why are aggregate data such as length of stay (LOS) and cost per case less desirable APN outcome measures?
2. Why is a control chart a valuable strategy for recording APN outcomes?
3. What are the key elements of APN outcome measures?

**A**dvanced practice nurses (APNs) are increasingly being asked to demonstrate the effectiveness of their roles. In some cases, the inability of an APN to do so results in the dissolution of the role. For many institutions, effectiveness is measured in financial outcomes, or some derivation of financial outcomes such as patient volume. Unfortunately, many APNs are not in revenue-generating positions and must be thoughtful in demonstrating their effectiveness and "value-added" benefit to the institutions in which they practice.

Well-controlled studies on APN outcomes continue to be relatively scant (Kleinpell, Ely, & Grabenkort, 2008; Newhouse et al., 2008). However, some do exist and suggest that APNs "provide safe, effective, quality care to a number of specific populations in a variety of settings" (Newhouse et al., 2008). The studies on APN outcomes are extremely helpful as guides to APN practice. While more studies are needed on APN roles in specific settings, clinicians in practice must continue to demonstrate the effectiveness of their roles in less labor-intensive ways than performing a research study. To that end, the purpose of this chapter is to describe a number of different methods and outcome measures that might be used to evaluate an APN's effectiveness. Examples of actual APN outcome projects will illustrate the methods and demonstrate the importance of determining appropriate outcome data for measurement.

## SELECTING APN ROLE-SENSITIVE OUTCOME MEASURES

A common approach used to determine APN outcomes is to attempt to link institutional aggregate data such as length of stay (LOS) and cost per case to APN practice. While these types of measurements are important and helpful in some cases, they are generally not sensitive enough to clearly demonstrate the APN's unique contribution. Rarely does aggregate data show the causal effect of an individual on a patient population; there are simply too many intervening variables that may have contributed to the effect (this is discussed in depth later in the chapter). Thus, it is important to consider other, more sensitive indicators. There is also a practical reason for carefully selecting outcome variables; APNs are busy and data collection takes time. The data that the APN collects should be easy to obtain prospectively (in the course of his/her daily role) and should be specific to the APN's role. Data collection should not be extensive but instead limited to carefully selected role-sensitive indicators. If the data collection burden is too great, it is unlikely that the required metrics will be routinely collected.

Unfortunately, many APNs are averse to collecting data and believe that having to "prove" their worth is unjustified since their roles are not revenue generating. In addition, the APNs may feel that data collection distracts them from their primary roles as clinical experts. But, if the outcome measures are carefully selected, the data will not only help to clarify the APN's value to the institution and beyond, but may also be used to focus the role accordingly.

When an APN is hired, the manager, administrator, and physician (if applicable) to whom the APN will report will generally have a specific role or function in mind (educator, case manager, clinical nurse specialist [CNS], clinical coordinator, nurse practitioner [NP], etc.). Following role negotiation, the APN begins the role focusing on the negotiated objectives. Outcome measures should be specific to the role and should be mutually agreed upon by the APN and the individual who hired the APN. Examples of role-specific outcome measures follow and an example of an APN "outcome planning, tracking, and reporting worksheet" is found in Exhibit 3.1.

## ACUTE CARE NURSE PRACTITIONER FOR A MEDICAL ACUTE CARE FLOOR

If the role is that of acute care nurse practitioner (ACNP) for a medical acute care floor, the collaborating physician may be interested in the number of ACNP-managed patients requiring readmission within a selected time interval. These data are relatively easy to collect and can be obtained from institutional clinical data repositories. The ACNP will need to maintain a secure database of his/her discharged patients in order to query the system on a regular basis (e.g., every 2 months, quarterly, yearly). It may be desirable to compare these to other health care provider data as well, while being mindful that readmissions to outside facilities may not be easy to determine and are important for the accuracy of the report.

## UNIT EDUCATOR

Another example is that of an APN hired to be a unit educator. In this case the manager and educator may agree that educational offerings and evidence-based practice (EBP) changes designed and implemented by the educator are the outcome measures of interest. These are relatively easy to document as they are accomplished. Descriptions of these initiatives, including the time required to complete them, will help clarify the complexity of the projects as well as the efficiency and effectiveness of

**Exhibit 3.1** *APN Outcomes Planning, Tracking, and Reporting Worksheet*

**APN Name** _____ **APN** ☐ 1 ☐ 2 ☐ 3

**Date** _____

**Manager**_____ **Administrator** _____

**Area of Outcomes Focus:** Brief title summarizing the activities described below.

**Problem Statement:** Briefly describe needed practice change and rationale.

**Process / Methods / Interventions:** Describe intended approach and evolution of plans, if any.

Describe the data collection method:
   ☐ existing data source _____
   ☐ data prospectively collected _____

IRB Approval Number: ____ (if needed for your initiative)

**Specific Goals**: The APN and administrator meet to mutually agree on the goals for each evaluation time period.

| Describe Measurable Goals | Source for Measurement | Timeline |
|---|---|---|
| 1. (add rows as needed) | | Progress by: Completion by: |

**Progress Reports:** As appropriate, APN should log and date periodic notes for each goal.

**Measurement and Reporting of Outcomes:** Brief summary of findings and lessons learned. Graphical representation of the outcome variable of interest pre- and post intervention/initiative is encouraged.

Outcomes Apply to:
   ☐ Metrics important to the institution (e.g., LOS, UTI). Describe:
   _____

*(continued)*

**Exhibit 3.1** *continued*

---

☐ Implement and sustain an evidence-based unit or institutional practice change. Describe: _____
☐ Improve metrics over time in a patient population. Describe: _____
☐ Improve satisfaction, knowledge, adherence to guidelines, and development of others. Describe: _____
☐ Other. Describe: _____

**Staff Assisting With Outcomes Activities:** Give names and credentials.

**References:** Evidence-based literature/guideline that supports the change.

---

Adapted for use with permission of University of Virginia Professional Nursing Staff Organization, University of Virginia, Charlottesville, VA (copyright 2011).

the educator. For some initiatives, the educator may also consider assessing the degree of knowledge learned and applied to practice as well as design periodic audits to ensure adherence with the EBP changes.

## CLINICAL NURSE SPECIALIST (CNS)

The role of CNS generally encompasses all the domains of advanced practice (e.g., clinical management, education, research, consultation, and change agency). However, it may be that outcome measures may focus on only one or two measures of role effectiveness and that these may change over time. For example, the manager and CNS may agree that one key objective for the year is to improve medication safety (i.e., medication errors). The CNS in this example might partner with the quality assurance (QA) department to track unit medication errors following the implementation of a CNS educational and practice change initiative. A control chart might be used to graphically demonstrate the change in percentage of medication errors per time interval. In this case, the APN does not actually need to collect data but instead partners with the QA department to ensure that the intervention date (e.g., training of staff) is marked accurately on the control chart. Very few examples like this one would be needed to demonstrate the APN's worth to the institution. More importantly, the APN can use the data to readjust or change the intervention if necessary. See Exhibit 3.2 for examples and an explanation of control charts.

The CNS may also monitor the effect of a change initiative on practice and patient outcomes. Perhaps the initiative is one designed to incorporate prone positioning into the care management protocol for patients with acute respiratory distress syndrome (ARDS). A prospective audit by the CNS following implementation of the educational and competency-based initiative would be relatively easy to

### Exhibit 3.2   *Control Charts*

Most data used to monitor the effect of system interventions in health care are displayed as numerical comparisons (lists or tables of data, etc.). Unfortunately these approaches have serious drawbacks. The comparisons made with lists of numbers are often narrowly focused, weak, and difficult to interpret because they rarely help us understand the context (e.g., how stable the historical data have been). Tables, on the other hand, often present too much data and are hard to interpret. Graphs provide a solution to these problems because they include previous data by which to compare the effect of the intervention. Essentially, the context for interpreting the current value is integrated into the chart. Additionally, the charts are easier to understand because the data are represented visually rather than numerically.

Control charts start with a time series graph but control limits and a central line are added to visually delineate the variability of the measure of interest. By having control limits, the tendency to inappropriately intervene (called "tampering"), which is costly, and time and effort intensive, may be avoided. Generally, three consecutive points above the upper or lower control limit are considered significant (e.g., where action should be taken). This approach may help prevent the often counterproductive response of many to "random variation" in the system. Refer to Wheeler (2000) for a more in-depth discussion of control charts.

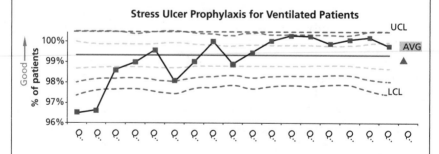

In this example, the percent of patients receiving appropriate stress ulcer prophylaxis is being monitored over time. The benchmark for the lower control limit has been derived from regulatory agency benchmark goals of 90%. As demonstrated in the chart, this critical care unit easily meets the benchmark with an average goal attainment over time of greater than 96%. Note: The dotted lines represent the corresponding percent. The undulations reflect the differences in the total patients for the sample (i.e., the denominator).

*(continued)*

**Exhibit 3.2** *continued*

Time series (or running record graphs) are especially helpful to trend the effect of an intervention over time.

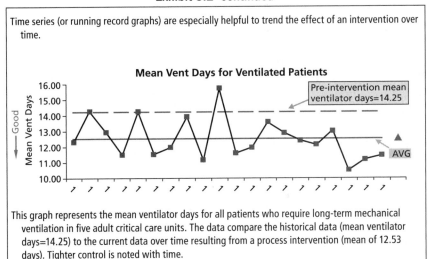

This graph represents the mean ventilator days for all patients who require long-term mechanical ventilation in five adult critical care units. The data compare the historical data (mean ventilator days=14.25) to the current data over time resulting from a process intervention (mean of 12.53 days). Tighter control is noted with time.

accomplish while the CNS is on the unit. Elements to track would be protocol adherence (i.e., was it implemented), accuracy (i.e., was it done correctly), and what was the patient's response (e.g., $PaO_2$ following prone positioning, physiologic tolerance). Little data collection would be necessary since the maneuver is generally used infrequently. The reason such an initiative is a reasonable one to use as a CNS outcome is because the procedure is potentially risky and is almost entirely nurse managed. The CNS's effectiveness in safely implementing such a protocol is essential as it speaks to integration of all the CNS role components and demonstrates effective leadership and follow through. In addition, the CNS can use the data to quickly adapt and adjust the protocol as needed. This "real-time" monitoring with short cycles of intervention, evaluation, and correction ensure quality.

Some specific categories of outcome measures and the attendant-associated issues with each are discussed below.

## CATEGORIES OF APN OUTCOME DATA

A variety of indicators may be used to demonstrate the effectiveness of an APN. The strengths and weaknesses of the indicators are described.

## Satisfaction (Patient, Family, Caregivers, Physician)

Satisfaction is a variable that speaks directly to the institution's "market share" of customers. If customer satisfaction is not good, the customer will not return. In addition, the customer's negative advertisement of the hospital will have far-reaching implications for the institution. As noted by Digby (2011), 91% of unhappy customers will leave without complaining and never come back, and 13% of dissatisfied customers will tell 20 more people about their negative experience. Few hospitals exist today that are arrogant enough to ignore satisfaction as an outcome measure. However, as we know, satisfaction is not always synonymous with quality. Regardless, it is an important variable to monitor. The satisfaction of other staff and physicians with the APN practice may also be of interest as an outcome measure.

Most institutions routinely measure patient satisfaction in a global manner. Like other aggregate data, it is hard to specifically attribute the outcomes to APN practice. For example, in many cases, the satisfaction instrument will not distinguish the APN from the bedside nurse or the physician. Further complicating the matter, many institutions only collect data related to service line (i.e., medicine or surgery). Thus, for satisfaction to be linked to APN practice, a separate survey may be necessary. However, even this may be a stumbling block. In some institutions, patient satisfaction surveys are closely controlled and may only be distributed via the institutional mechanism in place. There are good reasons for this; the institution does not want the patients and families "bothered" with numerous forms and questionnaires. Further, more specific and detailed questions are difficult to design, take the patient additional time to complete, and often require interpretation. If satisfaction is a desired APN outcome measure, it is necessary to determine whether the existing institutional survey is sensitive enough. If not, the APN may need to design his/her own survey, if permissible within the institutional structure.

If an institutional survey is used to measure APN satisfaction outcomes, it is best to directly target a specific question(s). This is exemplified by an ACNP who wanted to improve patients' pain management satisfaction scores. She identified the following survey questions as targeted outcome measures for unit: "how well was pain controlled" and "nurses kept me informed." She designed a project to address these specific satisfaction measures by providing education about medication availability, timing, and by involving patients in their own pharmacologic pain management regimen. This nursing intervention provided patients with the information they needed to improve their pain management and empowered them to control the discomfort. The intervention was successful. Using the institutional survey data, the ACNP was able to demonstrate a sustained improvement in satisfaction scores, a valuable institutional outcome (Figure 3.1).

However, there are times when a broad institutional survey cannot address the unique attributes of a particular customer service initiative. Although difficult as described, it may be possible to use a separate survey to determine customer satisfaction with a specific intervention without overtaxing the survey process or overburdening patients and families. A key to success lies with introducing a well-timed, brief, and focused survey. For example, an operating room clinical research team implemented a new perioperative communication plan to evaluate the effect on family member anxiety and satisfaction. The communication plan included regularly scheduled OR nurse updates to a designated family member from the perioperative team on his/her loved one's status throughout the surgery. With minimal intrusion, family members who were receiving the status updates responded to a short questionnaire about the experience. The survey participation rate was high. The satisfaction data directly demonstrated customer satisfaction with the new communication plan (Figure 3.2). Such interventions can directly contribute to an increased overall customer service rating but the outcome cannot be attributed to the APN-led project without specific data.

Surveys of staff and physician satisfaction may also be an effective and useful measure of APN practice. The satisfaction of caregivers is important because their dissatisfaction can affect recruitment, retention, quality of care, and other financial outcomes. Institutional costs of nursing turnover are cited to be $22,000 to over $64,000 (United States) per nurse (Jones & Gates, 2007). Additionally, frequent turnover makes the assurance of quality care difficult. It is costly (in time and money) to provide enough training to ensure the basic competency of "safe" care delivery following orientation. In this time of a "nursing shortage," retention is essential, and nurses' satisfaction with their work environment, professional development opportunities, and ability to "make a contribution in a collaborative manner" are important variables to consider. The APN may well have an important part to play in satisfaction as it relates to one or more of these variables. Satisfaction surveys related to these and other specific aspects of APN practice may be useful and relatively easy to accomplish via mechanisms such as the unit or service line intranet.

Physician satisfaction is another variable that may be measured. The physician generates revenue and the APNs with whom they work

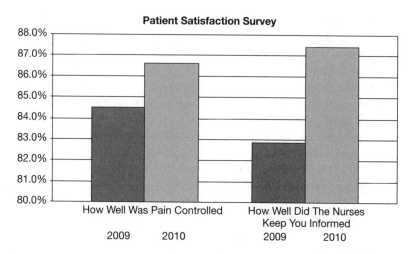

Figure 3.1 *APN-Directed Pain Management Intervention: Results of Patient Satisfaction Survey*

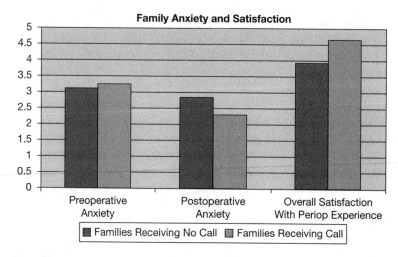

Figure 3.2 *Survey Results Comparing Pre operative and Post operative Satisfaction of Patients' Families Related to Communication Intervention*

contribute to the efficiency and effectiveness of the physicians' practice. In these cases, physician satisfaction with the collaborative relationship and the results of the same are important to follow.

Additional considerations for the APN with regard to the development and use of satisfaction surveys include decisions related to whether or not the project must be reviewed and approved by the hospital's institutional review board (IRB) before implementation.

If the information received from the survey is deidentified, it is likely that the project will receive an "exempt status" approval from the IRB. However, in some institutions, a satisfaction survey must seek approval via the QA department or sometimes a nursing research department. It is the responsibility of the APN to proceed via appropriate channels. A second and important consideration when designing satisfaction surveys is that of the validity and reliability of the instrument. If it is not a tested instrument, the survey may provide inaccurate and erroneous answers. To avoid this potential stumbling block, use of an existing tested instrument is preferable.

### Clinical Outcomes Measures

APN-sensitive clinical outcomes may be difficult to identify because many factors may potentially affect them. It is important to remember that clinical outcome measures need not be inclusive of everything the APN practice may affect, but rather those that are the most easily and clearly attributed to the APN practice. For example, consider the NP charged with managing the care of a neurosurgical patient population. Because in this case the NP's role is focused on managing the medical aspects of care of the patients, selected aspects of care may yield sensitive indicators of effectiveness. Examples include such indicators as urinary tract infection (because the NP is responsible for ordering catheter removal), decubitus ulcer formation (secondary to initiation of mobilization), and selected discharge outcomes.

A common error made by APNs who manage large groups of patients is to collect a large data set in the hope that it will show something. This approach, "fishing in the data," is unnecessary and a poor use of the APN's time. A rule of thumb, as with any research study, is that the question should be clear and the variables of interest, measurable. For example, perhaps the APN's role is focused on improving the outcomes of patients who require prolonged mechanical ventilation. It is important that the APN have benchmark data available on ventilator duration so that a comparison may be made. Length of stay (LOS), though sometimes related to ventilator duration, may not be directly affected by the APN since the clinician's role may not extend to the unit to which the patient is transferred following successful weaning. In contrast, duration of ventilation may be attributable if the APN is the one charged with ensuring proper application of, and adherence to, a weaning protocol. In this example, the data are relatively easy to collect because they are congruent with the role of the APN and can be easily collected in the course of a practice day.

Another outcome directly attributable to an APN may be defined through attention to the details of medication reconciliation. The National Patient Safety Goals for Hospitals includes a requirement to "maintain and communicate accurate patient medication information" (The Joint Commission, 2011). For one inpatient ACNP who works in an academic medical center, managing medication orders placed by different care providers is a daily activity. As the ACNP accurately verifies or properly adjusts medications to meet the needs of an individual patient, she records these data points and demonstrates her unique contribution to patient safety. By presenting her daily work in terms of her effort to meet regulatory requirements and enhance patient safety, she is actively showcasing her influence on institutional outcomes (Figure 3.3).

Similarly, an APN who contributes to the identification and treatment of patient complications is directly influencing patient outcomes and can measure this involvement. One example is a CNS on a medical intensive care unit (MICU) who noted low compliance with delirium assessment and developed an action plan for improvement. The CNS repeatedly focused intense efforts on educating staff about delirium assessment using multiple modalities. She continued the educational strategies and audited adherence until compliance with the intervention improved from 84% to 100%. Obtaining adherence with delirium assessment is an essential step in aggressively targeting interventions. The APN can readily measure their effectiveness in educating staff and obtaining compliance through audits.

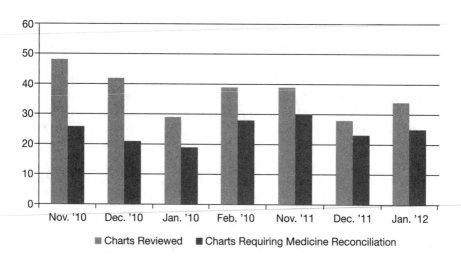

Figure 3.3 *ACNP Medicine Reconciliation Chart Review*

As with any selected outcome measure, it is essential that monitoring be done long enough that the effect can be evaluated accurately. As noted earlier, clinical outcomes should be those that are directly attributable to the APN intervention.

### Efficiency (Timesaving) Outcomes

Time and efficiency are appropriate outcome measures for APNs and can be measured in a number of different ways. Again, the appropriateness of the measures is dependent on the specific role of the APN. For example, if the role of the APN is to coordinate care of transplant patients, the APN might keep a log of telephone conversations with patients and categorize them into different content areas. Representative categories such as medication advice, updates on lab and other tests, consultations about when to come in to the hospital or clinic, or other topics might be selected. The conversations can be monitored in time segments. Once summarized, the time elements may represent a significant portion of time caring for patients and providing continuity of care. It also may prevent unnecessary clinic visits and "free-up" clinic time for other patients to be seen. It must be recognized, however, that the time elements must all have value to the physician or administrator paying for the APN, or be acknowledged as important additions to the practice. By monitoring these data, the aggregate data related to patient volume may be more accurately interpreted. In addition, this kind of "availability" of the APN is very attractive to worried patients and families. The element may also be measured in a satisfaction survey.

In another example, an ACNP was hired to manage congestive heart failure (CHF) patients in the cardiology clinic. Prior to the ACNP's practice in the clinic, clinic patients would learn of test results upon returning to the clinic or would call the secretary or doctor to learn the results. The ACNP quickly identified that this practice was not optimal and assumed responsibility for this component of the practice, as well as management of the patients during clinic visits. Her collaborative practice allowed for an increase in the total volume of patients cared for in the clinic. She also began to maintain a log of phone consultations, both by time allotment and by category (medication adjustment, information, symptoms, etc.). Patient and family satisfaction have increased (as evidenced by unsolicited comments and letters) and the collaborating physician has noted that his efficiency has been enhanced. The NP is able to translate the time log into patient interactions. The combination of increased physician efficiency and patient satisfaction in combination with a decreased readmission rate and increased patient volumes since the NP began her practice is convincing evidence that she is effective in her role.

Other time-related measures may demonstrate the APN's effectiveness as well. An example might be an initiative that emerges because emergency department patients are not being seen in a timely manner and satisfaction has suffered. APNs are frequently charged with system initiatives like this one but often do not measure the effects of the initiatives. In this case it would be appropriate to measure satisfaction and waiting times resulting from the initiative. Though in any system initiative there are numerous people who also play a role in making the approach successful, the APN heading the project could use the results as an indication of his/her effectiveness.

Time is money, and the translation of time to money (i.e., cost savings) is relatively easy to do. This type of measure is underused by APNs who frequently play a very important role in improving the quality and efficiency of care initiatives.

### Financial Outcomes

While virtually any outcome measure can be translated into financial outcomes, some financial data are especially of interest to institutions. An example is the use of cost and profit data. As noted earlier, the data are difficult to ascribe to any one APN; however, it can be used to trend the effect of an intervention coordinated or spearheaded by the APN. An example is an initiative such as the "outcomes manager" (OM) role for patients who require long-term mechanical ventilation. In this case, the OM is charged with managing and coordinating selected elements of care of patients assigned to a multidisciplinary clinical pathway. All key stakeholders are recognized as important to the initiative; however, improvements in the variables of interest (generally using retrospective/prospective data comparisons) speak strongly to the effectiveness of the APN in managing the program of care (Burns et al., 1998, 2003).

Financial outcomes can also be presented in terms of dollars saved. Although aggregate data are difficult to relate to an individual intervention, there are times when these measures are appropriate for the situation. For example, when an acute care CNS introduced a guideline to manage patients with pancreatitis, improving LOS without increasing readmissions was a natural outcome to track. Once adherence was determined through chart audits, the CNS was able to use an institutional database to measure the influence of the guideline. The CNS was able to demonstrate an association between the decreased LOS and stable readmission rate with guideline use because she also had a strong understanding of additional variables that might contribute to these data. Although other factors were at play during the time of the guideline introduction, the guideline was the most influential change and had the largest influence on the 19.1 to 14.7 day decrease in LOS. A LOS change can be converted into institutional dollars saved.

### Aggregate Data and/or Hospital Benchmark Data

As noted earlier, aggregate data are defined as data collected and reported by organizations and/or departments (e.g., QA, clinical data repositories) as a sum or total over a given time period (i.e., monthly or quarterly; Ryan & Thompson, 2002). The data are helpful and attractive to organizations because they can be translated into financial savings (or in most cases estimates of financial savings). Despite the common use of such outcome data, it is rarely possible to attribute such data to any one source unless the outcome element is carefully selected as in the examples provided previously. For example, if the APN begins an educational initiative aimed at decreasing ventilator-associated pneumonia (VAP) in a MICU population, it is important to first determine whether the institutional data may be used to track the outcome. In some cases this would be possible and all that would be necessary is that the APN intervention be marked so that a control chart might be developed to demonstrate effect over time. However, this example using aggregate data can also be illustrative of how such institutional data are fraught with problems. Unless the APN can ensure that adherence to the VAP preventive strategies is good and that all other interventions that may potentially affect the outcome are controlled (meaning they are stable and unchanging during the study period), outcomes may not be attributed to the APN practice initiative. Instead the outcomes may be the result of an attending physician's practice, introduction of a continuous subglottic suctioning endotracheal tube in patients admitted through the emergency department (ED), a hospital-wide "increased awareness campaign," or a new sinusitis prophylaxis regimen.

As described above, for the APN to clearly demonstrate his/her effectiveness in successfully initiating a practice change that positively affects VAP rates, an understanding of how well the intervention was implemented and followed by clinicians is essential. In this case, the APN's educational initiative was to teach every bedside caregiver to maintain the head of the bed in a 30-degree "head up" position. An audit prior to the intervention of head of bed elevation in the units, and on different shifts, demonstrated that adherence was very low (less than 20%). These data served as a baseline for comparison following the intervention. At intervals of 1 and 3 months, adherence was again audited and found to be improved (more than 70%). Being able to identify that the VAP intervention was occurring allowed for greater assurance that the APN initiative might be linked to the VAP rate improvement. Control charts may be used to mark the beginning of the initiation and subsequent "re-teaching" episodes as they relate to the VAP rate over time. The financial results of a successful initiative such as this one are easily calculated, and the APN may be recognized as having contributed to the positive results.

Aggregate data are also referred to as hospital benchmark data and are often used to compare institutional outcomes to those of other similar type facilities (academic medical centers, community hospitals, etc.). Given the volume of data available in institutional data banks, it is easy to understand why administrators and clinicians alike attempt to assign causality to this type of aggregate outcomes data. The assumption, that the data represent the effect of specific interventions or care, is often unwarranted. This is especially a problem when an attempt is made to infer the reasons for the outcomes and impose solutions. Those upon whom the solutions are to be imposed comment that the data are not representative of their patients, that they are "sicker" or "different," and that the data are not sensitive enough to stratify appropriately. In fact, the approach often engenders irritation, frustration, and lack of buy-in for the initiative. For example, say the APN has been charged with a hospital-wide initiative on wound care. The APN learns that pressure ulcer rates can be retrieved from the institutional data banks by service center. Unfortunately, when the APN tries to separate the data by specific units, she/he learns that the data are not available in that form. In fact, the data do not distinguish which patients had pre-existing ulcers (and where they originated) or where the majority of the care was delivered when the ulcer developed since the "service line" designation is by discharge unit, not the unit in which the pressure ulcer developed. Thus, the data may be helpful to look at overall hospital trends but will be less useful if a targeted intervention is to be developed. In this case, unless the APN can "drill down" by examining site of origin or use prospectively collected data to find the answers, the intervention might be applied to all the units though it may only be warranted in one.

The use of aggregate data may be helpful to follow trends but requires an in-depth understanding of the variable of interest to ensure accurate interpretation. An example is the use of LOS data. Take, for example, LOS data related to patients with tracheostomies. If one institution is able to transfer patients to discharge facilities with the tracheostomies in place (and requiring mechanical ventilation), the data on LOS may be inaccurately compared to an institution where similar transfer facilities do not exist. If this fact is not understood, erroneous comparisons between the two hospitals may be made. Instead a more sensitive indicator of quality for these patients may be weaning, reintubation rates, and ventilator duration.

Profit per case and cost per case may also be misleading since the factors affecting the numbers may have little to do with the intervention of interest. Consider the example of the ventilator-weaning initiative mentioned above. Cost of care may be higher in patients transferred to an MICU from a cardiovascular critical care unit than for patients who originate in the MICU. This may inaccurately assign cost per case to the MICU since all costs are attributed to the discharge unit (in this case the MICU) versus the unit in which the larger proportion of the costs was accrued. Thus, if these financial measures are used to chart progress, they may easily be misinterpreted unless appropriate "drill down" is accomplished.

Institutional aggregate data are useful in some cases; however, a thorough understanding of the data is necessary if the outcomes are to be attributable to APN practice.

## SUMMARY

The effectiveness of APNs has been called into question many times in the past. Often, when financial shortfalls are realized, constraints are placed on practicing clinicians. APNs whose practice in the past has not easily been linked to outcomes are often targeted. While these solutions may "save money" in the short term, their impact on quality, and ultimately finances, may be significant. APNs are essential to the quality system initiatives that occur in hospitals. Their work is important but is too often not recognized because it is "invisible." Using carefully selected data to demonstrate the APN's effect on some of these system initiatives is possible and important if APNs are to demonstrate their "value-added" contributions. Though system outcomes may be hard to ascribe to any one individual, the contributions of APNs are more likely to be acknowledged if data are available.

This chapter provides some examples of outcome measures that may be selected and used to accurately demonstrate the impact of APN practice. It is essential that APNs recognize that the measures should be selected carefully and be clearly linked to the APN role. Aggregate data are perhaps the least sensitive in being able to demonstrate the effectiveness of individuals but may be used to demonstrate trends in system approaches lead by the APN. While financial data are an appropriate indicator of APN "value-added" in some cases, it may be less so in others, especially if the role is not specifically linked to direct patient management.

## CONCLUSION

APNs are essential to the provision of quality patient care. Not only are they responsible for a wide variety of EBP changes and system initiatives, they are also responsible for the direct provision of evidence-based care. APN practice outcomes can and should be monitored to more strongly demonstrate the APN's positive contributions to health care.

### Answers to Chapter Discussion Questions

1. Aggregate data are often relatively easy to obtain but are rarely associated with the specific APN intervention under examination. Aggregate data are influenced by multiple factors. It is very difficult to relate these large and variable groupings to individual interventions because the effect of the intervention cannot be appreciated on such a hefty scale. An APN who is striving to demonstrate the value of his or her practice by using aggregate data is not accurately demonstrating his or her contributions. Smaller, more specific outcome measures are better able to capture an APN's influence.

2. Patterns of normal variation exist in every practice setting. Control charts take normal variation into consideration. Control charts include a target goal as well as upper and lower limits so that normal variation is accounted for. If the APN does not include upper and lower limits among the target goal, she or he will be constantly adjusting the intervention to meet the normal variation. She or he will never truly be able to evaluate the true effect of the intervention over time.

*3.* APNs need to identify outcome measures that are specific to their daily practice. The outcome measures must also be important to the institution in terms of patient care, satisfaction, efficiency, or dollars saved. It is important that outcome measures be derived from data that is easy to collect and the data should account for a period of time so that the outcomes may be translated into sustained improvement as a direct result of APN practice. The outcome measures may be unique to the APN, his or her role, and practice setting, but the key elements should be included.

## REFERENCES

Burns, S. M., Earven, D., Fisher, C., Lewis, R., Merrel, P., Schubart, J., ... Bleck T. (2003). Implementation of an institutional program to improve clinical and financial outcomes of patients requiring mechanical ventilation: One year outcomes and lessons learned. *Critical Care Medicine, 31,* 2752–2763.

Burns, S. M., Marshall, M., Burns, J. E., Ryan, B., Wilmoth, D., Carpenter, R., ... Truwit, J.D. (1998). Design, testing and results of an outcomes managed approach to patients requiring prolonged mechanical ventilation. *American Journal of Critical Care, 7,* 45–57.

Digby, J. (2011). 50 facts about customer experience: retrieved 8/7/12 from: http://returnonbehavior.com/2010/10/50-facts-about-customer-experience-for-2011/

Jones, C. B., & Gates, M. (2007). The costs and benefits of nurse turnover: A business case for nurse retention. *OJIN: The Online Journal of Issues in Nursing, 12*(3), Manuscript 4. Retrieved from: www.nursingworld.org/MainMenuCategories/ANAMarketplace/ANAPeriodicals/OJIN/TableofContents/Volume122007/No3Sept07/NurseRetention.aspx

Kleinpell, R., Ely, E. W., & Grabenkort, R. (2008). Nurse practitioners and physician assistants in the intensive care unit: An evidence-based review. *Critical Care Medicine, 36,* 2888–2897.

Newhouse, R. P., Stanik-Hutt, J., White, K. M., Johantgen, M., Bass, E., Zangaro, G., ... Weiner, J. P. (2011). Advanced practice nurse outcomes 1990–2008: A systematic review. *Nursing Economics, 29,* 230–250.

Ryan, S., & Thompson, C. (2002). The use of aggregate data for measuring practice improvement. *Seminars in Nurse Management, 10*(2), 90–94.

The Joint Commission. (2011). *Hospital: 2012 National patient safety goals.* Retrieved August 1, 2012 from: http://www.jointcommission.org/assets/1/6/NPSG_Chapter_Jan2012_HAP.pdf

Wheeler, D. J. (2000). *Understanding variation: The key to managing chaos* (2nd ed.). Knoxville, TN: SPS Press.

# Chapter 4: General Design and Implementation Challenges in Outcomes Assessment

*Ann F. Minnick*

## Chapter Objectives

1. Ensure that the design can meet the project's purpose.
2. Select outcomes.
3. Maximize the ability to link cause and effect.
4. Select a design that is amenable to resolving analytic quandaries.

## Chapter Discussion Questions

Identify an outcome of interest to you and then answer the following questions:

1. Outline the five steps you would take to ensure saliency of the outcome.
2. Describe the three steps that will help achieve the necessary qualities of reality and "common currency" for your project.
3. Describe the seven challenges to establish cause and effect in non-experimental designs.
4. Considering your outcome of interest, what analytic issues do you anticipate?

5. Identify four implementation challenges existing within outcomes assessment projects. Suggest a solution for each challenge.

***

*T*he conduct of outcomes assessment (OA) studies is expensive, especially in terms of human resources that might be applied to any number of other important activities. The results of OA projects are needed to determine public policies and institutional efforts. Both of these uses of OA results make it imperative that the studies be designed to avoid common design flaws and make parsimonious use of resources during their execution. Simply put, you need to avoid wasting your time and someone else's money while producing valuable information.

This chapter is based on the assumption that few practitioners want to simply describe a single outcome but rather are trying to devise assessments that will help them improve care in multiple ways. This chapter discusses solutions to the four most common design problems and four implementation challenges to achieving this goal. Recognition of these basic problems and challenges will lead to the discovery of other issues that can be threats to the execution of OA studies. Although the list of potential solutions presented in this chapter is not exhaustive, it is designed to arm the person embarking on such projects with a basic set of effective responses.

## SOLVING DESIGN PROBLEMS

Four common design problems in OA are (1) ensuring that the design can meet the project's purpose, (2) selecting outcomes, (3) maximizing the ability to link cause and effect, and (4) selecting a design that is amenable to resolving analytic quandaries.

### Linking Purpose and Design

#### Common Problems

The first and perhaps most important step is to determine what question(s) the OA project seeks to answer. Many novices have found themselves implementing a design only to discover that they never determined specific questions they sought to answer. This occurs most often when clinicians note that some naturally occurring event, such as a change in practice at one site, will result in what seems like experimental and control groups. They then begin to track outcomes, but, because specific questions were never posed, find that they neglected to collect data on some important variable or that the pre-/postintervention design they used cannot really capture the additional ongoing practice changes at the sites.

A second problem in linking purpose and design is the failure to plan a project that could have answered, with only a few design changes, many more questions that are of interest to the larger world of institutional and public policy making. Many practitioners can verbally explain the larger issues for which OAs are needed, but they design studies that do not help inform the important debates over outcomes and how best to achieve them. At a minimum, any OA usually needs to include some exploration of patients' physical and psychosocial outcomes as well as some elements of service costs and impact on provider.

### Solutions

Persons planning to embark on OAs can take the following steps to avoid these two problems:

1. Write the *questions* your OA project seeks to answer. Next, answer the question: How will answering these questions lead to actions that will improve outcomes for patients, the practice and/or institution, and the public?
2. For each project question, identify who cares about the answer and the level at which each person/agent functions in terms of making decisions that might influence changes your project might suggest. For example, is it a professional nurse practitioner group, the practice manager for your group, or a state agency? Or could it be all of them if the design were changed? You will need resources for your study, even if your plans encompass only an assessment of outcomes within your own practice. These people/agencies could be sources of support. The first rule of sales (and gaining support for any type of project) is to meet the customer's needs. Be sure your project does so.
3. If in step 2 you could not identify more than one audience of interest, reconsider the questions. OA projects are too expensive to be one-trick ponies. If you identify someone who has resources but whom

you believe will not be supportive, consider how at least one question of interest to him/her can be included and be answered as *part* of the assessment. In providing an answer for what the individual or institution may think is the most important aspect of an OA, you will have the opportunity to bring these other questions (and findings!) to his or her attention.

4. Verify through literature review and consultation with persons at each of the specified levels that these are the most important questions. "Important" means those questions that arise because there are great gaps in understanding and for which solutions are most urgently needed.

5. Seek consultation to ensure that it is possible to design an assessment that produces data that can answer the questions.

### Selecting Outcomes

#### Problems

Once the above five steps are taken, it becomes easier to address the problem of defining outcomes. Each outcome must have the three attributes to make a project worth the investment: *salience, objectivity,* and *common currency.*

Salience is the quality of being related to the phenomenon of interest. By meeting the five steps already mentioned, salience can be achieved. Objectivity is the ability of an outcome to be measured without bias. For an outcome to be said to be based in reality, it must be one that has the quality of being true to life. One example of a bias problem is illustrated by a seemingly simple outcome: Rehospitalization within 60 days after treatment. In one study, we had to grapple with the bias inherent in defining rehospitalization as having occurred only if it happened at the single hospital where most nurse practitioners had privileges. There was the chance that some patients were being rehospitalized at several other hospitals at which a few of the nurse practitioners also had privileges.

Another example of this problem involves physical restraint use as an outcome. Once the physical restraint is defined, it should be fairly easy to determine if someone is restrained. The issue arises in counting restrained persons. If patients are transported to a unit in restraints, should they be counted against the receiving unit in a project seeking to assess the outcomes of a restraint-reduction program? If not, how long should the unit be given to use restraint alternatives before patients are counted as restrained? Should there be another outcome such as "duration of restraint use for patients admitted in restraint"? How much detail is necessary?

Reality can be defined as the extent to which the outcome definition has some fidelity to nature, that is, is true to life. Depression, quality of life, and spiritual health are examples of outcomes for which there are readily acknowledged problems in capturing the reality of the situation. Other outcomes, although seemingly immune to this problem because they are behaviorally based, are just as vulnerable. Consider the outcome "ambulation sufficient to accomplish five activities of daily living." If the outcome is operationalized as the ability to do this in a setting assumed to be a one-story home, but many patients live in multistory dwellings, there is little that is true to life about the study because many people need to be able to not only just ambulate but also climb stairs. Resources to consult in the definition and measurement of common outcomes are listed at the end of this chapter. The books listed highlight the advantages, disadvantages, and design issues associated with each approach.

A final problem revolves around what outcome researchers often assume is "common currency" in defining outcomes. For example, if death is an outcome and the performance of numerous hospitals is being measured in the OA, the death rates will be very different in the hospital that includes its hospice unit in the report versus those that do not have such a unit. A hospital may include deaths in the emergency department and another may not. If a hospital is the public receiving facility for the pronouncement of death in police and fire cases, should these deaths be included in the operationalization of the definition of death? Responsible persons at each hospital often believe everyone at other hospitals uses the same definitions for outcomes when in fact there is no common currency.

### Solutions

Solutions lie in rigorous definitions:

1. Each time an outcome is mentioned in the project's questions, underline it. Within the context of each question, define the outcome in terms that can be objectively applied within the context of the study. It is important that you do this with each question independently. You may find that the outcome you are referring to as "mobility" in question 1 may be very different by question 4. To define is to choose outcomes.

2. Discuss your definitions at sites where you plan to conduct the assessment to determine if data are currently amassed using your definition. Ask the responsible parties to describe any special situations they may have that could influence their outcomes, even when their definition is the one you propose. Be prepared to give examples of situations. Remember, most people do not believe their situation is the exception.

3. Simultaneous with step 2, complete a review to determine what definitions were used in the most important outcomes studies published to date. Although you may choose to define an outcome in a new way and may, in reality, be developing a new outcome of interest, an OA is strengthened if there can be some comparison with findings from previous studies. For example, in a study of physical restraints, we measured prevalence and incidence, although earlier studies had relied almost exclusively on the latter. We were thus able to ascertain that the lower usage we documented was in fact a decline based on comparisons with earlier reports, as well as demonstrate that there were very great differences between incidence and prevalence. Consult the Agency for Health Care Policy and Research Web sites listed at the end of the chapter to learn how outcomes of interest to your project have been defined and measured.

### Tracing Cause and Effect

As students of traditional research know, a well-executed, double-blind, randomized pretest–posttest design is effective when one seeks to establish that a particular intervention produces measurable effect(s). In OA projects, this approach is usually not an option because of real-life issues. For example, it is often not possible to randomize patients or blind providers to treatment. It is rare to find a project that seeks only to measure one outcome. The science of improvement drives the desire to identify variables associated with the outcome. Seven challenges to the ability to make conclusions about causation and to identify interventions that might result in outcomes improvement are common. These seven challenges are:

1. Patient autonomy. The patient may be following the recommended treatment on a continuum ranging from "entirely" to "not at all." The patient may be following one aspect of the treatment entirely and another not at all. The patient may follow a treatment plan one day and not at all the next.

2. Multiplicity of health problems in a single individual. Almost no patient presents with a single health challenge. Multiple system failures are common and the simultaneous presence of physical and mental disorders has been well documented. This makes assessment of a single outcome related to a particular disorder difficult.
3. Nonclinical characteristics. Income, education, insurance coverage, geographical location, exposure to violence, and many other variables can influence outcomes.
4. Multiplicity of health providers. This includes known as well as unknown providers who, in turn, use many different types of treatments. Some of these treatments may have been obtained from ethnic healers. Some medications may have been obtained illegally. Other providers might be recognized in foreign countries and their advice obtained by the autonomous patient through the Internet. Even if the providers are known, their skill in providing a specific treatment may vary. Depending on the schedule, the patient may have received each treatment in a repetitive series from different providers.
5. Unknown time delay between intervention and expected outcome. The classic example of this challenge is the difficulty in determining the outcomes of providers' health-promotion activities because many years (and many intervening messages and experiences) will often pass before a condition manifests itself.
6. Lack of baseline measurements. Patients often change providers, and accumulating good baseline measures of health status, quality of life, and other variables are expensive to collect de novo. Even if there is support for de novo measures, it is often impossible to collect a full record that captures the rich and complex changes in human life that may influence an outcome.
7. The complexity of nonpatient, nonindividual provider variables. These variables include labor (overall staffing quantity and quality) and capital inputs (e.g., equipment), as well as conditions of employment and leadership. In studies of whether or not a particular activity influences outcomes, these types of variables rather than the activity itself may be paramount. For example, staff may have the same beliefs and knowledge about ways to avoid extubation accidents, but a shortage of supplies or staff may make the execution of these steps impossible. Merely assessing extubations by practice group or before and after an educational session with the staff will not assist in tracing why an outcome is occurring.

## Solutions

All of the solutions depend on the outcomes assessor having a broad knowledge of patients, providers, and system variables. Consultants for each of these areas during the design phase can be worthwhile. They may ensure that the potential effects of these variables are at least considered.

Through interviews with providers and patients as well as review of clinical documents, such as medical records, determine what the potential is that aspects 1 through 4 may influence the OA. During this process, attempt to determine if these aspects are evenly distributed across cases or if only select groups are influenced. For example, many patients at one clinic site may visit a traditional healer down the street, and patients at another site might not. As with the issue of defining outcomes, patients and providers will not necessarily think that their situations are unique. During the project-planning phase, you will need to ask questions that will provoke a wide-ranging discussion, such as "Tell me about some of the things you do for your arthritis besides coming to the clinic."

Plan on multiple measurement over time. Multiple measures over time will help to ascertain any change/attenuation of effect on outcomes. This is especially important if the OA is part of an intervention effort. An outcome may at first seem to be favorably influenced, but there may be rapid attenuation. Conversely, it may take an unknown period of time for full effects to be realized.

After reviewing the availability of baseline data, recognize that significant OA resources may need to be assigned to build a database. The project budget needs to reflect this expense. Make it a priority to explore how to maintain the elements of these data after the assessment project is complete. Experience has shown that once providers and institutions have access to such a database, they are willing to devote the resources necessary for its maintenance because a well-designed database can be used for many OA projects, as well as to meet accreditation demands.

Use a framework such as the one in Figure 4.1 to ascertain that you have assessed the system variables that are most likely to influence outcomes. Many times the key to improving outcomes is to attempt to modify system—rather than individual provider or patient—variables. For example, in the last century, anesthesia outcomes were improved significantly when the tubing connection ends of various gases provided during surgery were made compatible only with the appropriate delivery device.

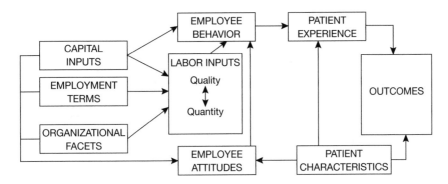

*Figure 4.1  A Framework of Variables Influencing Patient Outcomes*

*Source.* Developed in preparation of Minnick, Roberts, Young, Kleinpell, and Marcantonio (1997).

### Analytic Issues

#### Problems

As can be deduced from the discussion of the many variables that need to be accounted for in an OA project, multivariate analysis becomes a necessity. Any outcome may be affected by attribute variables, contextual variables, and specific treatment effects. The problem in executing such an approach is that one usually does not know at the beginning of a project if the variables of interest are orthogonal to one another (an assumption of many statistical techniques). This problem is known as collinearity. A second problem is the definition and treatment of attribute and contextual variables. More analytic problems occur when an outcome is rare or infrequent. Finally, the third problem is that data of interest are drawn from different levels. For example, an outcome may be drawn from individual patient records, but variables such as staffing may be unit based with others drawn from an institutional level. Special techniques are needed for the analysis.

#### Solutions

Few practitioners are equipped to deal with these problems. The following steps are advisable for practitioners who do not have advanced statistical and design expertise:

*1.* Recognize what one does not know and consult experts during the design phase. The timing is essential because many of the solutions to these problems are rooted in selecting the proper design and definitions. For example, in the case of rare outcomes, a case-control approach may be advised.

2. The practitioner should, however, be knowledgeable enough to recognize the possibility that all three problems exist and to ask a statistician how the problems can be addressed. In asking the statistician for advice, the practitioner should enquire about the advantages and disadvantages of each proposed solution.

## ADDRESSING IMPLEMENTATION CHALLENGES

### Issues

Having considered the complexity of the design issues described above, thoughtful practitioners may be tempted to run from the very idea of launching a systematic OA. This section is devoted to providing "doable" solutions for the four major implementation challenges: (1) assembling a competent and productive team, (2) securing the resources to complete the project, (3) obtaining institutional cooperation, and (4) enlisting the cooperation of providers and patients.

### Solutions

The solutions are based on the belief that the process of getting this type of project done is no different than the steps one would take in any type of project, from remodeling one's home to opening a new clinic. You would neither attempt to do either of these projects alone nor would you attempt to go forward without adequate resources.

1. Assemble a team of people who are as interested in the idea as you are. If no one is interested, begin building interest one person at a time. Put yourself in that person's position. What responsibilities or needs would this type of project help that person address? Use these points in discussion. Try to include formal resource allocators as well as informal opinion makers in this effort.

2. Consider all sources of support, including those outside of your institution. Your well-designed project and its findings could serve as a model for others. Foundations as well as federal agencies are interested in models and in projects that are large enough to produce generalizable findings about the outcomes. Once you

have ascertained why your institution or an outside agency should be interested, prepare a short (no more than three-page) discussion paper that explains the need for the project, the answers it will produce, and why the results will be valuable to the funder. Include an estimate of the general costs. This is a major marketing tool. People who are asked for resources need to know what they are buying, why they need it, and what it is going to cost.

3. Build alliances with the database, statistical, and design experts whose help you will be able to afford once step 2 is accomplished. You will need to begin building these alliances before approaching resource holders to get a general idea of costs and to amass the technical expertise that will make the proposal a solid one.

4. Consider banding together with like-minded providers, institutions, professional associations, or healthcare systems. This cooperation can drive down costs by spreading the fixed expenses (e.g., statistical help) over a greater number of supporters. It also is a wonderful way to gather data on rare events and to develop a database that allows for exploration of multiple factor influences on outcomes. For example, if you are in Nebraska, you may not have sufficient population to explore the effect of a specific ethnicity on patient outcomes. A project that includes sites in Illinois, New York, or California may make this possible.

As noted in the beginning of this chapter, OAs are important sources of information on which public policies and private actions are based. Given this fact and the expense of these assessments, an OA can truly be said to be one of those activities in which "if it is worth doing, it is worth doing well." A poor OA can be worse than none at all because it will lead to poor decisions. With an awareness of the design pitfalls and access to solutions and experts, practitioners can help ensure that OAs are truly worth the investment.

## Answers to Chapter Discussion Questions

1. The five steps are listed on pages 95 and 96.
2. (a) Check that the same outcome is used throughout the questions. (b) Discuss definitions at sites to determine if data are amassed using these definitions. (c) Complete a literature review of the definitions.

3. (a) Patient autonomy, (b) provider multiplicity, (c) nonclinical characteristics, (d) multiplicity of health problems, (e) unknown time of delay between interventions and expected outcome, (f) lack of baseline measurements, and (g) complex systems variables.

4. Your answer should include assessment of the likelihood that the following issues might arise: colinearity, treatment of attribute and contextual variables, and how multiple levels of data will be addressed.

5. Your answer should revolve around specifics individualized to your project steps to address: (a) assembling a competent and productive team, (b) securing resource, (c) securing institutional cooperation, and (d) enlisting the cooperation of providers and patients.

## REFERENCE

Minnick, A. F., Roberts, M. J., Young, W. B., Kleinpell, R. M., & Marcantonio, R. J. (1997). What influences patients' reports of three aspects of hospital services? *Medical Care, 35*(4), 399–409.

## RESOURCES—BOOKS AND WEBSITES

AHRQ, the Agency for Healthcare Research and Quality (http://www.ahrq.gov/), is "the nation's lead Federal agency for research on health-care quality, costs, outcomes, and patient safety" and is a key source for information about national outcomes assessment efforts.

CAHPS, the AHCPR's Consumer Assessment of Healthcare Providers and Systems program (https://www.cahps.ahrq.gov/default.asp), is "a public–private initiative to develop standardized surveys of patients' experiences with ambulatory and facility-level care." The CAHPS website provides free information and AHRQ tools to measure consumers' assessment of their health care experiences. Survey tools can be downloaded and technical advice is available.

Doran, D. M. (Ed.) (2011). *Nursing outcomes. The state of the science.* Sudbury, MA: Jones and Barlett. (This work reviews outcome categories, their measurement and use within the framework of nursing accountability.)

Frank-Stromborg, M., & Olsen, S. J. (Eds.). (2004). *Instruments for clinical health care research* (3rd ed.). Sudbury, MA: Jones and Bartlett.

Kane, R. L., & Radosevich, D. M. (2011). *Conducting health outcomes research* (2nd ed.). Sudbury, MA: Jones and Bartlett. (Although aimed at researchers, this classic work points out many issues that could influence outcomes assessments.)

McDowell, I., & Newell, C. (Eds.) (2006). *Measuring health. A guide to rating scales and questionnaires* (3rd ed.). New York, NY: Oxford University Press.

*Medical Care Research and Review.* (2007). In April 2007, this journal sponsored a special supplement (Vol. 64, No. 2 Suppl.) on Performance Measurement and Outcomes of Nursing Care. The contents for this supplement, with downloadable PDFs of separate articles, is available online: http://mcr.sagepub.com/content/vol64/2_suppl

Moorhead, S., Johnson, M., Maas, M. L., & Swanson, E. (Eds). (2013). *Nursing outcomes classification (NOC): Measurement of health outcomes* (5th ed.). St. Louis, MO: Mosby.

Muennig, P. (2008). *Cost-effectiveness analyses in health. A practical approach* (2nd ed.). San Francisco, CA: Jossey-Bass. (Although assessing cost effectiveness as an outcome requires specialized skills, this book is a good basic primer toward understanding this complex outcome.)

# Chapter 5: Locating Instruments and Measures for Advanced Practice Nursing Outcome Assessments

MARILYN WOLF SCHWARTZ AND ROGER GREEN

## Chapter Objectives

1. Provide a guide for finding instruments, including questionnaires, scales, and tools, to measure treatment outcomes.
2. Remind the reader of the value of using library resources, not just Google or the Internet. There is also value in consulting a professional medical librarian to find the appropriate instruments in a timely manner.
3. Emphasize the importance of requesting permission to use instruments, whether standard or unpublished. Permission to use an instrument is an ethical issue related to copyright and proper research method.

## Chapter Discussion Questions

1. What two databases are appropriate to start a search on an instrument to use for diabetes primary care outcomes? What terms and strategy were used to do the search? List a measurement tool found

in the database search that an advanced practice nurse (APN) could use in practice.

2. In what reference books would you find a review and description of the Minnesota Multiphasic Personality Inventory? Find a local medical, nursing, or university library's online catalog to see if a few books listed in the Suggested Readings—Books at the end of this chapter may be found in a local library.

3. List two university websites looked at to learn about requesting permission to use an instrument. List an instrument on pain assessment/scale and where to request permission to use it, if there is training required to use it, and if there is a cost.

4. What are some of the mobile applications to access resources discussed in this chapter to find information on an instrument that could be used to measure the physician–nurse professional collaboration?

5. List resources that are most promising for a future outcome assessment nursing or medical problem that needs to be studied.

**A**dvanced practice nurses (APNs) and researchers need to know how to find surveys, questionnaires, or other measurement instruments to determine if a treatment is effective. In the evidence-based health care era, APNs as well as researchers need to study, measure, and report significant changes in interventions. When APNs report evidence-based findings in the literature, they are improving the quality of health care and contributing to the professions. This chapter is intended to help APNs find the instruments that measure the impact of APN care and interventions.

Providing information on finding instruments would not be complete without mentioning the responsible use of tests and measures. Many university library websites explain the ethical use of measurement tools or instruments. Authors doing authentic research must prove validity and reliability. Textbooks on developing measurement tools emphasize the importance of testing and validating tools. Consequently, respected instruments are copyrighted, costly to develop, and need to be used appropriately. In the section Suggested Reading—University Library Websites, several websites listed note the importance of requesting permission and how to make such inquiries. For starters, following is a website to read a summary of ethics of use and why permission should be requested: http://info.library.okstate.edu/tests (retrieved August 9, 2012).

The authors present major resources that librarians and clinicians can use to find instruments. The terms "instruments," "questionnaires," "surveys," and "tools" are used interchangeably. "Instrument" is the preferred term, however, because that is what the database Cumulative Index to Nursing and Allied Health (CINAHL) uses in indexing the field that has the descriptor for the tools mentioned in articles.

In this chapter, readers will find:

1. Books: The books described herein are standard reference texts regarded as the first sources to check in finding instruments.
2. Bibliographic databases: These are defined in the order of importance to nursing applications. Examples are given for the kinds of instruments that might be found in the CINAHL and the Health and Psychosocial Instruments (HaPI) databases. Some suggestions are given on fields to search in these databases for the instruments. The reader may then apply some of the same techniques to searching other databases. It is important to consult a medical librarian, when available, to process searches, especially when doing an evidence-based study or publishing or presenting papers. Using the controlled vocabulary or thesauri for retrieval in databases is important, and medical librarians are adept at using them effectively.
3. Internet resources: Those listed include professional organizations and government sites as well as library guides to tools. University librarians, especially in medical settings, are placing descriptions of mobile applications (apps) used on iPads, iPhones, Blackberrys, and other handheld devices to access literature searching. Library websites are good places to check for mobile apps to access literature databases and electronic books. Note the Internet Resources and Online Library Resources section for more details on apps. The Internet resources listed are by no means exhaustive but considered selective.

## STANDARD BOOKS

In this age of technology, using standard textbooks is not the most popular source of information. However, following are some tried and true measurement tool books. Note the additional books listed in the bibliography at the end of this chapter, many of which are more specific to nursing and medicine. The books to consult are too numerous to describe individually. Many nursing and medical libraries own the books listed in the Bibliography. Of course, most books may be purchased from online book vendors, such as Amazon. Where websites are given, all sites were active as of August 9, 2012.

### Mental measurements yearbooks (MMYBs) by Buros Institute of Mental Measurements

Check the website (http://www.unl.edu/buros) to see that this group has been around for 70 years and are experts.

This standard reference text is available in most university and public libraries on reference shelves. It is updated every 2 years and may be accessed online through many library online database menus. It has been published since 1938. The book lists tests in alphabetical order with descriptive information with purpose, intended population, acronyms, authors, scores, time, prices, publishers, and cross references. Each volume provides information on reliability, validity, and includes reviews of tests and test materials. Many libraries have access to this book online. Buros also publishes *Test Reviews Online*. There is also a link to test reviews through http://buros.unl.edu/buros/jsp/search.jsp. This Buros site contains only reviews for tests, which the user decides whether to purchase.

### Tests in Print (Tip) by Buros Institute of Mental Measurement

TIP lists target audience, length, score(s), and cost and is a companion to the Buros MMYB. The TIP and the MMYB are the main sources for finding information on published tests.

### Tests: A Comprehensive Reference for Assessments in Psychology, Education, and Business, edited by Taddy Maddox. PRO-ED, Inc., published from 1983 to the present, with a 2008 edition.

Descriptions are brief and contain information on test population, purpose, format, scoring, and cost and do not include reviews or evaluations of tests.

### Test Critiques, Kansas City, Missouri, Test Corporation of America, published since 1984

This multivolume set is the companion to *Tests* and includes reliability and validity information. For a complete description of *Test Critiques*, see the American Psychological Association's website at http://www. apa.org/science/testing.html. It publishes in-depth reviews of frequently used psychological, education, and business tests, and provides descriptions, practical applications, technical aspects, and critiques of tests. Each volume has a cumulative index.

*Directory of Unpublished Experimental Mental Measures, edited by B.A. Goldman and D.F. Mitchell, published by the American Psychological Association since 1970 (latest volume 9 published 2008)*

Volume 9 lists tests published in the 2001 to 2005 issues of the 36 journals covered. This directory includes information on recently developed or noncommercial, experimental tests in 24 categories. The entries cover 36 relevant professional journals published in the United States. The measures described in dissertations are not included. Volumes do not include reviews. Check the category index. However, the volumes do not have title indexes. Some of the categories of measures are achievement, adjustment, aptitude, attitude, behavior communication, concept meaning, development, motivation, perception, personality problem solving and reasoning, values, vocational interest and evaluation, and trait measurement.

Please note the many additional books listed in the bibliography. The McDowell book, with a guide to rating scales and questionnaires, in particular, is an excellent source for finding health-related instruments and is cited in the bibliography at the end of the chapter. University libraries usually have the books listed and some are in reference sections. Remember that most university libraries now have their catalogs available online so that if a library has a collection of tests or instruments, the information on the tests may be found through the catalogs. Library staff may request interlibrary loans for books not owned. Reference and selection librarians usually welcome requests for purchase of instrument resource books when not owned by the library.

## BIBLIOGRAPHIC DATABASES

Searching bibliographic databases retrieves references to articles about instruments, but the articles do not always print copies of the instruments. However, remember that searching databases may provide references to articles that occasionally include the instruments. Finding full-text journal articles online in databases may show instruments in the articles. In the Internet Resources section of this chapter is a description of how to find dissertations, which usually include instruments used in doctoral or PhD work.

## LEVELS OF EVIDENCE

The MEDLINE and the Cochrane databases contain references to the highest quality journals or peer-reviewed literature as do CINAHL, PsychINFO, and Educational Resources Information Center (ERIC). The database producers, especially MEDLINE, publish on their websites statements of the criteria required for the journals to be indexed. APNs reviewing the instruments and articles describing the tools need to critically appraise the literature to make sure the evidence created in using the instruments is sound.

CINAHL is available from EBSCO Publishing database vendor and journal subscription agency. For access information, go to http://www.ebscohost.com. EBSCO and other vendors now provide tutorials, offered on YouTube or other media formats, to explain the use of search strategies for their databases.

A starting point for finding any instrument is the CINAHL because instruments may be searched directly in the instrumentation field of the bibliographic record. Once the user logs into CINAHL, search directly on the "instrumentation" field from the "indexes" on the main screen. If you search the "Publication Type" field and choose "research instrument," you may actually find the full text of an instrument. This database is not free to the public, and users must request codes from institutional libraries, ask a librarian, or pay for a service to process searches. Remember that as technology changes for the vendors, screens may change. Call the technical support number or email the vendor to learn how to search the indexes or fields as some vendors call them.

## HEALTH AND PSYCHOSOCIAL INSTRUMENTS (HaPI)

HaPI is produced by Behavioral Measurement Database Service (BMDS), Pittsburgh, PA 15232–0787. This database lists evaluation and measurement tools, questionnaires, and test instruments. HaPI is available through the database vendor Ovid, a Wolters Kluwer Publishing division. Go to http://www.ovid.com/site/index.jsp for access information. Ovid databases are available through many medical libraries and major university libraries. Contact the HaPI publisher for direct access and to find other database vendors who provide access.

The HaPI database does not provide copies of instruments. However, this database shows information on where to find the tool/ instrument and often gives the address and phone number. This database is bibliographic, meaning that it retrieves references to articles about the instrument. The references are indicated as secondary sources, then below the citation, the primary sources tell where the instruments were originally described and usually where to call or write to get a copy. This database is not free to the public, and users must request codes from institutional libraries, consult a librarian, or pay for a service to process searches.

## MEDLINE/PUBMED

PubMed.gov is the National Library of Medicine's databases, which include MEDLINE (Medical Literature Analysis and Retrieval System Online). APNs may search this database for reference to articles on a specific instrument. The references often discuss the reliability and validity of the instrument. The articles, at times, provide a copy of the instrument discussed. In MEDLINE, email addresses are provided with the authors' names making it easier to find an author to write for further information about an instrument that may have been discussed in the article. One of the limiters available for searching is the publication types, including questionnaires.

This database is free to the public at http://pubmed.gov. Check with local medical resource libraries and librarians for instructions in using PubMed. Note that this database has brief tutorials at http://www.nlm.nih.gov/bsd/disted/pubmed.html (retrieved August 9, 2012), as well as a detailed tutorial that may take several hours to complete. The time invested in looking at the tutorials usually pays off in terms of saving time in using the database.

## COCHRANE DATABASES

The Cochrane databases are excellent sources to find the highest level evidence-based studies that may describe instruments used. These databases are usually available through libraries or institutions, such as hospitals or drug companies. Ovid and EBSCO are two vendors providing access to many of the databases, including:

- Cochrane Database of Systematic Reviews
- Cochrane Database of Abstracts of Reviews of Effects
- Cochrane Central Register of Controlled Trials
- Cochrane Methodology Register
- Health Technology Assessment
- ACP Journal Club

The website of the Cochrane collaboration, http://www.cochrane.org (retrieved August 9, 2012), gives free access to a few references containing reviews. Another website that has free information from the Cochrane Database of Systematic Reviews is http://www.mrw.interscience.wiley.com/cochrane/cochrane_clsysrev_articles_fs.html (retrieved August 9, 2012). Also, try a Google search at http://www.google.com or a Google Scholar search at http://scholar.google.com (retrieved August 9, 2012) on Cochrane Databases to read more. Use the Advanced Search button on Google to narrow your search because basic searches often retrieve thousands of entries. Many university library sites have information on the databases and how to search them.

When searching the Cochrane databases on Ovid or EBSCO, limit the topics by using the terms instrument(s), questionnaire(s), scale(s), or survey(s). Use the truncation symbol of a dollar sign $ at the ends of root words for Ovid and the asterisk * for EBSCO to retrieve various spellings. For example, type in Instrument$ or instrument* to retrieve instrument, instruments, or instrumentation. Results in searching the Systematic Reviews will provide fewer references than in literature searches because the subject may not have been studied. In retrieving actual reviews, load up the printer with plenty of paper because reviews often can be over 50 pages or download the review onto a thumb drive.

## EDUCATION RESOURCES INFORMATION CENTER

ERIC is produced by Institute of Education of the U.S. Department of Education, Washington, DC. This database lists evaluation and measurement tools, questionnaires, and test instruments. ERIC's Clearinghouse on Assessment and Evaluation (AE) has a Test Locator at http://ericae.net/testcol.htm (retrieved August 9, 2012), which includes free tests. This site also has a link to Buros Institute of Mental Measurements and allows shopping and purchase of tests (http://buros.unl.edu/buros/jsp/search.jsp) (retrieved August 9, 2012). The *Test Reviews Online* is on this link.

APNs often participate in educating patient or staff in treatments or procedures. The challenge in the educational process is to show that what was presented caused a change in knowledge and practice. Although the ERIC database contains a limited amount of health or medical literature references, it does provide references to general educational concepts that may be applied to measure whether educational interventions are working.

This database is free to the public at http://www.eric.ed.gov/ (retrieved August 9, 2012).

## PSYCHINFO

PsychINFO is produced by the American Psychological Association and contains references to articles about various psychological instruments. Many database vendors offer PsychINFO, including Ovid, EBSCO, and ProQuest (formerly Dialog Knight-Ridder), and each has its own search engine

Depending on what the APN is studying, the PsychINFO database may include references to articles relevant to measure psychological changes. This database covers professional and academic literature in psychology and related disciplines, including medicine and nursing. PsychINFO is international in scope and includes abstracts for citations in over 2,150 journals, dissertations, books, and book chapters. Some university libraries allow access to this database for users in the library or for students and staff remotely. Some libraries may require you to access via a professional librarian.

The strategy is different from CINAHL or HaPI. A search hint in using PsychINFO is to use the thesaurus and use the "measurement" heading to find related topics that may be of use. In PsychINFO, retrieval may be limited to "test & measures" using the limit button on Ovid. Retrieval will be for article references, and possibility of the full instrument being in the article may occur occasionally. Rely on PsychINFO to find articles on validity or reliability of particular measures. Articles may be found on various measures used for a particular health or psychological issue. Note the American Psychological website listed in the Bibliography under Internet Resources as an excellent source for finding the actual instruments.

## DISSERTATION ABSTRACTS INTERNATIONAL

Dissertation Abstracts is the index of doctoral dissertations and master's theses written at most North American graduate schools. The CINAHL database also contains dissertations. The dissertations may be searched and ordered through UMI/Proquest company. Go to the following website to order a dissertation online: http://www.proquest. com/products_umi/dissertations/disexpress.shtml (retrieved August 9, 2012). This site's name is Dissertations Express and in 2012, the cost for a dissertation varied with the format. PDF format is $37.00; unbound, $39.00; and microfiche, $51.00 for a 357-page dissertation. Pricing is given for soft cover, hard cover, and microfilm when ordering. On this database, the user may order a dissertation as an individual for the stated fee, or if your library/institution subscribes to this database, library service may request it for you.

If a dissertation is not available through Dissertations Express, check with a local medical librarian to request an interlibrary loan from the institution from which the dissertation was required and published.

## PROQUEST DIALOG

ProQuest Dialog provides access to hundreds of databases that most universities and many hospitals use to conduct searches for library patrons. Individuals usually need to use these databases through their libraries because of the expense. The Bluesheets list the databases and their descriptions. Check the following website to view relevant database descriptions for finding instruments at http://library.dialog.com/ bluesheets/ (retrieved August 18, 2012). Librarians access ProQuest/ Dialog to help library patrons search the appropriate databases.

## INTERNET RESOURCES AND ONLINE LIBRARY RESOURCES

Please note that the Bibliography at the end of this chapter is where to find the links to library websites that have guides to finding instruments. This list is not exhaustive but has quality sites. Use Google to find other websites that may be helpful (Google and Google Scholar, http://www.google.com and http://scholar.google.com, respectively).

Google may be used as a starting point or last resort. In using Google, try to use advanced search if the basic search does not retrieve information needed. Use Google Scholar (http://scholar.google.com) for articles about an instrument. A Google Scholar search on the Visual Analog Pain Scale Faces retrieves several articles discussing uses of the scale, some with pictures of faces rating pain. This is only one of many pain scales that are visual.

## UNIVERSITY LIBRARY WEBSITES

Note sites listed in the Bibliography. Some of the university sites have charts and tables describing databases and step-by-step methods for finding instruments. Most of these websites include most of the information in this chapter.

## MOBILE/HANDHELD DEVICES AND MEDICAL APPLICATIONS (APPS)

Practitioners often use mobile devices for medical "apps" to access patient records, drug information, and bibliographic databases, to name a few. To see lists of databases or other medical apps, many university libraries are providing information in chart format on their websites to make it easy for users to see what is available. For example, Texas A&M University Libraries has a list of mobile databases that are accessible through various devices. Specifically, the guide shows that "CINAHL Plus with Full Text Mobile" is available from EBSCO. Check the URL http://msl.library.tamu.edu/services/mobile-resources.html. With the latest handheld technology, APNs could check CINAHL in a patient setting or when not near a laptop to look up information on an instrument. Another well-presented example of mobile apps is from the University of Washington Health Sciences Library, entitled "Handheld Accessible Resources," available at URL: http://libguides.hsl.washington.edu/mobile. San Jose State University library staff, in 2010, used the term "Appography" to describe a bibliography for apps. The term is "iPhone Appography," and the URL is http://libguides.sjsu.edu/print_content.php?pid=109524.

Many popular mobile or handhelds (the term the National Library of Medicine uses) are used to access databases and websites to search outcome measures. The APN may use CINAHL, Medline/PubMed, HaPI, MMYB, TIP, and PsychInfo with handhelds. Many other resources are searchable via mobile. The reader may do a Google search on each resource followed by the term "mobile" or "handhelds" to retrieve university or vendor sites that describe how to access. Sometimes apps are free through local universities.

To learn about the National Library of Medicine's Gallery of Mobile Apps, check the URL www.nlm.nih.gov/mobile. Read about PsychINFO Mobile at URL: www.apa.org/pubs/databases/news/2011/03/mobile-apps.aspx. A Google search can also be done using "PsychINFO mobile."

## PROFESSIONAL ASSOCIATION SITES

American Nurses Association publishes books and pamphlets that may help in finding instruments. Note the URL site for one such publication is http://nursingworld.org (retrieved August 11, 2012). Other specialized, advanced practice nursing sites may have clues to instrument information. For example, check the sites for the American Academy of Nurse Practitioners, the American Academy of Clinical Nurse Anesthetists, National League of Nursing, American Nephrology Nurses, Emergency Nurses Associations, or others. If an APN is part of a special professional association, encourage the website manager to include dissertations or articles of members who may have used or developed instruments.

The Sigma Theta Tau International Honor Society of Nursing Virginia Henderson Library may be another source of information for instruments. The website describes their evidence-based practice publication at http://www.nursinglibrary.org/vhl (retrieved August 11, 2012).

Many professional health and medicine associations now provide measurement tools on their sites. A well-respected site is the Institute of Medicine at www.iom.edu with lists of reports, projects, and topics. When looking through the lists, abstracts of some of the projects describe measurement tools that might be available for use.

The Medical Library Association offered the course, Measure for Measure: Locating Information on Health Measurement Tools, developed and taught by Ester Saghafi, MEd, MLS, and Rebecca Abromitis, MLS, from the Health Sciences Library System of the University of Pittsburgh. This course was taught at the annual meeting in Chicago, IL, in May 2008. The information provided by the librarians was thorough and is highly recommended for review. This course is neither currently offered nor is the syllabus available. However, the authors are developing a library guide for finding measures with content from the course. This guide will be published on the university library's website and may be live by the publication of this book. The reader may check the website for the library at http://www.hsls.pitt.edu/about/libraries/falk.

## CORPORATE WEBSITES

The Health Measurement Research Group has some standard instruments with some free and others for purchase. The Health Measurement Research Group is a collaborative program of research for evaluating health-related quality of life. The URL for the group is http://www.healthmeasurement.org/Measures.html (retrieved August 12, 2012). For example, a copy of the Minnesota Living with Heart Failure Questionnaire is available free along with scoring information. Remember, if this questionnaire is being used and reported in a publication, the reader needs to request permission to use and publish.

ProQolid is a patient-reported outcome and quality of life instruments database. Go to URL http://qolid.org (retrieved August 11, 2012) to learn about this database. Two access points are available on this website. A free access section shows an alphabetical list of instruments available and listed also by author's name, by targeted population, and by pathology/disease. There is a member charge to subscribe and is priced in euros because of its Lyon, France, origin. There is an online payment option.

Survey Monkey is a site that helps you develop your own survey and lists other programs available to help do your surveys. Go to URL http://www.survey monkey.com (retrieved August 11, 2012).

The Rand Corporation publishes, on its website, many summaries of research projects and reports with a special section on health instruments. Check Rand Health Surveys and Tools at www.rand.org/health/surveys_tools.html. Note that the space between "surveys" and "tools" in the URL has an underline.

## GOVERNMENT SITES

Some government agencies have sections on their sites that contain useful instruments. Instruments developed by government agencies may be found in the government documents departments of university, and law libraries. Tax dollars pay for these agencies' work, are free to use, and sites can be searched using terms: surveys, question-naires, measures, tools, and instruments. Check with the librarians to help find the publications cited. Please note the following (all retrieved August 11, 2012):

Agency for Healthcare Research and Quality (AHRQ): Tools and Resources for Better Health Care (http://www.ahrq.gov/qual/tools/toolsria.htm).

Health Resources and Services Administration (HRSA) U.S. Department of Health and Human Services: The HRSA has a wealth of information by searching its website http://www.ahrq.gov with terms, measures, tools, and instruments. If you go specifically to http://www.ahrq.gov/qual/tools/toolsria.htm, the reader may click on "clinical quality measures" and find information on screening for various conditions. It is a great website to explore.

National Guideline Clearinghouse published by the Agency for Healthcare Research and Quality of the U.S. Department of Health and Human Services: The site, http://www.guideline.gov, has a section on measures and tools relevant to specific health problems.

National Technical Information Service http://www.ntis.gov/search/index.aspx Springfield, Virginia, Department of Commerce: This database is free and contains many reports of government-supported research. Searching the site using the term "health surveys" in the database yielded 153 references. Using the term "health question-naires" provided 53 references. This database is a stretch for finding a copy of an instrument but is worthwhile to check.

## SUMMARY

In locating instruments, a search on Google occasionally may retrieve a copy of an instrument or scale. Librarians refer to such searches as a "quick" and "dirty" way of finding what is needed. Searching through the print books suggested is a good starting point for standard instruments. Many of the books cited in the text and in the bibliography should be readily available in major university libraries.

The databases suggested starting with CINAHL, HaPI, PubMed, Cochrane Databases, PsychINFO, and ERIC may all need to be searched methodically to find articles on validity and reliability. It is hoped that with the suggested terms given in this chapter, the APN may practice basic search strategies and use the techniques in other databases to construct meaningful strategies. Luckily, some authors include the instrument in the article. If a dissertation contains an instrument, the document may be ordered online or through library service.

In using the Internet Resources section, take time to look at the university library websites to supplement the information in this chapter. It is worthwhile looking at these for more step-by-step approaches that are not covered here. And finally, medical librarians are usually good resources to help find measurement instruments.

### Answers to Chapter Discussion Questions

1. The two best databases to start searching are CINAHL and HaPI. In CINAHL, when doing a search use the "Select Field" drop down menu, choose "instrumentation" from the list. Type in the term, "diabetes" in the box to left of instrumentation. Using the limiters on the left of the screen, under "Publication Type," scroll down to choose both "questionnaire/scale" and "research instrument." Other limiters were English and references published within the last 6 years. In CINAHL, the strategy retrieved, Kiblinger, L. (2007) Tool chest. Diabetes Risk/Improvement Scale, *Diabetes Educator,* 33 (4), 628,630,632 passim. In the HaPI database, using the strategy of entering diabetes in the box and selecting field "measure," then "and-ing" nursing in all text fields, many references were retrieved. Limits included 2000–2012 publication years. One of the references retrieved was Lin, C., et al. (2008). Diabetes Self-Management Instrument, *Research in Nursing & Health, 31, 370–380.* EBSCO and some university websites have videos on their own players or on YouTube that explain how to use the CINAHL database.

2. To find details about the MMPI, check MMYB as well as test critiques. If in a library, check the other books in the reference collection around the MMYB to become familiar with these standard sources. This reference is also online in many libraries. Details on the MMYB are found in this chapter under Standard books. To check what local library has these books, the online catalog may be found by a Google search of the name of the university or public library. A good source to check is the *WorldCat* at the URL www.worldcat.org. This amazing site provides information on the libraries that own the book in the area where the reader lives. For example, search the *WorldCat* for *Handbook of Disease Burdens and Quality of Life Measures;* scrolling down shows several locations in the state. *WorldCat* also has a mobile app for a fee.

3. In the Suggested Reading—University Library Websites section, check different sites to see which ones have information on responsible use of tests. Dan Chaney, Librarian, at Oklahoma State University has succinct descriptions, "Suggestions for Getting a Copy of That Test or Measurement." Also, listed are three points about "Responsible Use of Tests and Measures." URL for this work is in the Bibliography at the end of this chapter. Miriam Joseph, Librarian at Saint Louis University, has created a lengthy list of "Test-Related Companies." The URL for this information is in the Bibliography at the end of this chapter. Also, look at the tab on "Access and Use Issues." Permission was granted to use her link for this chapter, as was the work by Dan Chaney. Article references often have the author's e-mail address, which can be used to find out about using the test/instrument described. Many instruments cannot be used except by social workers or psychology professionals or by special training. In the HaPI database is a primary source article entitled "Worst Pain Intensity Scale," in *Oncology Nursing Forum*, 38 (1), 33–42 by M. J. Dodd. Checking PubMed for a recent article by M. J. Dodd, the email address was listed because of being the first author. To find out about the scale and how it is used, email the author. Researchers are flattered that their work may be used and duplicated with their knowledge. The assumption might be made that this author would explain use and could give permission and training for use of the instrument.

4. For information on physician–nurse professional collaboration, the PsychINFO, CINAHL, HaPI, and PubMed Handheld are all available on mobile/handheld devices. The PsychINFO app is available from EBSCOHost and the American Psychological Association site. CINAHL and HaPI are also available through EBSCOHost. PubMed Handheld is available from the National Library of Medicine. A search of PsychINFO provides many references on nurse–physician professional collaboration using keywords, such as "practice environment, nurse physician communication, job satisfaction, nursing role effectiveness model, teamwork, and interprofessional education." The CINAHL database keywords for searching might be "work environment, nurse–physician relations, collaboration, occupational stress, professional autonomy, questionnaires, psychological tests, and theoretical nursing models." In PubMed, Medical Subject Headings to use are "attitude of health personnel, physician–nurse relations, cooperative behavior, questionnaires, medical staff, hospital, and nursing staff, hospital."

5. The most promising resources for the reader are subjective. However, a list of databases most promising would be CINAHL, PubMed, HaPI, PsychINFO, and ERIC. All university websites listed at the end of this chapter are relevant. For books, library catalogs usually may be checked online, and university libraries assign passwords to students and faculty for access to electronic books.

## WEB LINKS

For bibliographic databases, most charge a fee and are accessed via universities, hospitals, or other places of employment. Following are some free access databases:

National Library of Medicine's Medline ■ http://Pubmed.gov

Education Resources Information Center ■ www.ERIC.ed.gov

Cochrane Collaboration for evidence-based medicine free summaries ■ www.Cochrane.org

Search through Google often retrieves references from Medline and other databases. ■ http://google.com

Provides some full text articles ■ http://scholar.google.com

American Psychological Association's site on tests provides ethics research information and proper use of psychological tests ■ http://www.apa.org/science/programs/testing.html

Educational Testing Service (ETS) database with descriptions of 25,000 tests and research instruments. ■ http://www.ets.org

Please use the additional websites provided at the end of this chapter on Suggested Reading—University Library Websites.

MMYB has free Test Reviews Online at URL: http://buros.unl.edu for all publications by the Buros Institute, go http://buros.org

To check a local library collection, consider using www.WorldCat.org. An added feature when using the mobile app, WorldCat Mobile, allows typing in the zip code to locate the nearest library. In conjunction with WorldCat Mobile, the app RedLaser (purchase from iTunes) uses the iPhone camera to scan the ISBN to check on books in bookstores and to discover the books in library locations. Libraries are beginning to develop their own handheld apps so that users may access their catalogs.

## BIBLIOGRAPHY WITH SUGGESTED BOOKS AND UNIVERSITY WEBSITES

### BOOKS

Aday, L., & Cornelius, L. J. (2006). *Designing and conducting health surveys* (3rd ed.). San Francisco, CA: Jossey-Bass.

American Psychiatric Association. (2000) *Handbook of psychiatric measures.* Washington, DC: Author.

Bowling, A. (2001). *Measuring disease: A review of disease-specific quality of life measurement scales.* Philadelphia, PA: Open University Press.

Bowling, A. (2005). *Measuring health: A review of quality of life measurement scales.* New York, NY: Oxford University Press.

Clayton, G. M. (1989). *Instruments for use in nursing education research.* New York, NY: National League for Nursing, pub. No 15–2248.

Dana, R. H. (2005). *Multicultural assessment: Principles, applications, and examples.* Mahwah, NJ: Lawrence Erlbaum Associates.

*Directory of Unpublished Experimental Mental Measures* published by the American Psychological Association since 1970 is edited by B. A. Goldman & D. F. Mitchell. Washington, DC: American Psychological Association, latest volume published 2007.

Frank-Stromborg, M. (2004). *Instruments for clinical health-care research.* Boston, MA: Jones and Bartlett.

*Handbook of Disease Burdens and Quality of Life Measures.* (2010). In V. R. Preedy & R. R. Watson (Eds.). Vol. 6. New York, NY: Springer. [Note: This is a $3,000.00 set, available in medical and university libraries, some have the electronic version. See website under Suggested Reading—Internet Resources]

Kane, R. L., & Radosevich, D. M. (2011). *Conducting health outcomes research.* Sudbury, MA: Jones and Barlett Learning.

Kleinpell, R. M. (2001). *Outcome assessment in advanced practice nursing* (3rd edition in press 2012). New York, NY: Springer Publishing.

Lewis, C. B. (1997). *The functional tool box: Clinical measures of functional outcomes* (Vol. 2). McClean, VA: Learn. Tools to aid in measuring patient outcomes in rehabilitation interventions. Each tool has simplified instructions with population, descriptions, completion time, interpretation, reliability, validity, and complete references. (2000 edition out of print)

McDowell, I. (2006) *Measuring Health: a guide to rating scales and questionnaires* (3rd ed.). New York, NY: Oxford University Press.

*Measurement of nursing outcomes.* (2nd ed.) (3 vols.) [Vol. 1: Waltz, C.F., & Jenkins, L. (Eds.). (2001). *Measuring nursing performance: Practice, education and research;* Vol. 2: Strickland, O. L., & Dilorio, C. (Eds.). (2003). *Client outcomes and quality of care;* Vol. 3: Strickland, O. L., & Dilorio, C. (Eds.). (2003). *Self-care and coping*]. New York, NY: Springer Publishing.

*Mental Measurements Yearbook.* (2007). (17th ed.). (published every two years). In L. L. Murphy, R. A. Spies, & B. S. Plake. Lincoln, NE: Buros Institute of Mental Measurements.

Miller, D. C., & Salkind, N. J. (2002). *Handbook of research design and social measurement* (6th ed.). Newbury Park, CA: Sage.

Peterson, K. W., Travis, J. W., Dewey, J. E., Framer, E. M., Foerster, J. J. & Hyner, G. C. (Eds.). (1999). *SPM handbook of health assessment tools.* Pittsburgh, PA: Society of Prospective Medicine, & Irving, Texas: Institute for Health and Productivity Management (published jointly). [This book discusses and lists various types of scales; also has addresses and validity/reliability remarks about them; contains life-style tools.]

Redman, B. K. (2003). *Measurement tools in patient education.* New York, NY: Springer Publishing.

Schutte, N. S., & Malouff, J. M. (1999). *Sourcebook of adult assessment strategies.* New York, NY: Plenum.

Shelton, P. J. (2000). *Measuring and improving patient satisfaction.* Gaithersburg, VA: Aspen [Appendices include: Appendix A – Focus Group Moderator's Guide; Appendix B – Patient Satisfaction Survey Instrument; Appendix C – Principles of Continuous Quality Improvement: Presentation slides.]

Streiner, D. L., & Norman, G. R. (2008). *Health measurement scales: A practical guide to their development and use.* USA: Oxford University Press. [Note Appendix B: Where to find tests. This appendix contains 16 categories including general, on-line sources, health and clinical conditions, quality of life and nursing and patient education.]

*Test critiques.* (1984-present). Kansas City, Missouri, Test Corporation of America, 10 vols. [This multivolume set is the companion to *Tests* and includes reliability and validity information. For a complete description of *Test Critiques*, see the American Psychological Association's website at http://www.apa.org/science/testing.html]

*Tests: A comprehensive reference for assessments in psychology, education and business.* (2008). (6th ed.). T. Maddox Pro-Ed. (Ed.), Texas. [Includes descriptions of tests, purpose of tests, cost, and availability. Does not contain evaluative critiques of data on reliability and validity.]

*Tests in Print* (TIP). (2011). (8th ed.). Lincoln, NE: Buros Institute of Mental Measurement. [Murphy, L. L., Geisinger, K. F., Carlson, J. F. & Spies, R. A. (Eds.)].

Thompson, C. (1989). *Instruments of psychiatric research.* Somerset, NJ: John Wiley. – this is a $595 book)

Waltz, C. F., Strickland, O. L., & Lenz, E. R. (2010). *Measurement in nursing and health research.* (4th ed.). New York, NY: Springer Publishing.

## SUGGESTED READING—INTERNET RESOURCES

American Psychological Association (APA) has an excellent section on their home page entitled: *Frequently Asked Questions (FAQ) on Psychological Tests* at http://www.apa.org/science/testing.html

*Educational Testing Service (ETS)* Test collection database http://www.ets.org/testcoll/index.html contains descriptions of over 10,000 tests and research instruments with information indicating either a person or institution to contact or a journal citation for an article describing or including the test.

## SUGGESTED READING—UNIVERSITY LIBRARY WEBSITES

Consider checking your favorite local university website in starting your search for instruments. Many librarians have created extensive, detailed guides to finding instruments because this is a common question asked of librarians. Below is a list of some good sites, but by no means is this an exhaustive list. These may be starting points, and a Google search may retrieve many other university sites. *These sites were all active when accessed/retrieved August 9, 2012.* The year given after the titles on the sites refers to the last update of the page. If websites have gone inactive by the time you access them, try to do a Google search of the university library.

Bardeen, A. (2011). *Finding tests, surveys and measurements.* Chapel Hill, NC: University of North Carolina, Chapel Hill. URL is http://www.lib.unc.edu/subjectguides/FindingTests/

Chaney, D. (2011). *Guide to finding psychological tests and measurements.* Stillwater, OK: Oklahoma State University. URL is http://www.library.okstate.edu/hss/chaney/psychology/test.htm or http://info.library.okstate.edu/tests

Hough, H. (2012*) Tests and measures in the social sciences*: Tests available in compilation volumes. Arlington, TX: University of Texas at Arlington. URL is http://uta.edu/helen/test&meas/testmainframe.htm. This guide is a good supplement to the material in this chapter. The library websites linked on this library guide is more comprehensive than the list provided here.

Joseph, M. (2012). *Instrumentation: Tests and measures.* St. Louis, Missouri: Saint Louis University. URL is http://libguides.slu.edu/tests. This website has an excellent list of test-related companies for requesting copies and permission to use. The author is in the process of updating the information. The site is not specifically for nurses but has valuable information for researchers.

Rich, J. (2012). *Measurement tools/reseach instruments.* URL: http://libguides.hsl.washington.edu/measure Seattle, Washington: University of Washington.

San Diego State University Library has a website that has a section *SDSU Test Finder.* It was developed by librarian M. Stover and may be accessed at http://www-rohan.sdsu.edu/~mstover/tests. On this site, you will find an index of complete tests and instruments found in scholarly journal articles.

Sathrum, R. (2011). *Finding psychological tests and measures.* Arcata, CA; Humboldt State University. http://library.humboldt.edu/infoservices/psychedtests.htm

Teno, J. M., Okun, S. N., Casey, V., & Welch, L. C. (2001). *Toolkit of instruments to measure end of life care resource guide* (TIME). *Resource guide: Achieving quality of care at life's end.* URL: http://www.chcr.brown.edu/pcoc/resourceguide/resourceguide.pdf. This text, which includes many appendices with tools, is considered free to use but not to publish.

University of Maryland Libraries *Tests and measurements guide.* (2011). URL: http://www.lib.umd.edu/guides/tests.html [This guide is designed to serve as a tool to help one get information about published and unpublished educational, psychological, and vocational tests and measurements. This site has a step-by-step description of the process of finding tests.]

University of Michigan Taubman Medical Library. (2012). *Finding tests and measurement instruments.* URL: http://guides.lib.umich.edu/tests [Note: This site provides a reference to a textbook on responsible test use.]

University of Pennsylvania. *Tests and measurements—Research guide.* URL: http://gethelp.library.upenn.edu/guides/educ/tests.html [Note: Includes good section on getting tests.]

# Chapter 6: Measuring Outcomes in Cardiovascular Advanced Practice Nursing

ANNA GAWLINSKI, KATHY MCCLOY, VIRGINIA ERICKSON, TAMARA HARRISON CHAKER, ELIZABETH VANDENBOGAART, JULIE CREASER, NANCY LIVINGSTON, AND DARLENE ROURKE

## Chapter Objectives

1. Identify outcomes of concern to advanced practice nurses (APNs) and compare these to the nurse-sensitive outcomes currently being measured in your institution and your patient population.
2. Discuss advantages and disadvantages of each of the methodologies that are used for outcomes measurement projects (i.e., research, research utilization, evidence-based practice, and quality improvement frameworks).
3. Analyze the relative effectiveness of interventions that have been shown to decrease medication discrepancies.
4. Discuss the role of the APN in reducing medication discrepancies in patients with cardiovascular disease, as well as other vulnerable patient populations.

## Chapter Discussion Questions

1. Discuss the definition of the medication reconciliation process described in the chapter. Compare this definition to the inventions implemented by the APNs in the exemplar medication reconciliation outcomes measurement project.
2. Compare and contrast examples of outcomes of concern to APNs listed in Exhibit 6.1 with nurse-sensitive outcomes currently being measured in your institution and your patient population.
3. Identify two to three clinical issues and related outcomes in your practice. Discuss which research designs or other frameworks would be most appropriate to use in an outcomes measurement project. Why?
4. Discuss the relative effectiveness of interventions described in the literature to decrease medication discrepancies. Design a study to address the medication discrepancy issue for your patient population and discuss why you chose that design.
5. Discuss why the heart failure population is more vulnerable to medication discrepancies. Compare and contrast these reasons to your own patient population.

National health care policymakers and health care professionals have increasingly advocated for the measurement and monitoring of patient safety, quality improvement, and health care outcomes. The development and implementation of national practice guidelines that are based on the best available research have provided clinicians with interventions that can improve patients' outcomes (Dykes, 2003; Titler, 2004). Yet these practice guidelines are not consistently used, and practices vary from clinician to clinician and from institution to institution, resulting in poor outcomes for patients (Centers for Medicare & Medicaid Services, 2012; Institute of Medicine, 2001; McGlynn et al., 2003; Titler, 2008; Ward et al., 2006).

This emphasis on evidence-based practice (EBP) has resulted in increased focus and incentives for those institutions and providers that perform well on indicators of safety and quality, with measurable outcomes. For example, The Joint Commission (TJC) has set standards for performance measurement that include measures of use of research-based therapies, such as aspirin, beta-blockers, and statins, in patients posthospitalization for myocardial infarction (TJC, 2011).

Cardiovascular disease in particular lends itself to measurement of such quality indicators and outcomes. Cardiovascular disease is the leading cause of mortality and health care cost for men and women in the United States (Kosiborod & Spertus, 2009). These statistics along with the high acuity and chronicity of cardiovascular disease, and the availability of published national guidelines outlining "best practices," contribute to the pressing need for outcomes measurement in the field of cardiovascular nursing (Deaton, 2001; Paul, 2000).

Although a great deal of effort has been devoted to developing EBP guidelines for cardiovascular disease, more data are needed to demonstrate how these guidelines can be translated into practice and what their subsequent effect is on outcomes in everyday clinical settings. Cardiovascular advanced practice nurses (APNs) are in a key position to use their expert knowledge of research-based practices and outcome measurement to generate data that demonstrate successful translation of these guidelines into the clinical setting.

The purpose of this chapter is to provide an overview of outcome measurement in advanced practice nursing, discuss methodologies that can be used for outcome measurement, and describe the role of the cardiovascular APN in outcome measurement. An outcome measurement project will be presented to demonstrate the unique role of the APN in using an EBP approach to implement changes that result in positive measurable outcomes. The contributors' aim is to present an exemplar of an outcomes project and share processes that can be replicated to reduce variations in practice and improve outcomes in cardiovascular patients.

## CLINICAL OUTCOMES

Clinical and patient outcomes are defined as the end results of care that can be attributed to the health care services provided (treatments, interventions, and care; Oermann, & Floyd, 2002; Urden, 1999). Outcomes are the consequences of treatment or interventions (Oermann & Floyd, 2002; Urden, 1999). They can be used to characterize the results (effect) of an intervention, treatment, or provider (cause). Clinical outcomes demonstrate the value and effectiveness of care and can be assessed for individuals, populations, and organizations (Hughes, 2008).

Outcomes are often quantified or measured through the use of indicators, which are referred to as metrics. Outcome indicators or metrics provide estimates that reflect the degree to which patients are affected by their care (Stanik-Hutt, 2012). Indicators must be valid and reliable measures that are related to the outcome of interest. For example, to measure the adequacy of cholesterol management (a clinical outcome) in a patient with coronary artery disease, indicators of this outcome would include levels of various components of a patient's blood lipid panel such as the total cholesterol, the low density lipoprotein (LDL), and the high density lipoprotein (HDL). Indicators provide a picture of the progress toward achievement of the outcome, whereas outcomes can be considered predictors of end-performance (Parse, 2006).

Indicators or metrics that are reported to agencies outside the internal organization are referred to as performance measures (Dennison & Hughes, 2009). Over the past two decades, a wide array of standardized health care performance measures have been developed, and a large number of these have been endorsed by the National Quality Forum (NQF). The NQF is a private, not-for-profit membership organization whose purpose is to develop a national strategy for health care quality measurement and reporting. The NQF currently develops, reviews, and measures performance standards for health care, and promotes national standardization of these quality performance measures (Stanik-Hutt, 2012).

A substantial growth has occurred in the number of entities using health care performance measures for a variety of purposes. For example, quality and efficiency performance measures are now embedded throughout the U.S. health care system. The purposes for their widespread use are: (1) quality improvement, (2) public reporting, (3) regulation (e.g., accreditation, certification, credentialing, and licensure), and (4) payment applications (e.g., financial incentives, tiered payment; Damberg et al., 2012).

Performance measures are often benchmarked or compared with other institutions. Benchmarking is a process to identify best practices, which, when implemented, can lead to superior performance (DesHarnais, 2013). It is the use of external comparisons to understand how one is doing compared to one's peers and/or one's competitors (practitioners or institutions). Data of performance measures are compared between health care systems or within a single health care system (DesHarnais, 2013). These comparisons allow the APN to identify areas of strengths and weaknesses in relation to best practice.

## NURSING OUTCOMES

The care of patients often requires the expertise of several health care professionals. When many health care providers interact with patients and contribute to their care, it may be difficult to attribute successful clinical patient outcomes to only one provider or treatment. Thus, identifying outcomes that can be attributed only to nursing care can be a challenge, because attribution requires a high level of confidence that the outcome is a direct result of that provider's care (Dennison & Hughes, 2009).

For example, a heart failure (HF) patient who was discharged and begins to experience symptoms of increasing dyspnea and weight gain at home, may be treated by several health care providers (RN, APN, and registered dietitian [RD], etc.). At hospital discharge, the RN provided the patient with detailed discharge instructions regarding the important aspects of HF management, including specific instructions regarding symptoms to immediately report to their health care provider (i.e., dyspnea and/or weight gain, 2 pounds in 24 hours or 5 pounds in 4 days). The RD counseled the patient in-hospital and reviewed the recommended guidelines for a low-sodium diet, and provided instructions about reading labels and interpreting sodium content.

The cardiovascular APN was notified of the new onset of the patient's symptoms and requested the patient to schedule a clinic appointment. During the clinic appointment, the APN assesses for contributing factors, such physiologic changes in cardiac function, medication nonadherence issues, and dietary indiscretion. Based on the assessment, the APN orders additional diagnostic tests (i.e., brain natriuretic peptide, echocardiogram), reinforces education regarding the need for the patient to adjust diuretic therapy based on daily weight, and reinforces specifics about medication and dietary regimens. A referral is also made to the RD. The RD reviews the recommended low-sodium diet and helps the patient make better food selections. Upon follow up, when the patient reports less dyspnea and decreased weight, the question arises as to which health care professional was responsible for the achievement of these positive outcomes. Was it the RN, the APN, or the RD, or the whole team (Stanik-Hutt, 2012)?

Attempts to measure outcomes that can be attributed to nursing care have resulted in a definition of nurse-sensitive outcomes. Nurse-sensitive outcomes are defined as outcomes that are sensitive enough to measure the effect of nursing practice (Joseph, 2007). They represent the impact of nursing interventions and describe the effect of what nurses do in response to the patient's condition. Several nursing care outcomes that reflect nursing performance have been selected for national reporting. These nursing care outcomes include measures of patient-centered outcomes such as mortality among surgical inpatients with treatable serious complications, prevalence of pressure ulcers, falls (with and without injury), use of restraints, and hospital-acquired infections such as catheter-related urinary tract infections, central line catheter-associated blood stream infections, and ventilator-associated pneumonias. Additional measures include nursing-centered intervention processes, such as smoking cessation counseling, and system-centered structures and processes such as nursing staff skill mix and nursing care hours per patient day (Kurtzman & Corrigan, 2007; Stanik-Hutt, 2012).

Researchers at the University of Iowa have provided leadership in the area of nurse-sensitive outcomes by creating the nursing interventions classification (NIC) and nursing outcomes classification (NOC) that link nursing interventions to diagnoses and outcomes. This research team has contributed to identifying outcomes and related measures at the individual patient, family, and community levels, which can be used to evaluate nursing care across the patient care continuum. Individual patient outcome data can be aggregated in a number of ways to assess nursing care effectiveness within an organization and across various settings (Moorhead, Johnson, Mass, & Swanson, 2012). This research team is disseminating and publishing their work to facilitate more consistent documentation of nursing interventions and outcomes.

## CLASSIFICATION OF OUTCOMES

Historically, the classification of health care outcomes used medical definitions known as the "five Ds": death, disease, disability, discomfort, and dissatisfaction (Lohr, 1988; Nolan & Mock, 2000; Urden, 1999). But classification of outcomes varies. They can be categorized as generic and broad-based outcomes that pertain to all patients and health care providers (i.e., quality of care, access, cost, patients' satisfaction and utilization of service).

Outcomes have also been categorized in other ways, such as patient/care related, system related, practitioner or performance related, and cost/financial related (Kleinpell-Nowell & Weiner, 1999). Other categories of outcomes are clinical, psychological, functional, and satisfaction related (Urden, 1999).

## OUTCOME MEASURES USED IN ADVANCED PRACTICE NURSING

APNs are often faced with the dilemma of what constitutes an outcome and which outcomes should be measured. The outcomes that best reflect clinical practice and the goals of treatment are the most meaningful and most amenable to measurement (Gawlinski, 2007; Kleinpell & Gawlinski, 2005). Several websites (Table 6.1) and publications provide APNs with excellent resources on selected health outcome information,

### Table 6.1 *Selected Health Outcome Information Websites*

| Organization | Website |
| --- | --- |
| Academy for Healthcare Research and Quality | http://www.ahrq.gov/clinic/outcomix.htm |
| American Nurses' Association: The National Database of Nursing Quality Indicators | http://www.nursingworld. org/MainMenuCategories/ ThePracticeofProfessionalNursing/ PatientSafetyQuality/Research-Measurement/ The-National-Database.aspx |
| Centers for Medicare & Medicaid Services | http://www.hce.org |
| IHI: Transforming Care at the Bedside | http://www.ihi.org/IHI/ Programs/StrategicInitiatives/ TransformingCareAtTheBedside.htm?TabId=3 |
| Institute for Healthcare Improvement | http://www.ihi.org |
| Institute of Medicine of the National Academies | http://www.iom.edu/?id=18795 |
| The Joint Commission on Accreditation of Healthcare Organizations | http://www.jointcommission.org |
| National Committee for Quality Assurance | http://www.ncqa.org |
| National Patient Safety Foundation | http://www.npsf.org |
| Nursing Quality Forum | http://www.qualityforum.org/Home.aspx |
| Registered Nurses Association of Ontario—"Implementation of Clinical Practice Guidelines" Toolkit | http://rnao.ca/sites/rnao-ca/files/BPG_Toolkit.pdf |
| University of Alberta—"Evidence-Based Medicine Toolkit" | http://www.ebm.med.ualberta.ca/ebm.html |
| University of Iowa College of Nursing | http://www.nursing.uiowa.edu/cncce/nursing-outcomes-classification-overview |
| U.S. Department of Health and Human Services—Hospital Compare | http://www.hospitalcompare.hhs.gov |

and specific outcome measures and instruments (Kleinpell, 2003, 2007; Kleinpell-Nowell & Weiner, 1999; Moorhead et al., 2012). For example, Fulton and Baldwin (2004) published an annotated bibliography reflecting clinical nurse specialist practice and outcomes. Urden (1999) published a list of a broad spectrum of outcomes using clinical, physiological, psychological, functional, fiscal, and satisfaction categories. Kleinpell (2003) provided a list of sources for identifying outcome measures and outcome instruments for analyzing the impact of APN care. Exhibit 6.1 provides a listing of outcome measures that can be used by APNs based on these published literature reviews.

### Exhibit 6.1  *Outcomes for Advanced Practice Nursing*

**Clinical (Care-Related) Outcomes**

Mortality

Morbidity

  Infection: nosocomial, urinary tract infection, ventilator or catheter related

  Hand hygiene compliance rates

  Medical conditions such as heart failure

  Loss of function

  Physiological response

   Blood pressure, heart rate

   Temperature

   Lung sounds

   Hemodynamic pressures

   Weight and weight management

   Serum/urine level of glucose

   Wound healing, skin integrity

  Symptom management

   Pain

   Fatigue

   Nausea, vomiting

  Constipation

*(continued)*

## Exhibit 6.1 *continued*

Nutritional status/management

Sleep maintenance

Restraint use

Smoking cessation

Low birth weight, preterm infants

Rates of adherence to best practices

**Psychosocial Outcomes**

Coping, stress management

Mentation

Return to work

Role functioning

Family functioning/coping

Anxiety

Depression

Sexual functioning

Caregiver strain/burden

Knowledge: medications, diet, treatment regime, motor skills, condition specific

Staff nurse knowledge

**Functional Outcomes**

Quality of life

Self-care: bathing, eating, dressing self, administration of nonparenteral medication

Mobility

Communication

Return to

   Work

   School

   Normal activity/social interaction

Symptom control

*(continued)*

**Exhibit 6.1** *Outcomes for Advanced Practice Nursing* *(continued)*

| |
|---|
| **Fiscal Outcomes** |
|   Length of stay |
|   Readmission rates to hospital, home care, other services |
|   Emergency department visits |
|   Health care services utilization |
|   Cost per episode of care |
|   Resource utilization: ancillary services, community/other services |
|   Staff nurse retention rates |
| **Satisfaction** |
|   Consumer |
|     Care provided |
|     Services provided |
|     Care provider |
|   Family |
|     Care provided to family member |
|     Services provided/available |
|   Payor |
|   Provider |

*Source*: Adapted from Urden (1999) and Kleinpell-Nowell and Weiner (1999).

APNs are at the forefront of improving care through outcomes measurement. They serve as critical members of the health care team. Because of their key role in the health care system, APNs frequently lead outcomes measurement and quality improvement initiatives. By virtue of their educational preparation, clinical knowledge, and critical thinking skills, APNs have an essential role in evaluating outcomes for improvement efforts. For these reasons, as well as the APNs' consistent presence with patients and their patient advocacy role, APNs frequently possess an integrated, holistic, and broader view of what constitutes important outcomes. Using this view, APNs not only measure traditional physiologic outcomes, but also include outcomes related to psychosocial, functional, behavioral, symptoms, quality of life (QOL), knowledge, and satisfaction. Because a change in one outcome may influence changes in another outcome, APNs are interested in the interaction and relationship of these outcomes. For example, exacerbation of a patient's symptoms can interfere with a patient's physiologic, psychosocial, functional status, and the QOL. APNs are especially interested in the management and control of symptoms.

In APN practice, examples of physiologic outcomes of concern may include pulse, blood pressure, lipid levels, blood glucose levels, weight, and other physiologic parameters. Psychosocial outcomes of concern may include the patient's mood, attitudes, and abilities to interact with others. For functional outcomes, a patient's mobility, physical independence, and ability to participate in desired activities of daily living would be considered important. Behavioral outcomes of concern may include adequacy of coping with health care needs or a patient's ability to follow (adhere) to recommended care. Symptoms, such as pain, dyspnea, and fatigue would require an assessment and evaluation independent from the diseases that cause them. QOL is another natural outcome of interest for APNs. QOL is defined as a patient's general perception of his or her physical and mental well-being that can be affected by many factors including disease and injury, stress and emotions, symptom control and functional status, as well as others. Finally, the patient's knowledge level may be an important outcome to APNs. This includes the individual's understanding of health-related information. Although patient satisfaction is a quality indicator for all health care providers, patient satisfaction with the care, communication, and compassion provided by the APN would be particularly important feedback for the individual practitioner (Stanik-Hutt, 2012).

Outcomes specific to the role of the APN are also of interest. These types of role-based outcomes are frequently related to the health care system and to cost. They may include clinic wait times, hospital length of stay, bed occupancy rate, timely discharge, and cost per adjusted discharge, and so forth.

Generally, outcome measures in the cardiac population have focused on phenomena such as the effect of an aggressive cholesterol management program implemented by an APN, the effect of applying EBPs to manage HF, the effect of APN practice on management of postoperative complications, interventions to promote QOL, and evaluation of a spectrum of physiological responses to APN interventions (e.g., blood pressure, heart rate, hemodynamics, urine output, daily weight, nutrition, and symptom control; Meyer & Miers, 2005; Paul, 2000). Sample outcome measures that are of concern in the cardiovascular population are listed in Exhibit 6.2.

**Exhibit 6.2** *Selected Outcomes for the Cardiovascular Population*

**Reduction of Cardiac Risk Factors**

Control of hypertension (blood pressure)

Diabetes control (blood glucose, glucose A1C)

Weight loss

Lipid (cholesterol, high- and low-density lipoproteins, triglycerides)

Frequency of aerobic exercise

Fat intake

Knowledge: medications, diet, treatment regimen, motor skills, condition specific

Risk control

  Chest pain/angina

  Activity level

  Smoking cessation

  Alcohol status

**Acute Myocardial Infarction**

Cardioprotective medication regimen

  Frequency prescribed

  Frequency of reaching target lipid levels

Chest pain

Arrhythmias

Depression

Resource utilization

  Electrocardiograms, blood tests, chest radiographs, etc.

Length of stay

Cost per case

Functional status

See *outcomes for Reduction of Cardiac Risk Factors*

**Heart Failure**

Readmission rates

*(continued)*

## Exhibit 6.2 *continued*

Symptom management

EBPs and medications

   Frequency prescribed

   Compliance with medication regimen

   Daily weight

   Fluid limit

Compliance with low-sodium diet

Functional status

Anxiety

Depression

See *outcomes for reduction of cardiac risk factors*

**After Percutaneous Transluminal Angioplasty/Stent Placement**

Reocclusion rates

Hematoma rates

Bleeding requiring transfusion

Other vascular complications

EBP medications

   Antiplatelet and antilipid therapy

Functional status before and after

Sheath removal techniques and products

See *outcomes for reduction of cardiac risk factors*

**After Coronary Artery Bypass Graft**

Pain management

Sedation

Hemodynamic management

Early extubation

Blood transfusion

Early mobility (fast track)

*(continued)*

**Exhibit 6.2** *Selected Outcomes for the Cardiovascular Population* *(continued)*

| |
|---|
| Infections (sternal, nosocomial pneumonia) |
| Wound healing, skin integrity |
| Cardioprotective meds |
|   Prescribed |
|   Compliance |
| Functional status |
| Quality of life |
| Depression |
| Cognition |

For example, in evaluating the effect of advanced practice nursing in managing patients with HF, important outcomes to be measured may include the following:

- Patients' knowledge of their medications, dietary guidelines, and adjustment of diuretics based on daily weight
- Symptom management
- Functional status before and after therapy
- Patients' perception of QOL
- Resource utilization (diagnostic and laboratory tests, procedures, medications)
- Number of inpatient admissions
- Overall length of stay
- Overall cost per case

## INSTRUMENTS AND APPROACHES TO OUTCOMES MEASUREMENT

The use of valid and reliable measures and instruments is important in an outcome project and contributes to the level of confidence that one can have in the results (Clochesy, 2002). Many valid and reliable instruments can be used to measure common health care outcomes such as QOL and functional status (Clochesy, 2002); such instruments include self-report questionnaires or scales, symptom checklists, visual analog scales, and numeric rating scales (Kleinpell, 2003; Nolan & Mock, 2000).

In general, three major approaches can be used for outcomes measurement: (1) outcomes measurement evaluation, (2) outcomes management, and (3) outcomes research. Outcomes evaluation is the monitoring and/or measuring of the extent to which providers meet the clinical or cost outcome goals of their patients or institutions. Outcomes management is a systematic improvement of outcomes by acting on information gained from outcomes measurement, often using the tools of continuous quality improvement. Outcomes research is a type of controlled, empirical assessment of the effect of a given intervention, product, or technology on patient, cost, or service outcomes (Prevost, 2005; Windle, 2006). The determination of which approach is used is dependent on the outcome of interest, available resources, and feasibility. Within these three major approaches, several methodologies can be used for outcome measurement projects, and are discussed in the following section.

## METHODOLOGIES FOR OUTCOMES MEASUREMENT

There are several methodologies that can be used for outcomes measurement in advanced practice nursing using research, EBP, or quality improvement frameworks. The APN can use any of these methodologies to evaluate the impact of a new intervention on patient, system, and fiscal outcomes. Each of these methodologies has its advantages and disadvantages. There is no single set of research designs or methods that are uniquely appropriate for outcome studies. The design and methods used will depend on the state of knowledge about a particular phenomenon and the resources available to the investigator. The APN will choose among these methodologies depending on the variables under study, the outcome measures under study, the instruments used for measurements, and the feasibility in terms of time and resources (Gawlinski & McCloy, 2006).

This section first reviews the most common research designs used by APNs for outcomes measurement projects (Figure 6.1) and discusses the strengths and weaknesses of each of these methodologies (Table 6.2). A discussion follows that describes other methods for outcomes measurement, such as the research utilization process, EBP models, and quality improvement frameworks.

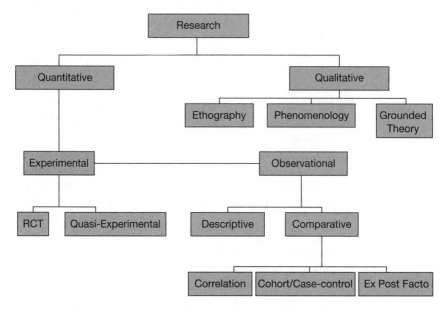

**Figure 6.1** *Research Designs Used by APNs for Outcomes Measurement Projects*

**Table 6.2** *Research Designs Advantages and Disadvantages*

| Design and Description | Advantages | Disadvantages |
|---|---|---|
| Randomized Controlled Trial (RCT)<br><br>Requires:<br>  Randomization<br>  Manipulation of independent variable<br>  Control group<br>Aim: Determine causation | Strong internal validity (confidence that effect was caused by manipulated variable)<br>Most powerful design to test cause-and-effect relationships<br>Provides strong evidence of a cause-and-effect relationship<br>Confounding variables controlled for by randomization<br>Clear measure of efficacy of intervention | Poor external validity (generalizability)<br>Can study only a limited number of variables<br>Complicated and time-consuming<br>Expensive<br>Difficult to maintain integrity of intervention unless done by the research team<br>Ethical and/or logistical issues with randomization<br>May not be able to manipulate variables of interest<br>Does not measure effectiveness of intervention in clinical practice |

*(continued)*

## Table 6.2  *continued*

| | | |
|---|---|---|
| Quasi-Experimental<br>Lacks either:<br>    Randomization or<br>    Control group<br>Aim: Determine causation | More amenable to real-life<br>    clinical situations<br>Practical, inexpensive, feasible<br>Strong external validity<br>    (generalizability)<br>Confounding variables may<br>    be able to be controlled by<br>    statistical means | Weaker internal validity (less<br>    causal attribution; i.e., less<br>    confidence that outcome<br>    was caused by manipulated<br>    variable)<br>Confounding variables may be<br>    unknown or unable to be<br>    controlled for<br>If there is no control group,<br>    alternative explanations<br>    cannot be ruled out |
| Descriptive<br>Complete picture of current<br>    state<br>Aim: Description | Simple<br>Relatively unlimited number of<br>    variables | Does not address relationships<br>    between or among<br>    variables<br>High risk of confounding and<br>    bias |
| Correlation<br>Examine relationship(s) between<br>    and among variables<br>Aim: Comparison/association | Test relationships between and<br>    among variables<br>Can collect a large amount of<br>    data<br>Can predict, as well as describe,<br>    association(s)<br>Relatively simple<br>Can study the relationship<br>    between many variables | Unable to determine cause-<br>    effect relationship<br>Due to complex interactions<br>    of patient characteristics,<br>    tendency for variables to be<br>    related to one another (e.g.,<br>    anxiety, coping, compliance) |
| Case-Control<br>"Case" has **outcome** of<br>    interest, "Control" does not<br>Aim: Retrospective comparison<br>    over time | Can use with relatively small<br>    sample sizes<br>Time saving because design<br>    is retrospective: Research<br>    begins with outcome and<br>    searches for antecedent<br>    variable ("cause"), which has<br>    already occurred | May be difficult to select an<br>    appropriate control group<br>Confounding variables may be<br>    unknown<br>Limited to one outcome<br>Confounding variables and bias<br>    are a concern<br>Need to demonstrate<br>    comparability between cases<br>    and controls |
| Cohort<br>Follow groups of subjects over<br>    time—exposure of interest<br>Aim: Prospective comparison<br>    over time | Can assess several outcomes<br>Temporal sequence is known<br>Can be used to evaluate<br>    effectiveness in other<br>    populations of interventions<br>    found to be efficacious in RCT<br>Stronger than retrospective<br>    comparison | Requires large sample size<br>More resources needed to follow<br>    subjects over time, especially<br>    if lengthy follow up<br>Results may not be identified<br>    for years<br>Danger of attrition/dropout of<br>    subjects<br>Confounding variables may be<br>    unknown |

*(continued)*

**Table 6.2** *Research Designs Advantages and Disadvantages* *(continued)*

| Design and Description | Advantages | Disadvantages |
|---|---|---|
| Ex Post Facto<br>Evaluate effect of a naturally occurring event on subsequent outcome<br>Aim: Identify possible causation | More realistic setting<br>Can be used where a more rigorous experimental approach is not possible<br>Can be a valuable exploratory tool to identify possible cause-and effect relationships for further study<br>May be able to control for some antecedent variables with statistical procedures | May be unable to identify all relevant variables, unknown if the causative factor has been identified<br>Poor internal validity if unknown or unidentified variables provide an alternative explanation of relationship<br>The antecedent variable may be a combination of multiple factors<br>Outcome may result from different antecedents on different occasions |
| Qualitative<br>Develop concepts and themes<br>Use words to explain phenomena<br>Natural setting and context<br>Inductive process (use specific data to elaborate theory and concepts)<br>Aim: Explanation/understanding | Used when phenomena are poorly understood<br>Requires a small number of subjects in comparison to quantitative studies<br>Richness of understanding lived experiences<br>Can complement quantitative research<br>Used to explore complex phenomena | Unable to determine causality or comparison<br>Requires extensive training<br>Time consuming |

## Designs

### Randomized Controlled Trials

The "gold standard" for evaluating the efficacy of drugs and other treatments and interventions in health care is the randomized controlled trial (RCT), or true experiment. RCTs must meet the following three criteria: (1) random assignment to the treatment or control group, (2) manipulation of the independent variable (treatment), and (3) a control or comparison group (Melnyk & Cole, 2011). RCTs are concerned with efficacy, that is, with the question of whether a treatment works under ideal conditions. Since efficacy is most easily determined in a homogeneous study sample, RCTs typically have strict inclusion and exclusion criteria and are conducted under highly controlled conditions (Horn, Gassaway, Pentz, & James, 2010). However, the same homogeneity that allows the researcher to determine the impact of the intervention in a well-defined population also limits the extent to which the findings of an RCT apply to the diverse patients usually seen in clinical practice (Ho, Peterson, & Masoudi, 2008). Thus, these studies have strong internal validity (attribution of causality), but weak external validity (generalizability).

Despite their significant strengths, RCTs also have important limitations. They are typically expensive, time consuming, and designed to answer a single research question or test a small number of hypotheses. Additionally, the intensive follow up necessary for most study protocols often bears little resemblance to follow-up patterns in usual clinical practice (Ho et al., 2008). Finally, the importance of clinical significance versus statistical significance cannot be overlooked. Results that do not reach statistical significance do not exclude the possibility of a clinically important relationship (Purssell & While, 2011; Rosenberg, Bass, & Davidson, 2012). Thus, although rigorous RCTs establish the efficacy of a specific therapy in a limited patient population receiving close follow up, they often leave remaining questions about the impact of therapy in populations not resembling those enrolled in the trial.

### Quasi-Experimental

In some situations, a true experimental design is not feasible because of ethical or logistical constraints. In such circumstances, nonrandomized quasi-experimental studies are often the most appropriate design with which to test cause-and-effect relationships (Ho et al., 2008). Quasi-experimental designs are differentiated from experimental designs by lack of random assignment and/or lack of a control or comparison group. However, they are similar to an experiment in that a variable is manipulated and comparison is made to a group not receiving the intervention (Sullivan-Bolyai & Bova, 2010).

Quasi-experimental designs do not have the rigor created by random assignment and control groups for comparison; rather, comparisons are made with nonequivalent groups or with periodic measurement of the same group (Powers, 2011). Quasi-experimental designs are at risk for threats to internal validity, that is, factors that provide an alternative explanation for associations between the independent and dependent variables, and therefore have limited ability to make cause-and-effect statements (Sullivan-Bolyai & Bova, 2010). Attributing causation is strengthened if the researcher is able to account for alternative explanations of intervention–outcome relationships.

Many nursing outcomes studies use a pretest/intervention/post-test methodology. These research designs can collect data from the same subject over time (within-subjects), or from different participant groups (between-subjects) at the same or different times. A within-subject design, also known as a repeated measure design, tests the same subject at two or more time points. In between-subjects designs, each participant participates in one and only one group.

### Nonexperimental/Observational

Many studies measuring health care outcomes are observational in nature, in contrast to studies that recruit patients in a controlled fashion, as with RCTs. The advantage of an observational methodology is that patient circumstances and outcomes of interventions are studied in a heterogeneous population, which better reflects actual practice environments. The obvious disadvantage is that without the controls imposed by an experimental study, observational results are subject to error and can be misleading or misinterpreted (Carson, 2010). Threats to validity, such as bias, or confounding or random error, can provide an alternative explanation other than the effect of the independent variable for changes in the dependent variable after intervention.

Bias is any factor or influence that produces a systematic distortion or error in the study results (Polit & Beck, 2012). Selection bias is especially problematic in nonrandomized studies, that is, that subjects who elect to participate are systematically different from those who decline participation. Two main factors that can contribute to selection bias are self-selection, when the sample selects itself, and convenience sampling, when individuals are selected because they are easy to obtain (http://gollum.lib.uic.edu/nursing/node/22). For example, in a study of caregivers of terminally ill patients, the researcher may choose a sample of subjects who responded to a recruitment flyer (self-selection) or a sample of caregivers who attend a support group (convenience sample). Either sample is probably not representative of the total population of caregivers of terminally ill patients.

Confounding variables are variables that are associated with both the independent and the dependent variable in such a way that the relationship between the intervention and outcome is actually due to a third (known or unknown) variable, and the nature of the association between the independent and dependent variable is misrepresented (O'Mathúna, Fineout-Overholt, & Johnston, 2011). The effect of a confounding variable can offer an alternative explanation for a relationship between an intervention and an outcome (Carson, 2010). For example, researchers may find an association between consuming a vegetarian diet and lower body mass index (BMI) and draw the conclusion that the diet is the cause of lower BMI. However, this association may be confounded by the fact that vegetarians are perhaps more health conscious in general and exercise more regularly. Thus, exercise may be the true cause of the difference in BMI. The use of multivariate statistical models such as linear or logistic regression may be able to "adjust" for confounding variables in some situations (Carson, 2010).

Random error is essentially nonsystematic bias, that is, the factor or influence that produces error is as likely to influence results in one way as another (Polit & Beck, 2012). Random error is due to variability in the data that occurs purely by chance. Because of random error, one cannot unequivocally state that the results obtained in a study are real rather than arising by chance. The probability that the outcome variable has occurred purely by chance is expressed as the "$p$" value. The most effective way of minimizing random error in a study is to increase the sample size (Akobeng, 2008). The classic example of correcting random error is the coin toss. When tossing a coin, we expect heads to occur 50% of the time. If the coin were tossed 10 times, it is likely that the number of heads–tails would not be 5–5, but may be for example 6–4 or 3–7. However, if the coin were tossed 1,000 times, we would be more likely to approach 50–50 on heads coming up.

## Descriptive

The descriptive research design is the most basic. It simply describes the nature of the phenomenon of interest. Newell and Burnard (2006) identify three ways in which data are gathered for descriptive research: observation of actions, appraisal of records or documents, and results of surveys specifically designed to measure variables of interest. Descriptive research involves observing, describing and documenting events or phenomena and then organizing, tabulating, depicting, and describing the data elements. Descriptive studies also report summary data such as measures of central tendency (mean, median, mode) and measures of dispersion (range and standard deviation). These designs describe what actually exists, determine the frequency with which it occurs, and categorize the information (Sousa, Dreissnack, & Mendes,

2007). Descriptive statistical techniques allow very large amounts of data to be made meaningful to the researcher.

Descriptive data are the foundation of any quantitative study and can serve as a foundation for theory generation or hypothesis testing in a qualitative study (Melnyk & Cole, 2011). The fact that descriptive studies are "simple" and one cannot infer causality from them does not diminish the value of the descriptive study design. An example of an important, purely descriptive research is the decennial U.S. Census, the purpose of which is to accurately and precisely describe the population of the entire country.

### Correlation

Correlation determines whether, and to what degree, a relationship exists between two or more variables. This design is used to determine if changes in one or more variables are related to changes in another variable (Sousa et al., 2007). Correlation can only tell you that two or more phenomena are related, not that a causal relationship exists. The degree of the relationship between variables is expressed as a correlation coefficient. The correlation coefficient indicates the strength of relationship (strong, weak, or none) as well as the direction of the relationship, that is, positive, in which variables move in the same direction, or negative, in which variables move in opposite directions. Correlation coefficients range in value from –1.0 (strongly negative) to +1.0 (strongly positive), with 0 indicating no relationship.

Correlation designs can be either descriptive or predictive. Descriptive correlation simply describes the variables under study and the relationship(s) between and among them. Predictive correlation predicts the amount of variance in one or more variables based on the amount of variance in other variable(s), given that the predictor variable occurs earlier in time (Sousa et al., 2007).

### Case-Control and Cohort

In the case-control study design, "cases" with a disease or condition are identified within a population of patients, and investigators go back a period of time before onset of the disease or condition and assess the presence of potential risk factors or other influences preceding the disease or condition (Ho et al., 2008). For example, Burns et al. (2009) conducted a case-control study to identify risk factors for delirium in patients undergoing elective heart surgery. The "cases" were the 11

(29%) patients who developed postoperative delirium, the "controls" were the 27 (71%) patients who did not. Numerous pre-, intra, and post operative variables were included in the analysis to determine risk factors for delirium. The factors most strongly associated with delirium were recent alcohol use, intubation time, time in the intensive care unit, and postoperative creatinine levels.

In the cohort study design, the presence of risk or predictor variables is measured at baseline within a selected population. Investigators then follow subjects over time to determine which patients develop the disease or condition of interest. Typically, cohort studies are prospective in nature, that is, subjects are followed forward in time (Euser, Zoccali, Jager, & Dekker, 2009). Perhaps the most famous cohort study in the United States is the Framingham Heart Study, begun in 1947 by the U.S. Public Health Service, and continued under the auspices of the National Heart, Lung and Blood Institute of the National Institutes of Health (NIH). The study initially enrolled a random sample of 5,209 subjects, aged 30 to 59 in the town of Framingham, Massachusetts (Dawber, Meadors, & Moore, 1951). Since 1948, the subjects have continued to return to the study every 2 years for a detailed medical history, physical examination, and laboratory tests. In 1971, the study enrolled a second generation, 5,124 of the original participants' adult children and their spouses, to participate in similar examinations. In 2002, enrollment of a third generation of participants was begun. Since 1951, investigators have published 2,346 studies based on Framingham Heart Study data in peer-reviewed medical journals (http://www.framinghamheartstudy.org/biblio/index.html).

### Ex Post Facto

Literally translated, "ex post facto" means "from what is done after." In ex post facto studies, the researcher retrospectively examines the effects of a naturally occurring event on a subsequent outcome for the purpose of establishing a causal link between them. Ex post facto studies are similar to case-control studies in that they begin by observing an existing condition or state of affairs. Subsequently, the researcher searches back in time for plausible causes, relationships, or associations between the variables (Giuffre, 1997). The study begins with preexisting groups that are already different in some respect(s) and searches in the past for the factor(s) that brought about the differences (Cohen, Manion, & Morrison, 2000).

By convention, the antecedent variable is often referred to as the "independent variable" or "cause," while the outcome variable is also called the "dependent variable," or "effect" (this despite the fact that ex post facto designs can only weakly predict cause and effect). For the purposes of clarity, the authors will use the terms "antecedent" and "outcome" variable.

Ex post facto designs are used when the researcher is interested in cause-and-effect relationships, but it is not possible to manipulate variables (i.e., to conduct an experimental study). Results of these ex post facto studies can provide a beginning sense of cause and effect relationships that can subsequently be tested with more rigorous research methods. It is an inexpensive study design in that the phenomena of interest have already occurred and no interventions are performed.

One of the major challenges for the researcher in using an ex post facto design is to identify preexisting groups that are comparable to a randomly assigned group, that is, that the only difference in the groups is the presence or absence of the outcome or "effect" variable (Giuffre, 1997). One of the most common means of achieving this comparability is to match the subjects in the "effect" and "no effect" groups on variables known or believed to influence the outcome variable. The difficulty with this strategy is that it assumes that the investigator knows what all the relevant factors are that may be related to the outcome variable. Similarly, factors that could influence the antecedent variable must be accounted for; again, there is the assumption that the investigator can identify all the relevant factors (Cohen et al., 2000).

Finally, the researcher must recognize that no single antecedent variable may be the "cause" of the outcome. Many antecedent variables may be interrelated or the result of more than one variable interacting with others. Likewise, a particular outcome may result from different antecedents on different occasions.

### Qualitative

Qualitative studies describe human responses in a particular situation and context and the meaning that human beings bring to the situation (Powers, 2011). Qualitative studies are often exploratory in nature and seek to generate new insight or understandings, using inductive (starting with data and developing hypotheses) rather than deductive (starting with hypotheses and testing them with data) approaches (Curry, Nembhard, & Bradley, 2009).

The three most often used qualitative designs are ethnography, phenomenology, and grounded theory (Miller, 2010). Ethnography is the direct description of a group, culture, or community; the culture as experienced by its members. Although ethnographic methods originated in cultural anthropology, they can also be used to describe the culture of a health care organization or patient care unit. Phenomenology uses in-depth interviews and open-ended discussion to describe and interpret the lived experience or phenomenon under study and to derive a depth of understanding and meaning from the experiences of participants.

Grounded theory uses data points (verbatim quotations) to gener-ate or modify a theory. Data are collected from in-depth interviews and open-ended discussion to understand processes and behaviors as individuals move through experiences over time. The purpose of this design is to generate a theory that is "grounded" in real-life empirical data (Powers, 2011). The developing theory evolves during data collec-tion and analysis as a part of the research process (Barroso, 2010) and the sample of participants is constantly developed to explore insights that emerge from the data (Curry et al., 2009).

The application of grounded theory is illustrated in a landmark study (Conrad, 1985) using data from 80 in-depth interviews of peo-ple with epilepsy. The study analyzed the meaning of medications in the lives of the subjects to determine why people did or did not take their medications. From the interview data, it was found that, from the patients' perspective, the issue was more of controlling dependence, and the practicalities of frequent medication administration. Conrad developed the theory of self-regulation from his belief that what appeared to be noncompliance (from a medical perspective) was actu-ally a form of asserting control over a disorder.

Qualitative research designs are often used in areas in which data or knowledge is inadequate or in which conventional theories may not be applicable. Qualitative methods can be used to understand complex social processes to capture essential aspects of a phenomenon from the perspective of study participants, and to uncover beliefs, values, and motivations that underlie individual health behaviors (Curry et al., 2009).

Qualitative research can be distinguished from quantitative research in several ways. First, quantitative research uses numbers (e.g., frequency or magnitude of variables) to describe phenomena, while qualitative research uses words to describe and understand the com-plexity and depth of phenomena or experiences. Second, quantitative research *tests* hypotheses with statistical methodology to determine statistical significance, while qualitative research seeks to *generate* hypotheses about a phenomenon, its antecedents, and its aftermath. Third, quantitative research is performed primarily in experimental settings and generates numeric data using valid and reliable instru-ments to measure predetermined variables. In contrast, qualitative research occurs in natural settings and produces word-based data through open-ended discussions, in-depth interviews, focus groups, observation, and document review (Curry et al., 2009).

## Mixed Methods

Mixed methods, in which quantitative and qualitative research designs are combined, are increasingly recognized as appropriate and important in health care research because they capitalize on the respective strengths of each approach (Curry et al., 2009). The NIH recently released a report on "Best Practices for Mixed Methods Research in the Health Sciences" (Creswell, Klassen, Plano Clark, & Smith, 2011). The report provides practical recommendations for researchers seeking to incorporate mixed methods research into their applications for NIH "R" series research grants as well as fellowship, career, training, and center grants.

Qualitative studies can generate theories and identify relevant variables to be studied subsequently in quantitative studies. They can also be used in a complementary fashion to yield findings that are broader in scope and richer in meaning than those derived from quantitative data alone (Ho et al., 2008).

Greenhalgh (2002) describes three ways in which qualitative research designs interact with quantitative methods: exploratory, explanatory, and evaluative. First, an exploratory process can be used to generate hypotheses and often serves as the first step in a sequence of research that includes a quantitative stage. Second, qualitative data can be used in an explanatory fashion to further inform relationships between or among variables in a quantitative study. While a quantitative study could answer the question of whether an intervention is efficacious, a qualitative study could answer the question of *why* the intervention was successful. Finally, after a quantitative study has demonstrated the efficacy of a particular intervention, qualitative data can be used to evaluate why this evidence may not become incorporated into practice, or be incompletely incorporated.

Approaches to mixed methods studies can vary based on the sequence of studies and the relative emphasis placed on each approach. The qualitative and quantitative elements may be performed concurrently or sequentially and, depending on the phenomena under investigation, one approach or the other may dominate the study design. For example, if a quantitative study yields unexpected or conflicting results, a qualitative follow-up study may help to ascertain important relationships that inform interpretation of the results. Likewise, qualitative studies may be performed to generate hypotheses or characterize a phenomenon about which little is known, that are then further studied using one or more quantitative methods. Strategies to enhance the validity of mixed methods studies include recognizing the role of each strategy and adhering to the methodological assumptions of each design (Curry et al., 2009).

## *Methods*

### Research Utilization and EBP

APNs may opt to use existing research to make a practice change and evaluate the effects of implementing a new innovation on specific outcomes. This type of project would use a research utilization approach or framework. Research utilization refers to the "process by which specific research-based knowledge (science) is implemented in practice" (Estabrooks, Walling, & Milner, 2003, p. 5). A disadvantage to using strictly research utilization methods is that traditional researchers use inclusion and exclusion criteria that restrict the subjects to a homogeneous sample, in order to decrease possible biases and variance and to increase the probability of identifying a statistically significant difference (Burns & Grove, 2007). Application of research findings to a population other than that studied may be problematic. One of the important steps in research utilization is to critique and synthesize research findings to determine relevance and feasibility in the APN's particular practice setting (Stetler, 2001). Increasingly, research utilization is being integrated into the larger concept of EBP (Killeen & Barnfather, 2005; Stetler, 2004).

EBP represents a broader concept than research utilization. When clinicians use the EBP approach, they can incorporate additional levels of evidence and consider the nurse's clinical expertise as well as the patient's preferences and values. Sackett et al. originally defined EBP as "the conscientious, explicit and judicious use of current best evidence in making decisions about the care of the individual patient. It means integrating individual clinical expertise with the best available external clinical evidence from systematic research" (Sackett, Rosenberg, Gray, Haynes, & Richardson, 1996, p. 71). Consideration of the individual patient's values and preferences was considered as part of the health care provider's clinical expertise (Sackett, Richardson, Rosenberg, & Haynes, 2000). Ingersoll (2000) proposed that EBP should also consider the importance of using theoretical foundations in the evidence-based decision making process.

There are a number of models for implementing an EBP methodology for outcomes research. Common elements of all EBP models include (1) identify a clinical problem, (2) gather evidence, (3) critique and synthesize evidence, (4) implement practice change, and (5) evaluate the impact of practice change on outcomes. These models can assist nurses to systematically approach clinical practice problems and proceed toward actual implementation in a specific practice setting. Use of an EBP model can prevent incomplete or unsuccessful implementations of the practice change, promote timely evaluation, and maximize use of time and resources (Gawlinski & Rutledge, 2008). EBP models that have specific stages or phases that can guide the APN in an outcomes measurement project are described in Table 6.3. EBP models that do not have

Table 6.3 *Selected EBP Nursing Models and Their Key Components*

|  | Iowa | Stetler | Rosswurm and Larrabee | Johns Hopkins | ACE Star |
|---|---|---|---|---|---|
| Emphasis | Organizational process | At individual nurse or organizational level | Organizational process | Organizational process | Knowledge transformation |
| Stages/phases | 1. Trigger: problem or new knowledge<br>2. Organizational priority?<br>3. Team formation<br>4. Evidence gathered<br>5. Research base critiqued and synthesized<br>6. Sufficient?<br>7. Pilot change<br>8. Decision?<br>9. Widespread implementation with continual monitoring of outcomes<br>10. Dissemination of results | 1. Preparation<br>2. Validation<br>3. Comparative evaluation<br>4. Decision making<br>5. Translation/application<br>6. Evaluation | 1. Assess need for change in practice<br>2. Link problem interventions and outcomes<br>3. Synthesize best evidence<br>4. Design practice change<br>5. Implement and evaluate change in practice<br>6. Integrate and maintain | 1. Practice question identified<br>2. Evidence gathered<br>3. Translation: plan, implement, evaluate, communicate | 1. Knowledge discovery<br>2. Evidence summary<br>3. Translation into practice recommendations<br>4. Integration into practice<br>5. Evaluation |

*Source:* Adapted from Gawlinski, A., and Rutledge, D. (2008).

specific stages or phases, but help describe and conceptualize the many variables and interactions that can occur when making an EBP change, are described in Table 6.4.

### Quality Improvement

Finally, a quality improvement (QI) process can be chosen to guide an outcomes measurement project. QI methodology involves systematic processes of data collection and inquiry and refers to activities that use data-based methodologies to bring about rapid improvements in health care delivery (Baily, 2008). A basic premise of QI is that measures of good performance reflect good-quality practice, and that comparing

**Table 6.4** *Select EBP Frameworks*

|  | ARCC Model | PARIHS Framework |
|---|---|---|
| Key focus | Organization of department or unit | Understanding key components of EBP |
| Key concepts | EBP mentor—an individual who has proficient knowledge and skills in EBP and the passion to help others practice daily from an evidence-based care | Evidence<br>Context<br>Facilitation |
| Major proposition | The development of APNs and other nurses as EBP mentors facilitates an organizational culture change toward evidence-based care | Practice changes are most likely when based upon robust evidence, conducted in a context "friendly" to change, and facilitated well |
| Utility—practical implications | Need to...<br>Assess and organize culture and readiness for EBP<br>Identify strengths and major barriers to EBP implementation<br>Implement ARCC strategies<br>Develop and use of EBP mentors<br>Interactive EBP skill building workshop<br>EBP rounds and journal clubs<br>EBP implementation<br>Improve patient, nurse, system outcomes | Need to...<br>Critically appraise evidence<br>Thoroughly understand the practice arena prior to implementing a change<br>Make a strategic plan for facilitation of any practice change—from development through implementation and evaluation |

ARCC = Advancing Research & Clinical Practice through Close Collaboration; PARIHS = Promoting Action on Research Implementation in Health Services.
*Source:* Adapted from A. Gawlinski and D. Rutledge (2008).

performance among providers and organizations will encourage better performance (Hughes, 2008).

The QI process includes developing indicators to assess progress toward certain predefined goals and reviewing performance against these measures. Data for QI investigation are derived internally and usually only reported internally. QI evaluates work processes in a cyclic fashion, benchmarks practice against established indicators and provides a means to continually evaluate and improve established practice (Hughes, 2008).

QI methods enable organizations to make change in a systematic way, measuring and assessing the effects of a change, feeding the information back into the clinical setting, and making adjustments until they are satisfied with the results (Baily, 2008). The APN is in an ideal position to implement and participate in QI activities through the roles of practitioner, teacher, researcher, and consultant. A thorough knowledge of the institution's QI methodology as well as skillful implementation of the QI process is required for the APN to monitor unit-based quality indicators of care, the performance of practitioners, and the overall quality of care provided (Altmiller, 2011).

There is no one "right" QI method that can be applied that will be effective in all organizations. Individual organizations have their own networks, structures, organizational histories, and challenges, which need to be considered in relation to the choice and implementation of QI methods. The specific approach (or combination of approaches) may be less important than the thoughtful consideration of the match and "best fit" for the particular circumstances (Powell, Rushmer, & Davies, 2008). There are a number of QI methodologies that have been adapted to the health care setting (Nicolay et al., 2012). A brief description of these methodologies is provided in Table 6.6.

## ROLE OF THE APN IN OUTCOMES MEASUREMENT

The role of the APN is to integrate education, research, management, leadership, and consultation into his or her clinical practice, making the APN well-suited to manage the complexities of HF patients and their evolving care needs. The following section describes an evidence-based outcomes measurement project initiated by the APNs employed in the Ahmanson University of California Los Angeles (UCLA) Cardiomyopathy Center, for the purpose of improving patient education and decreasing medication discrepancies during

## Table 6.6  *Quality Improvement Models*

| Model | Description |
|---|---|
| *Donabedian's Model of Quality Health Care* Donabedian was one of the founders of quality improvement and the model continues to serve as a unifying conceptual framework for quality improvement All steps are vital: process improvement is limited and temporary, when the structure is not also improved. | Structure: Availability, accessibility, and quality of resources Process: Delivery of health care services by clinicians Outcome: Final results of health care |
| *Total Quality Management and Continuous Quality Improvement (Deming)* Developed in Japan in the 1950s to rebuild and improve their manufacturing industry Terms are now also used to describe more general approaches to quality improvement Important concepts include: Continuous performance evaluation Involves management at all levels Quality is the responsibility of everyone Quality improvement is data driven | Process management: Focus on process and systems to improve, rather than individuals Problem solving: Use of structured approaches based on statistical analysis; data is a key tool Leadership: Management involvement at all levels Employee empowerment: Use of teams to identify problems and opportunities and to take the necessary action |
| *PDCA (Plan-Do-Check-Act)* Also known as rapid cycle QI; promoted by the Institute for Healthcare Improvement (IHI) Repeated short-cycle small scale changes Begin with easiest changes, repeat cycles to address more complex processes Cyclic and iterative | Plan: A change in process to improve quality Do: Implement the change with a strategic plan for implementation Check: Evaluate and analyze results Act: Adopt, adapt, or abandon |
| *Six Sigma* Developed by Motorola in the 1980s for QI Sigma is the statistical term for variance; 1 Sigma is one standard deviation, 6 Sigma is 6 standard deviations, which represents 99.99966% of possible events Goal is 3.4 failures per million "opportunities" Also cyclic and iterative | Define: Goal of improvement and key people involved Measure: Current system; may be challenging if data are not available for the processes of interest Analyze: Ways to close gap Improve: Implement and evaluate Control: Plans and process to maintain |
| *Toyota Lean* Developed by Toyota in 1940s Basic principle is to minimize waste, both in product and processes Focuses on value to the customer | Value stream map identifies exact steps of the work process and the value associated with the step Processes are aligned for continuous flow of work Create an environment of constant review Extensive use of visual cues to streamline processes and prevent error |

*(continued)*

Table 6.6 *Quality Improvement Models* *(continued)*

| Model | Description |
|---|---|
| *Root Cause Analysis*<br>Began as a way to evaluate industrial accidents<br>Systematic retrospective analysis to identify and understand the underlying cause of process failures<br>Extensive use of tools and diagrams of process require extensive training | Focus on systems and processes<br>Goal is to understand contributory factors that create an environment where errors can happen<br>Required by the Joint Commission (JCAHO) and other regulatory agencies for all sentinel events<br>Extensive use of tools and diagrams of process require extensive training |
| *Failure Modes and Effects Analysis (FMEA)*<br>Prospective risk assessment tool developed by the military and National Aeronautics and Space Administration (NASA) to evaluate potential failures and unrecognized hazards.<br>Can be used to evaluate both designs and processes<br>Goal is to identify process failures that would be the most significant and design preventive or mitigating measures before failure occurs<br>Flowcharts and brainstorming are useful tools | Identify the system to be analyzed and the individual processes within the system that are the most problematic or high risk<br>Create a process map (diagram) to describe each individual step in the process<br>Identify all potential failures in a process<br>Define and anticipate effect of each failure, cause, degree of seriousness, and possible solutions<br>Calculate a risk priority score for each potential failure<br>System or process redesign<br>Reanalysis |

the high-risk transition from hospital to home. Through a detailed plan of interventions, the APNs created a new process across the hospitalization to home continuum. APNs providing in-hospital patient education, facilitating and participating in the patient discharge process, and providing phone monitoring through to the outpatient follow-up clinic visit have resulted in a decrease in medication discrepancies posthospital discharge.

## Background

HF continues to be a major public problem resulting in substantial morbidity and mortality. A rapidly increasing aging population coupled with the advancement of life prolonging interventions has led to increasing rates of HF. HF prevalence rises with age, its incidence approaches 10 per 1,000 population after 65 years of age (Roger et al., 2012). A 2012 update from the American Heart Association (AHA) estimated that there were 5.8 million people with HF in the United States with an incidence of 550,000 new cases diagnosed annually. Projections indicate that by 2030, an additional 3 million people will have HF, a 25.0% increase in prevalence from 2010 (Roger et al., 2012). While survival after HF diagnosis has improved over time, the mortality rate remains unacceptably high: Approximately 50% of people diagnosed with HF will die within 5 years and about 1 in 5 people who have HF die within 1 year from diagnosis (Lloyd-Jones et al., 2010).

HF also accounts for a large burden in rising health care expenditures, translating into 3.4 million office visits, 668,000 emergency department visits, and 1.1 million hospitalizations per year (Roger et al., 2012). It is the most common diagnosis-related group discharge in persons older than 65 years (Roger et al., 2012). The indirect and direct costs of HF treatment in the United States are now up to $39.2 billion annually, a sobering statistic, driving 5.4% of all health care costs (Lloyd-Jones et al., 2010). With an average 6-day length of stay, hospitalization is the predominant contributor to HF costs, and is the largest single expense for Medicare. Unfortunately, nearly one third of HF patients are readmitted within 30 days of discharge (Landro, 2007).

The Center for Medicare & Medicaid Services (CMS), TJC, and the Hospital Quality Alliance (HQA) define core measures for patient care and HF management. Medication safety, patient education, and implementation of evidence-based HF guideline management are critical elements defined by these organizations. "Hospital Compare," created through the efforts of the CMS, the Department of Health and Human Services (DHS), and the HQA: Improving Care through Information, provides objective and verifiable data regarding HF outcomes. Thirty-day mortality rates and 30-day rehospitalization rates for HF are key outcome measures, as HF is the most frequent diagnosis-related group and has the highest readmission rate of any other common Medical or surgical condition in Medicare beneficiaries.

Due to the high mortality and tremendous costs associated with HF treatment, adherence to evidence-based therapy is critical. Literature supports the benefits of evidence-based guideline medical therapy and lifestyle modification in delaying disease progression and improving survival in patients with HF (Calvin et al., 2012; Fonarow et al., 2010). However, patient adherence to these treatment regimens show high variability with rates ranging from 10% to as high as 85% (Calvin et al., 2012; Fonarow et al., 2010; Foust, Naylor, Bixby, & Ratcliffe, 2012; Grady et al., 2000; Yancy et al., 2010). The most common factors associated with patient nonadherence to HF treatment recommendations and rehospitalization include complicated medical regimens, inappropriate medication reconciliation, poor discharge instructions, lack of patient understanding, poor communication among healthcare providers between sites of care, lack of a plan for appropriate medical follow up after discharge, lower socioeconomic status, minority status, psychosocial variables, and age (Calvin et al., 2012; Fonarow et al., 2010; Foust et al., 2012; Grady et al., 2000; Nielsen et al., 2008; Yancy et al., 2010).

## Clinical Issue

Maximizing evidence-based HF guideline therapy is part of the inpatient and outpatient management. Despite written hospital discharge instructions and prescriptions provided by the hospital critical care unit service, a large number of patients did not know what medications, purpose or indication, dose or frequency they were taking when interviewed at their 1-week hospital follow-up HF clinic visit. The patients and/or care providers were often confused regarding their medication regimens and changes made while in the hospital. Medication discrepancies can be detrimental to the control of HF symptoms for the patient resulting in ongoing HF progression, fluid overload exacerbation, hypertension, hypotension, hyperkalemia, hypokalemia, renal insufficiency, or liver dysfunction. It became apparent to the APNs that there was a need to bridge the education gap at the transition from hospital discharge to home. The APNs found that cardioprotective medications initiated, uptitrated, or changed in the hospital were often not continued after discharge. In an effort to improve the discharge transition to home, the APNs identified the factors contributing to medication discrepancies, which included:

- New prescriptions were not filled due to need for insurance authorization, high cost, or inability to go to pharmacy.
- Patients experienced side effects and discontinued the medicine without consultation with a practitioner.
- Patients used old prescriptions/medications available at home of same drug but dose or strength was not same as what was prescribed.
- Patients expressed that discharge paperwork was overwhelming or confusing.
- Elderly population with functional impairments; difficulty following and understanding dosing regimen.
- Patients unclear who to contact with medication questions (especially if discharged weekend/after hours).
- Lack of social support to assist with medication management.
- Knowledge deficit of the importance of their HF medications.

## REVIEW OF LITERATURE

To evaluate how to best improve the clinical problem, a review of evidence-based literature regarding the transition from hospital discharge to home and improving posthospital medication discrepancies was essential. The APNs began a literature-based patient improvement project to determine whether implementing a standardized in-hospital to outpatient transitional medication education and reconciliation process could improve the number of medication discrepancies at discharge.

Medication discrepancies at care transitions, such as from hospital discharge to home, are common and may lead to patient harm. A high burden of illness often accompanied by polypharmacy and variable health literacy creates greater vulnerability for medication discrepancies to occur during the transition from hospital discharge to home. The scope of this problem is well recognized with approximately 1.5 million preventable adverse medication events occurring annually at a cost of more than $3 billion per year (TJC, 2006). Effective interventions to decrease medication discrepancies need to be implemented to decrease the potential for medication errors, especially at high-risk transitions times. Medication reconciliation is a strategy that can reduce risk and ensure safe and effective medication use.

Medication reconciliation is a process that involves obtaining and maintaining accurate and complete medication information across the continuum of care (American Pharmacists Association and American Society of Health-System Pharmacists, 2012). The process requires members of the health care team to comprehensively evaluate a patient's medication regimen to avoid medication errors at all care transition points. The transition from hospital to home is an especially high-risk time because of changes in medication regimens that occur during an acute illness requiring hospitalization. Foust et al. (2012) reported a review of studies that indicated medication discrepancies commonly occured at hospital discharge (39.6%–70.7%) and during the posthospital transition (14.1%–94%). Among posthospital adverse events, medications were the most common problem (66%–72%), and nearly all posthospital adverse drug events (ADEs) involved a new medication or dosage change. Medication reconciliation, therefore, needs to be an integral part of the care transition process at hospital discharge.

Medication reconciliation at hospital discharge is a complex process, which can involve a multitude of critical elements such as: (1) case manager involvement, (2) use of discharge checklists that incorporate medication- and disease-specific information, and (3) designating a specific health care provider to review and reconcile medications at the point of discharge. Mueller, Sponsler, Kripalani, and Schnipper (2012) provide a systematic review of 26 studies in the hospital setting from 1966 through 2010. These studies involved various aspects of medication reconciliation interventions aimed at reducing medication discrepancies. The authors found that various interventions for medication reconciliation were associated with a decrease in ADEs. These interventions included involvement of a pharmacist, use of information technology, and the electronic medical record, as well as interventions such as use of a standardized medication reconciliation tool and staff education and feedback.

A number of relevant studies within the review highlighted the effectiveness of a dedicated pharmacist in the medication reconciliation process at hospital discharge (Gillespie et al., 2009; Kwan et al., 2007; Walker et al., 2009). Gillespie et al. (2009) evaluated the effectiveness of focused interventions by hospital unit-based pharmacists on reducing morbidity and rehospitalization in 368 elderly patients who were randomized to either usual care or an intervention by a hospital unit-based pharmacist. The pharmacist performed medication histories and medication reconciliation at hospital admission and discharge, provided patient and health care provider counseling during hospitalization, communicated with the primary care physician at hospital discharge, and communicated with the patient via a follow-up phone call 2 months post hospital discharge. The pharmacist-based intervention group demonstrated an 80% decrease in drug-related readmissions, a 47% decrease in visits to the emergency department, and a 16% decrease in all visits to the hospital.

Kwan et al. (2007) randomized patients who were undergoing surgical procedures to usual care or to an intervention utilizing a structured pharmacist-led protocol. The protocol included a medication history and assessment and generation of a postoperative medication form. Medication discrepancies at discharge were substantially reduced in the intervention group (20.3% versus 40.3% in the control group).

Eggnick et al. (2010) randomized 81 HF patients to a pharmacist intervention or usual care. The pharmacists provided medication education and medication reconciliation at hospital discharge and at the first follow-up visit posthospitalization. Patients randomized to the pharmacist-guided intervention demonstrated a reduction of almost half in medication discrepancies and prescription errors (68% pharmacist group versus 38% usual care).

Corbett et al. (2010) described and classified medication discrepancies as identified by nurses when high-risk patients transitioned from hospital to home. High-risk patient diagnoses included HF, coronary artery disease, myocardial infarction, diabetes, and others.

These nurse-identified medication discrepancies were classified as either patient level or system level. The most common patient-level medication discrepancies were intentional nonadherence, nonintentional nonadherence, and not filling a prescription. The most common system-level medication discrepancies were incomplete or inaccurate discharge instructions, conflicting information from different sources, and duplication of medications.

A research group at Boston University developed "Project RED" (Re-Engineered Discharge) to promote patient safety and reduce rehospitalization rates (Agency for Healthcare Research and Quality, 2011). The project tested strategies to improve the hospital discharge process for high-risk patient populations including patients with HF. Results of this project included development of a guideline that provided targeted actions aimed at improving the hospital discharge process. As part of "Project RED," Jack et al. (2009) randomized 749 medical patients to a nurse-led educational intervention with pharmacist follow up, compared to usual care. The nurse-taught intervention group demonstrated significantly lower rates of hospital utilization postdischarge compared to the usual care group (22% versus 27%, $p = .028$).

Some interventions that have been conceptualized to improve medication reconciliation at hospital discharge involve using a multidisciplinary approach in patients with HF (Holland et al., 2005). Discharge protocols and education by staff nurses at the time of discharge are also recognized as important components of the medication reconciliation process in patients with HF (Foust et al., 2012).

Foust et al. (2012) provide a retrospective chart review of nurse-identified rate and types of medication reconciliation problems in 162 older adults with HF. They found at least one type of medication reconciliation discrepancy 71.2% of the time and 76% of these discrepancies involved a high-risk medication. The most common issues identified were medication discrepancies (58.9%), incomplete hospital discharge summaries (52.5%), and partial discharge instructions (48.9%).

In summary, small studies using specific interventions to improve the medication reconciliation process, such as use of pharmacists or nurse-led education, have shown beneficial outcomes. However, further testing of these interventions and other innovative strategies are needed in larger populations and with more diverse groups of patients. Evaluation of the effectiveness of APNs in medication reconciliation is warranted because of the APN's unique role in coordination of clinical care and oversight at times of care transitions, such as hospital discharge.

## PROJECT FRAMEWORK, GOALS, AND CRITERIA

Using the Iowa Model of Evidence-Based Practice to Promote Quality Care (Titler et al., 2001), authors spearheaded an outcomes project to improve the medication reconciliation process. The goals of the project were to increase patients' knowledge about their HF medications and to decrease discrepancies related to HF medications when patients transitioned from hospital to home. Patient selection criteria for the project included: (1) being admitted for New York Heart Association class II to IV HF, (2) having more than 1 hospitalization for HF within the last year, and (3) requiring enhanced HF patient education based on the assessment of the APN.

### Interventions for Project Development and Implementation

The first intervention was to implement a thorough HF education teaching session where the APN met with the patient and caregiver(s) (pending caregiver availability), to review information in the *Heart Failure Handbook*. The contents of the handbook included important aspects of HF management, which are listed in Exhibit 6.3. The handbook was written at an eighth grade reading level and was available in Spanish. Spanish-speaking patients comprise a large portion of the HF patient population at our health care facility. When needed, an interpreter would be used for teaching sessions in other languages. The UCLA Health System has a robust interpreter service with 24-hour availability in all languages.

Based on APNs assessment, many patients/caregivers received more than one teaching session to reinforce information and to enhance adherence and compliance. If caretakers were not available in person, the teaching was done with them over the phone and then reinforced during the first follow-up phone call and the first follow-up clinic visit. HF patients who would not be returning to the clinic under the care of the HF service received all teachings and interventions for the medication reconciliation project. These patients, however, were excluded from the measurements of the project outcomes.

The second intervention was to develop an individualized typed medication list for each patient that included the name of each of their cardiac medications, the rationale for taking the medication, and the dose and frequency of the medication (Exhibit 6.4). The frequency section of the medication list included columns labeled breakfast, lunch, dinner, and bedtime. An "X" was used to indicate the time the patient was scheduled to take the medications. Other information on the medication list included patient's name, medical record number, the

**EXHIBIT 6.3 HEART FAILURE HANDBOOK: TABLE OF CONTENTS**

UCLA Health System
Ahmanson UCLA Cardiomyopathy Center

**Introduction to Heart Failure**

- What is the normal function of the heart?
- What is cardiomyopathy?
- What is heart failure?
- What are the signs and symptoms of heart failure?
- When to call your doctor?

**Prescribed Daily Routine**

- Two (2) liter fluid restriction
- Daily weights
- Adjustment of diuretic dose

**Important Changes to Your Diet**

- Two (2) gram sodium diet
- Low fat, low cholesterol diet
- How to read a food label
- Alcohol
- Caffeine
- Cigarette smoking

**Know Your Medications**

- Medical regimen
- Commonly prescribed heart failure medications
- Warfarin (Coumadin) and your diet
- Safe cold, flu, and allergy medications
- Dental procedures and preventive antibiotic therapy
- Medications to be cautious with (e.g., NSAIDs)

**Device Therapy for Heart Failure**

**Additional Patient Information**

- Exercise and heart failure
- What about sex?

*(continued)*

**EXHIBIT 6.3 HEART FAILURE HANDBOOK: TABLE OF CONTENTS** *(continued)*

▪ Travel tips
▪ Advance directive

**Diagnostic Tests**

▪ Echocardiogram
▪ Cardiopulmonary exercise test (CPX)
▪ Swan-Ganz catheter

**Appendices**

▪ Weight chart
▪ Chart of heart failure medications and doses
▪ Personal exercise schedule

*Source:* Used with permission from the Ahmanson University of California Los Angeles Cardiomyopathy Center.

**EXHIBIT 6.4 SAMPLE PATIENT MEDICATION LIST**

UCLA Health System
Ahmanson UCLA Cardiomyopathy Center

| Patient Name | | Medical Record Number | | Date |
|---|---|---|---|---|

| Drug name | Indication | Dose | Breakfast | Lunch | Dinner | Bedtime |
|---|---|---|---|---|---|---|
| Coreg/Carvedilol | protects heart/ lowers heart rate and blood pressure | 3.125 mg take twice a day | X | | X | |
| Lisinopril/Zestril | protects heart/ lowers BP | 10 mg take twice a day | | X | | X |
| Lasix/Furosemide | diuretic/increases urination | 80 mg take twice a day | X | | X | |
| Potassium Chloride | Potassium replacement | 20 mEq take twice a day | X | | X | |
| Spironolactone/ Aldactone | protects heart/ potassium sparing mild diuretic | 25 mg take once a day | X | | | |

*(continued)*

## Exhibit 6.4 *continued*

| Drug name | Indication | Dose | Breakfast | Lunch | Dinner | Bedtime |
|-----------|-----------|------|-----------|-------|--------|---------|
| Fish oil | lowers cholesterol | 1 g twice a day | X | | X | |
| Aspirin (baby) | mild blood thinner | 81 mg daily | X | | | |
| Coumadin/ Warfarin | thins blood / for LV clot | mg tabs—take daily as directed by clinic/doctor | Start Wed if labs OK 1mg daily | | | X |
| Amiodorone/ Pacerone | prevents heart arrhythmia | 200 mg take once a day | X | | | |
| Digoxin/Lanoxin | protects heart | 0.125 mg take once a day | | | X | |
| Magnesium oxide | supplement | 400 mg take once a day | X | | | |
| As needed meds | | | | | | |
| Tylenol/ acetaminophen | mild pain/ headache | 500–650 mg as needed 3–4 times per day | | | | |
| Docusate/Colace | stool softener | 100 mg twice a day | | | | |
| Magnesium hydroxide/MOM | laxative/relieves constipation | 30 mL = 2 tablespoons as needed | | | | |
| **UCLA Cardio- myopathy** | **Clinic address** | **Clinic phone number** | | | | |
| **Bring medication list AND bottles to clinic visit** | | **Cardiomyopathy physician name, and clinic appointment date/time** | | | | |

*Source:* Used with permission from the Ahmanson University of California Los Angeles Cardiomyopathy Center.

date last updated, the cardiomyopathy physician's name, and the next scheduled clinic appointment. Additionally, the patient was reminded to bring the medication bottles and the medication list to the first cardiomyopathy clinic appointment.

Medication lists were also tailored to each patient's specific needs. For example, if the patient could only read Spanish, the list was typed in Spanish. If a patient had problems with their vision, then all words were enlarged and bolded.

Patients were encouraged to view their medication list as an educational tool. The medication list included all HF-related medications, but did not consistently include all of their other condition-specific medications. Patients were educated about the need to follow all instructions written on their discharge medication prescription bottles. They were also encouraged to continuously update their medication list by writing in any additional changes to their medication regimen. When the APN assessed that a patient was confused by the medication list or had problems with understanding instructions, the medication list was given to a family member. Detailed instructions were then given to the family member regarding all aspects of HF medication use and management.

The third intervention was to review with the patients and caretakers a form titled the "Heart Failure Medication Management Patient Information" (Exhibit 6.5). The purpose of the form was to enhance patients' understanding of their medications, to facilitate patients' adherence and responsibility for their medication regimen, and to encourage self-care. The medication information sheet emphasized the importance of the following:

1. Ensuring all new discharge prescriptions were filled the day of discharge.
2. Bringing an updated medication list and medication bottles to the patient's clinic appointments.
3. Updating the patient's medication list with any changes in medications.
4. Including all regularly taken medications (herbs, vitamins, over-the-counter medications, etc.) on the patient's medication list.
5. Allowing at least a 2-day notice to their physician for any medication refills.

A statement was also included to indicate that adhering to the above recommendations would expedite the patient's check-in time at the clinic.

After the APN reviewed the medication sheet with the patient (or caregiver), the APN would ask the patient to identify the main person responsible for managing medications. This person, who was usually the patient him-or herself, would be asked to sign the medication information sheet indicating agreement with the guidelines for self-managing medications. When patients was not able to perform the functions listed in the medication management information sheet, then the caregiver would be asked to sign the form indicating agreement with performing the guidelines for managing the patient's medications.

## EXHIBIT 6.5 HEART FAILURE MEDICATION MANAGEMENT PATIENT INFORMATION

### UCLA Health System
### Ahmanson UCLA Cardiomyopathy Center

You have been provided a list of your medications, their doses, and why and when they need to be taken. As a patient, it is important that you have an understanding of your medications and take them as prescribed by your physician.

We request that you do the following:

- Have ALL new discharge prescriptions filled the day of discharge.
- Bring an updated medication list to all your appointments.
- Bring all medication bottles to your appointments.
- Keep a copy of your medication list in your purse or wallet.
- Whenever a medication change is made, update your medication list.
- Include all medications on your medication list (herbs, vitamins, and any over-the-counter medications, e.g., Advil, Tylenol) that you take regularly.
- Please allow us 48 hours notice for all refills.

"Check-in" at your clinic appointment may be delayed if you do not have your updated medication list/medications with you.

Name of the person who helps organize your medications:

_____

_____

Contact number:

_____

I, _____, have read the information above and will educate myself about the medications I take and take them as prescribed by my physician.

Patient Signature:

_____

Date:

_____

*Source:* Used with permission from the Ahmanson University of California Los Angeles Cardiomyopathy Center.

The fourth intervention was initiation of a follow-up phone call to the patient by the APN on the first business day after discharge to review medications and HF management. During the phone call, the person responsible for managing medications was asked to read out loud what was written on the discharge medication bottles. To verify that the patient was taking the correct prescriptions, the APN cross-referenced what medications the patient had at home to the hospital's documented discharge summary. If a medication discrepancy was identified, it would be documented and corrected with the patient. If a medication was missing, the APN would immediately contact the patient's pharmacy for a new prescription. The APN also asked about the patient's current weight, and compared it to their discharge weight to determine if adjustments in diuretics were needed. Signs and symptoms of HF and daily weight monitoring were reviewed, as well as the importance of following sodium and fluid restrictions. Lastly, the patient was reminded to bring the medication bottles and an updated medication list to the clinic appointment.

The fifth intervention occurred at the first clinic appointment. Here, the nursing assistant documented if the patient brought the medication list and bottles to the clinic visit. If the patient came without a medication list, the nursing assistant would provide a wallet-sized blank medication card for the patient to complete. After check-in procedures, the APN performed medication reconciliation for each medication. If a discrepancy was encountered, it was documented in the clinic chart and corrected with the patient. If the APN assessed that the patient needed further clarification regarding a medication discrepancy, the patient was called the next day and asked to verbalize the correct instructions listed on the medication bottle(s).

While the project was being implemented, the APNs collaboratively discussed problems they encountered and shared ways of improving the project. Ideas for improvement included having: (1) the administrative office staff remind patients to bring their medication list and bottles to their visit during appointment-confirmation calls, (2) the APNs update the patient's existing medication list at the first visit as needed, (3) the APNs demonstrate the process of writing down medications on the blank wallet-sized card when patients did not bring their medication list to the clinic.

Other important aspects of the project included ongoing education and reinforcement of project details to all staff nurses caring for these patients. The APN project leader attended unit staff meetings to discuss specific details of the outcomes project. For example, the APN described the purpose of the project, the rationale for providing patients with an individualized medication list, and the importance of the staff nurses, role in providing and reinforcing HF teaching during each patient and family interaction.

### Outcomes Measured

The outcomes that were identified for this project were selected based on problems that the APNs observed related to patients' accurate and safe medication use during the transition of care (i.e., from hospital discharge to home and the follow-up clinic visit). These outcomes included the percent of patients who (1) were provided with a medication list prior to discharge, (2) brought either their medication list or their medication prescription bottles to clinic, (3) experienced medication discrepancies that were indentified during the first follow-up phone call, and/or (4) experienced medication discrepancies identified at the first follow-up clinic visit.

Monthly, the APN project leader performed an audit on all patient charts (Exhibit 6.6). The audit consisted of documenting the number of patients discharged each month and the number who received the interventions previously discussed for this project. The audit tool tracked the important outcomes of the project such as the number of medication discrepancies, the type of discrepancies (e.g., correct drug, dose, frequency, or supply), and the number of patients who brought their medication lists and/or medication prescription bottles to their clinic appointment.

### Results Pre- and Postproject Implementation

After implementing the outcomes project, the APN evaluated the changes in outcome measures preimplementation versus postimplementation (Figures 6.2–6.5). Improvement in the outcomes occurred over time in areas of (1) patients consistently receiving their medication list (pre approximately 10%, increased post 71%–100%), (2) patients consistently bringing their medication list and/or prescription bottles to their first clinic visit (pre approximately 50%, increased post 86%–100% for the majority of months), (3) medication discrepancies, which markedly decreased during the first follow-up phone call (pre approximately 38%, decreased post over time to 0% for the majority of months), and (4) medication discrepancies which also markedly decreased at the first follow-up clinic visit (pre approximately 50%, decreased post over time to 0%). For the outcome related to patients bringing their medication list or medication bottles to clinic, an improvement occurred from 10%

## EXHIBIT 6.6 MEDICATION RECONCILIATION: MONTHLY AUDIT TOOL

UCLA Health System
Ahmanson UCLA Cardiomyopathy Center

*1.* Number of patients discharged.
*2.* Number of patients who were provided:
   A. HF Education / Medication review / HF handbook: ___ / ___
   B. Medication list: ___ / ___
   C. Medication contract / copy in chart: ___ / ___
   D. Phone call s/p hospital discharge: ___ / ___
*3.* Number of patients with:


   A. Medication discrepancy identified on phone follow up: total #
      ___ / ___

### Type of discrepancy

| Drug | ACE/ARB | BB | AA | Diuretic | K+ |
|------|---------|----|----|----------|----|
| Dose |  |  |  |  |  |
| Frequency |  |  |  |  |  |
| Supply |  |  |  |  |  |


   B. Medication list at first clinic visit s/p hospital discharge: total #
      ___ / ___
   C. Medications brought to first clinic visit s/p hospital discharge:
      total # ___ / ___
   D. Medication discrepancy at first clinic visit s/p hospital discharge: total # ___ / ___


### Type of discrepancy

| Drug | ACE/ARB | BB | AA | Diuretic | K+ |
|------|---------|----|----|----------|----|
| Dose |  |  |  |  |  |
| Frequency |  |  |  |  |  |
| Supply |  |  |  |  |  |

*Source:* Used with permission from the Ahmanson University of California Los Angeles Cardiomyopathy Center.

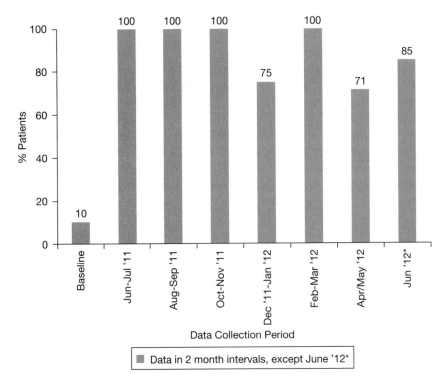

**Figure 6.2** *Percent of Patients Provided With Medication List Prior to Discharge*

pre to 100% for the first 10 months postintervention. During months 11 (April 2012) and 12 (May 2012), there was a decrease in the percent compliance of these measures due to a non-APN health care professional seeing the patient who was unfamiliar with the new medication reconciliation processes (Figure 6.3). There was also a missed opportunity in documenting whether a patient brought their medication list or bottles to the first follow-up clinic visit.

The overall improvements in project outcomes indicated an adoption of the new medication reconciliation processes by the patients, the caregivers, and the APNs. However, there was a need to identify additional strategies when non-APN health care professionals saw patients in the clinic. Additionally, reminders were needed for documentation by nursing assistants regarding whether patients brought their medication list or bottles to clinic.

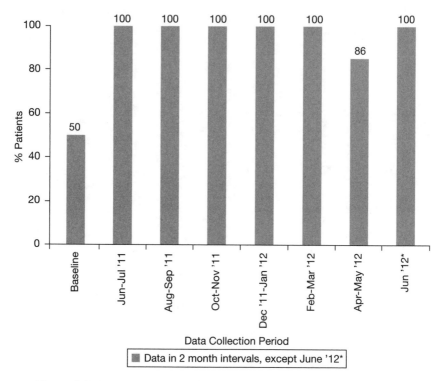

**Figure 6.3** *Percent of Patients Who Brought Either Medication List or Prescription Bottles to First Clinic Visit*

## Limitations

The design of the medication reconciliation outcomes project was based on current best evidence and patient-, clinic-, and APN-identified needs. Consequently, results and tools may be applicable only to similar patients, hospital, and clinic settings. Although medication discrepancies were frequently identified by APNs during patients' first postdischarge clinic visits, there was no standardized mechanism to consistently collect and summarize the frequency of medications discrepancies, and other outcome variables at the preintervention (baseline) period. However, the newly standardized medication reconciliation processes developed for this outcomes project have been effective in achieving project goals. Patients consistently received their medication list, brought their medication list or bottles to clinic, and medication discrepancies decreased.

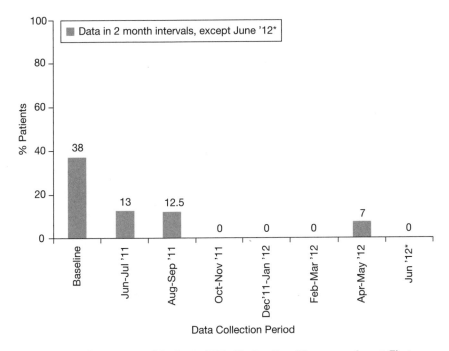

Figure 6.4 *Percent of Patients With Medication Discrepancies at First Follow-Up Phone Call*

### SUMMARY

Effective medication reconciliation is composed of multiple processes that together support safe medication use by patients. Medication reconciliation structures and processes can be improved by assessing current practices during transitions of care, developing an evidence-based process improvement intervention, and evaluating the impact on outcomes. In this project, cardiovascular APNs found that implementing an evidence-based medication reconciliation process for HF patients has improved the process of medication reconciliation in several ways. These processes and tools have been effective in increasing the consistency at which patients received an accurate medication list and brought their medication list or bottles to clinic. Additionally, medication discrepancies decreased during the first follow-up phone call and at the first follow-up clinic visit. Cardiovascular APNs, at the point of care delivery, play a key role in developing and successfully implementing an effective medication reconciliation process for high-risk HF patients.

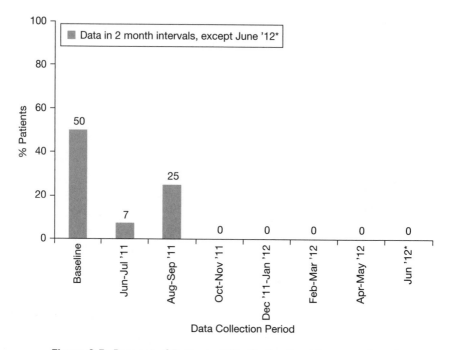

**Figure 6.5** *Percent of Patients With Medication Discrepancies at First Follow-Up Clinic Visit*

## Answers to Chapter Discussion Questions

1. The definition of the medication reconciliation is a process that involves obtaining and maintaining accurate and complete medication information across the continuum of care. The process requires members of the health care team to comprehensively evaluate a patient's medication regimen to avoid medication errors at all care transition points. The transition from hospital to home is an especially high-risk time because of changes in medication regimens that occur during an acute illness requiring hospitalization. The interventions implemented by the APNs in the exemplar provided in the chapter are consistent with this definition. Note: The APN and/or student should expand on how the interventions in the exemplar are consistent with the definition.

2. The outcomes of concern to APNs listed in Exhibit 6.1 are broad spectrum outcomes in categories of clinical, physiological, psychological,

functional, fiscal, and satisfaction outcomes. These outcomes may be similar, but may not include all nurse-sensitive outcomes that have been selected for national reporting. Nurse-sensitive outcomes represent the impact of nursing interventions and describe the effect of what nurses do in response to a patient's condition. These outcomes may be the result of direct care, non-APN practices, and thus may not all be listed in Exhibit 6.1.

3. The APN and/or student should review the advantages and disadvantages of various research designs illustrated in Table 6.2 and determine appropriate designs/frameworks in relationship to the clinical issue and outcomes they identify. The APN and/or student may be able to use more than one research design or framework. Note: Have the students provide rationales and support for their selection of various research designs and frameworks.

4. The APN and/or student should identify the relative effectiveness of interventions described in the review of literature section in the chapter. These interventions include, but are not limited to (1) case manager involvement, (2) use of discharge checklists that incorporate medication and disease-specific information, and (3) designating a specific health care provider to review and reconcile medications at the point of discharge. Review the advantages and disadvantages of various research designs and other methodologies for outcomes measurement projects.

5. The HF population is more vulnerable to medication discrepancies because of the complex medication regimen that patients are prescribed. Other factors also include inappropriate medication reconciliation process, poor discharge instructions, lack of patient understanding, poor communication among health care providers between sites of care, lack of a plan for appropriate medical follow up after discharge, lower socioeconomic status, minority status, psychosocial variables, and age.

### REFERENCES

Agency for Healthcare Research and Quality. (2011, October). *Preventing avoidable readmissions: Improving the hospital discharge process.* Retrieved from http://www.ahrq.gov/qual/impptdis.htm

Akobeng, A. K. (2008). Assessing the validity of clinical trials. *Journal of Pediatric Gastroenterology and Nutrition, 47*(3), 227–282.

Altmiller, G. (2011). Quality and safety education for nurses competencies for the clinical nurse specialist. *Clinical Nurse Specialist, 24*(4), 187–188.

American Pharmacists Association, & American Society of Health-System Pharmacists. (2012, March). *Improving care transitions: Optimizing medication reconciliation.* Retrieved from http://www.ashp.org/DocLibrary/Policy/PatientSafety/Optimizing-Med-Reconciliation.aspx

Baily, M. A. (2008). Quality improvement methods in health care. In M. Crowley (Ed.), *From birth to death and bench to clinic: The Hastings Center bioethics briefing book for journalists, policymakers, and campaigns* (pp. 147–152). Garrison, NY: The Hastings Center.

Barroso, J. (2010). Qualitative approaches to research. In G. LoBiondo-Wood & J. Haber (Eds.), *Nursing research: Methods and critical appraisal for evidence-based practice* (7th ed., pp. 100–125). St. Louis, MO: Mosby Elsevier.

Burns, K. D., Jenkins, W., Yeh, D., Procyshyn, R. M., Schwartz, S. K. W., Honer, W. G., & Barr, A. M. (2009). Delirium after cardiac surgery: A retrospective case-control study of incidence and risk factors in a Canadian sample. *BC Medical Journal, 51*(5), 206–210.

Burns, N., & Grove, S. (2006). *Understanding nursing research: Building an evidence-based practice* (4th ed.). Philadelphia, PA: Saunders Elsevier.

Calvin, J. E., Shanbhag, S., Avery, E., Kane, J., Richardson, D., & Powell, L. (2012). Adherence to evidence-based guidelines for heart failure in physicians and their patients: Lessons from the heart failure adherence retention trial (HART). *Congestive Heart Failure, 18*(2), 73–78.

Carson, S. S. (2010). Outcomes research: Methods and implications. *Seminars in Respiratory Critical Care Medicine, 31*(1), 3–12.

Centers for Medicare and Medicaid Services. (2012). Roadmap for quality measurement in the traditional Medicare Fee-for-Service Program. Retrieved September, 2012 from http://www.cms.hhs.gov

Clochesy, J. M. (2002). Research designs for advanced practice nursing outcomes research. *Critical Care Nursing Clinics of North America, 14*(3), 293–298.

Cohen, L., Manion, L., & Morrison, K. (2000). Research methods in education (5th ed.). London, England: Routledge Falmer.

Conrad P. (1985).The meaning of medications: Another look at compliance. *Social Science Medicine, 20*(1), 29–37.

Corbett, C. F., Setter, S. M., Daratha, K. B., Neumiller, J. J., & Wood, L. D. (2010). Nurse identified hospital to home medication discrepancies: Implications for improving transitional care. *Geriatric Nursing, 31*(3), 188–196.

Creswell, J. W., Klassen, A. C., Plano Clark, V. L., & Smith, K. C for the Office of Behavioral and Social Sciences Research. (2011). *Best practices for mixed methods research in the health sciences.* National Institutes of Health. Retrieved September 4, 2012, from http://obssr.od.nih.gov/mixed_methods_research

Curry, L. A., Nembhard, I. M., & Bradley, E. H. (2009). Qualitative and mixed methods provide unique contributions to outcomes research. *Circulation, 119*(10), 1442–1452.

Damberg, C. L., Sobero, M. E., Lovejoy, S. L., Lauderdale, K., Wertheimer, S., Smith, A.,…Schnyer, C. (2012). An evaluation of the use of performance measures in health care. *RAND Health Quarterly, 1*(4), 3.

Dawber, R. T., Meadors, F. G., & Moore E. F. (1951). Epidemiological approaches to heart disease: The Framingham Study. *American Journal of Public Health, 41*(3), 279–286.

Deaton, C. (2001). Outcomes measurement and evidence-based nursing practice. *Journal of Cardiovascular Nursing, 15*(2), 83–86.

Dennison, C. R., & Hughes, S. (2009) Reforming cardiovascular care: Quality measurements and improvement, and pay-for-performance. *Journal of Cardiovascular Nursing, 24*(5), 341–343.

DesHarnais, S. I. (2013). The outcome model of quality. In W. A. Sollecito & J. K. Johnson (Eds.), *McLaughlin and Kaluzny's continuous improvement in health care.* (4th ed., pp. 155–180). Burlington, MA: Jones & Bartlett Learning.

Dykes, P. C. (2003). Practice guidelines and measurement: State-of-the-science. *Nursing Outlook, 51*(2), 65–69.

Eggnick, R. N., Lenderink, A. W., Widdershoven, J. W. M. G., & van den Bemt, P. M. L. A. (2010). The effect of a clinical pharmacist discharge service on medication discrepancies in patients with heart failure. *Pharmacy World Science, 32*(6), 759–766.

Estabrooks, C. A., Walling, L., & Milner, M. (2003). Measuring knowledge utilization in health care. *International Journal of Policy and Evaluation, 1*(3), 3–12. Retrieved from http://hdl.handle.net/10755/153540

Euser, M. A., Zoccali, C., Jager, J. K., & Dekker, W. F. (2009). Cohort studies: Prospective versus retrospective. *Nephron Clinical Practice, 113*(3), 214–217.

Fonarow, G. C., Albert, M. N., Curtis, A. B., Sough, W. G., Gheorghiade, M., Heywood, J. T.,…Yancy, C. W. (2010). Improving evidence-based care for heart failure in outpatient cardiology practices: Primary results of the registry to improve the use of evidence-based heart failure therapies in the outpatient setting (IMPROVE HF). *Circulation, 12*, 585–596.

Foust, J. B., Naylor, M. D., Bixby, B., & Ratcliffe, S. J. (2012). Medication problems occurring at hospital discharge among older adults with heart failure. *Research in Gerontological Nursing, 5*(1), 25–33.

Fulton, J., & Baldwin, K. (2004). An annotated bibliography reflecting CNS practice and outcomes. *Clinical Nurse Specialist, 18*(1), 21–39.

Gawlinski, A. (2007). Evidence-based practice changes: Measuring the outcome. *AACN Advanced Critical Care, 18*(3), 320–322.

Gawlinski, A., & McCloy, K. (2006). Measuring outcomes in cardiovascular advanced practice nursing. In R. M. Kleinpell (Ed.), *Outcome assessment in advanced practice nursing* (pp. 139–186). New York, NY: Springer.

Gawlinski, A., & Rutledge, D. (2008). Selecting a model for evidence-based practice changes: A practical approach. *AACN Advanced Critical Care, 19*, 1–10.

Gillespie, U., Alassaad, A., Henrohn, D., Garmo, H., Hammarlund-Udenaes, M., Toss, H.,...Morlin, C. (2009). A comprehensive pharmacist intervention to reduce morbidity in patients 80 years or older. *Archives of Internal Medicine, 169*(9), 894–900.

Grady, K., Dracup, K., & Kennedy, G. (2000). Team management of patients with heart failure: A statement of healthcare professionals from the Cardiovascular Nursing Council of the American Heart Association. *Circulation, 102*, 2443–2456.

Greenhalgh, T. (2002). Integrating qualitative research into evidence based practice. *Endocrinology and Metabolism Clinics of North America, 31*(3), 583–601.

Guiffre, M. (1997). Designing research: Ex post facto designs. *Journal of Perianesthesia Nursing, 12*(3), 191–195.

Ho, P. M., Peterson, P. N., & Masoudi, F. A. (2008). Evaluating the evidence: Is there a rigid hierarchy? *Circulation, 118*(16), 1675–1684.

Holland, R., Battersby, J., Harvey, I., Lenaghan, E., Smith, J., & Hay. L. (2005). Systematic review of multidisciplinary interventions in heart failure. *Heart, 91*:899–906.

Horn, S. D., Gassaway, J., Pentz, L., & James, R. (2010). Practice-based evidence for clinical practice improvement: An alternative study design for evidence-based medicine. In E. J. S. Hovenga, M. R. Kidd, S. Garde, & C. H. L. Cossio (Eds.), *Health informatics* (pp. 446–460). Amsterdam, Netherlands: IOS Press.

Hughes, R. G. (2008). Tools and strategies for quality improvement and patient safety. In R. G. Hughes (Ed.), *An evidence-based handbook for nurses* (pp. 1–39). Washington, DC: Agency for Healthcare Research and Quality. Retrieved from http://www.ahrq.gov/qual/nursehdbk/docs/HughesR_QMBMP.pdf

Ingersoll, G. L. (2000). Evidence-based nursing: What it is and what it isn't. *Nursing Outlook, 48*(4), 151–152.

Institute of Medicine. (2001). *Crossing the quality chasm: A new health system for the 21st century.* Committee on Quality of Health Care in America. Washington, DC: National Academy Press.

Jack, B. W., Chetty, V. K., Anthony, D., Greenwald, J. L., Sanchez, G. M., Johnson, A. E.,...Culpepper, L. (2009). A reengineered hospital discharge program to decrease hospitalization: A randomized trial. *Annals of Internal Medicine, 150*(3), 178–187.

Joseph, A. M. (2007). The impact of nursing on patient and organizational outcomes. *Nursing Economics, 25*(1), 30–34.

Killeen, B. M., & Barnfather, S. J. (2005). A successful teaching strategy for applying evidence-based practice. *Nurse Educator, 30*(3), 127–132.

Kleinpell, R. M. (2003). Measuring advanced practice nursing outcomes: Strategies and resources. *Critical Care Nurse, 23*(1 Suppl), 6–10.

Kleinpell, R. M. (2007). APNs: Invisible champions? *Nursing Management, 38*(5), 18–22.

Kleinpell, R. M., & Gawlinski, A. (2005). Assessing outcomes in advanced practice nursing practice: The use of quality indicators and evidence-based practice. *AACN Advanced Critical Care, 16*(1), 43–57.

Kleinpell-Nowell, R., & Weiner, T. M. (1999). Measuring advanced practice nursing outcomes. *AACN Clinical Issues, 10*(3), 356–368.

Kosiborod, M., & Spertus, J. A. (2009). Careers in cardiovascular outcomes research. *Circulation, 102,* 76–81.

Kurtzman, E. T., & Corrigan, J. M. (2007). Measuring the contribution of nursing to quality, patient safety and health care outcomes. *Policy, Politics & Nursing Practice. 8*(1), 20–36

Kwan, Y., Fernandes, O. A., Nagge, J. J., Wong, G. G., Huh, J., Hurn, D. A., . . . Bajcar, J. M. (2007). Pharmacist medication assessments in a surgical preadmission clinic. *Archives of Internal Medicine, 167*(10), 1034–1040.

Landro, L. (2007, December 12). Keeping patients from landing back in the hospital. *Wall Street Journal.* Retrieved from http://www.inqri.org/newsitem/dec-12-2007

Lloyd-Jones, D., Adams, R. J., Brown, T. M., Carnethon, M., Dai, S., DeSimone, G., . . . Wylie-Rosett, J. (2010). Heart Disease and Stroke Statistics—2010 Update. A Report from the American Heart Association Statistics Committee and Stroke Statistics Subcommittee. *Circulation, 121*(7), 46–215. Retrieved from http://www.circ.ahajournals.org/content/121/7/e46

Lohr, K. N. (1988). Outcome measurement: Concepts and questions. *Inquiry, 25*(1), 37–50.

McGlynn, E. A., Asch, S. M., Adams, J., Keesey, J., Hicks, J., DeCristofaro, A., et al. (2003). The quality of health care delivered to adults in the United States. *New England Journal of Medicine, 348*(26), 2635–2645.

Melnyk, B. M., & Cole, R. (2011). Generating evidence through quantitative research. In B. M. Melnyk & E. Fineout-Overholt (Eds.), *Evidence-based practice in nursing & healthcare: A guide to best practice* (2nd ed., pp. 397–434). Philadelphia, PA: Lippincott Williams & Wilkins.

Meyer, S. C., & Miers, L. J. (2005). Cardiovascular surgeon and acute care nurse practitioner collaboration on post-operative outcomes. *AACN Clinical Issues: Advanced Practice in Acute & Critical Care, 16*(2), 149–158.

Miller, W. R. (2010). Qualitative research findings as evidence: Utility in nursing practice. *Clinical Nurse Specialist, 24*(4), 191–193.

Moorhead, S., Johnson, M., Maas, M. L., & Swanson, E. (2008). *Nursing outcomes classification (NOC)* (4th ed.). St. Louis, MO: Mosby.

Mueller, S. K., Sponsler, K. C., Kripalani, S., & Schnipper, J. L. (2012). Hospital-based medication reconciliation practices: A systematic review. *Archives of Internal Medicine, 172*(14), 1057–1069.

Newell, R., & Burnard, P. (2006). *Research for evidence-based practice.* Ames, IA: Blackwell Publishing.

Nicolay, C. R., Purkayastha, S., Greenhalgh, A., Benn, J., Chaturvedi. S., Phillips. N., & Darzi, A. (2012). A Systematic review of the application of quality improvement methodologies from the manufacturing industry to surgical healthcare. *British Journal of Surgery, 99*(3), 324–325.

Nielsen, G. A., Bartely, A., Coleman, E., Resar, R., Rutherford, P., Souw, D., & Taylor J. (2008). *Transforming care at the bedside how-to guide: Creating an ideal transition home for patients with heart failure*. Institute for Healthcare Improvement. Retrieved from www.IHI.org

Nolan, M. T., & Mock, V. (2000). *Measuring patient outcomes*. Thousand Oaks, CA: Sage Publications.

Oermann, M. H., & Floyd, J. A. (2002). Outcomes research: An essential component of the advanced practice nurse role. *Clinical Nurse Specialist, 16*(3), 140–146.

O'Mathúna, P. D., Fineout-Overholt E., & Johnston, L. (2011). Critically appraising quantitative evidence for clinical decision making. In B. M. Melnyk & E. Fineout-Overholt (Eds.), *Evidence-based practice in nursing & healthcare: A guide to best practice* (2nd ed., pp. 81–134). Philadelphia, PA: Lippincott Williams & Wilkins.

Parse, R. R. (2006). Outcomes: Saying what you mean. *Nursing Science Quarterly, 19*(3), 189.

Paul, S. (2000). Impact of a nurse-managed heart failure clinic: A pilot study. *American Journal of Critical Care, 9*, 140–146.

Polit, D. F., & Beck, C. T. (2012*). Nursing research: Generating and assessing evidence for nursing practice* (9th ed.). Philadelphia, PA: Lippincott Williams & Wilkins.

Powell, A. E., Rushmer, R. K., & Davies, H. T. O. (2008). *Systematic narrative review of quality improvement models in health care*. Edinburgh, Scotland: NHS Quality Improvement Scotland.

Powers, B. A. (2011). Generating evidence through qualitative research. In B. M.Melnyk & E. Fineout-Overholt (Eds.), *Evidence-based practice in nursing & healthcare: A guide to best practice* (2nd ed., pp. 435–448). Philadelphia, PA: Lippincott Williams & Wilkins.

Prevost, S. (2005). From evidence to outcomes: Did it work? [presentation abstract]. In *Proceedings of Sigma Theta Tau's 16th International Nursing Research Congress, Waikoloa, Hawaii.*

Purssell, E., & While, A. (2010). P = Nothing, or Why we should not teach healthcare students about statistics. *Nurse Education Today, 15*(2), 837–840.

Roger, V. L., Go, A. S., Lloyd-Jones, D. M., Benjamin, E. J., Berry, J. D., Borden, W. B., . . . Turner, M. B. (2012). Heart disease and stroke statistics—2012 Update: A report from the American Heart Association. *Circulation, 125*, 2–220.

Rosenberg, E. I., Bass, P. F., & Davidson, R. A. (2012). Arriving at correct conclusions: The importance of association, causality, and clinical significance. *Southern Medical Journal, 105*(3), 161–166.

Sackett, D. L., Richardson, W. S., Rosenberg, W., Haynes, R. B. (2000). *Evidence-based medicine: How to practice and teach EBM* (2nd ed.). Edinburgh, Scotland: Churchill Livingstone.

Sackett, D. L., Rosenberg, W. M., Gray, J. A., Haynes, R. B., & Richardson, W. S. (1996). Evidence based medicine: What it is and what it isn't. *British Medical Journal, 312*, 71–72.

Sousa, V. D., Driessnack, M., Mendes, I. A. C. (2007). An overview of research designs relevant to nursing: Part 1: Quantitative research designs. *Rev Latino-am Enfermagem, 15*(3), 502–507.

Stanik-Hutt, J. (2012). Translation of evidence to improve clinical outcomes. In K. M. White & S. Dudley-Brown (Eds.), *Translation of evidence into nursing and health care practice.* New York, NY: Springer.

Stetler, B. C. (2001). Updating the Stetler model of research utilization to facilitate evidence-based practice. *Nursing Outlook, 49*(6), 272–279.

Stetler, B. C. (2004). Evidence-based nursing: A long day's journey into the future. *Worldviews on Evidence-Based Nursing, 1*(1), 3–5.

Sullivan-Bolyai, S., & Bova, C. (2010). Experimental and quasi-experimental designs. In G. LoBiondo-Wood & J. Haber (Eds.), *Nursing research: Methods and critical appraisal for evidence-based practice* (7th ed., pp. 174–194). St. Louis, MO: Mosby Elsevier.

The Joint Commission. (2006). *Sentinel event alert, issue 35: Using medication reconciliation to prevent errors.* Retrieved from http://www.jointcommission. org/sentinel_event_alert_issue_35_using_medication_reconciliation_to_ prevent_errors

The Joint Commission. (2011). Acute myocardial infarction core measure sets. Retrieved September, 2012, from http://www.jointcommission.org/core_ measure_sets.aspx

Titler, M. G. (2004). Methods in translation science. *Worldviews on Evidence-Based Nursing, 1*(1), 38–48.

Titler , M. G. (2008). The evidence for evidence-based practice implementation. In R. G. Hughes (Ed.), *Patient safety and quality: An evidence-based handbook for nurses.* Rockville, MD: Agency for Healthcare Research and Quality. Retrieved from http://www.ahrq.gov/qual/nurseshdbk

Titler, M. G., Kleiber, C., Steelman, V. J., Rakel, B. A., Budreau, G., Everett, L. Q.,...Goode, C. J. (2001). The Iowa model of evidence-based practice to promote quality care. *Critical Care Nursing Clinics of North America, 13*(4), 497–509.

Urden, L. D. (1999). Outcome evaluation: An essential component for CNS practice. *Clinical Nurse Specialist, 13*(1), 39–46.

Walker, P. C., Bernstein, S. J., Jones, J. N., Piersma, J., Kim, H. W., Regal, R. E.,.... Flanders, S. A. (2009). Impact of a pharmacist-facilitated hospital discharge program: A quasi-experimental study. *Archives of Internal Medicine, 169*(21), 2003–2010.

Ward, M. M., Evans, T. C., Spies, A. J., Roberts, L. L., & Wakefield, D. S. (2006). National Quality Forum 30 safe practices: Priority and progress in Iowa hospitals. *American Journal of Medical Quality, 21*(2), 101–108.

Windle, P. E. (2006) Outcomes research: A paradigm shift for nursing research. *Journal of Stroke and Cerebrovascular Diseases, 15*(2), 64–65.

Yancy, C. W., Fonarow, G. C., Albert, N. M., Curtis, A. B., Stough, W. G., Gheorghiade, M.,...Walsh, M. N. (2010). Adherence to guideline recommended adjunctive heart failure therapies among outpatient cardiology practices (findings from IMPROVE HF). *American Journal of Cardiology, 105,* 255–260.

# Chapter 7: Ambulatory Nurse Practitioner Outcomes

*MARY JO GOOLSBY*

## Chapter Objectives

1. Review the purpose and importance of measuring and documenting outcomes of individual nurse practitioner (NP) practices.
2. Briefly summarize some of the literature on NP outcomes.
3. Describe the categories and examples of outcome measures relevant to ambulatory NPs.
4. Discuss practical considerations for selecting outcomes and a measurement approach.
5. Provide examples of how to approach outcome measurement in practice.
6. Discuss available resources relevant to primary care outcome measurement.

## Chapter Discussion Questions

1. Identify two potential measures in each of the following categories for a patient diagnosed with diabetes: physiologic, behavioral/ knowledge, and resource utilization.
2. Describe two enabling factors supporting NP entry into outcome measurement.

3. Describe an outcome measure plan for a patient diagnosed with a chronic illness, based on a national evidence-based clinical recommendation.
4. Provide a brief summary of how performance measures and outcome measures differ, with an example of each related to a specific condition.

T he potential outcomes of ambulatory care match the broad range of conditions and patients encountered in these settings, whether primary or specialty care. NPs in primary care settings manage patients with both chronic and acute conditions, while they also address health promotion and disease prevention for their patients. The incidence of many chronic conditions, such as hypertension, chronic obstructive pulmonary disease (COPD), and diabetes, is increasing and many of these patients routinely seek care in primary care settings, along with patients with acute conditions, such as pneumonia, urinary tract infections, and upper respiratory infections. In both primary and specialty ambulatory care, NPs will want to measure outcomes of routine management, as well as acute illnesses and exacerbations.

In the early 1980s, a newly prepared NP assigned to a military internal medicine clinic maintained a one-page form on each of her patients, most of whom had been referred for management of one or more chronic conditions. The forms allowed quick access to patient-specific information, such as blood pressure, lipids, blood glucose, and/or weight, recorded immediately following each encounter because the patients' health records were maintained outside the clinic. Before long curiosity prompted comparisons of the data over time. As the primary care provider for adults with chronic conditions, such as hypertension, diabetes, COPD, and heart failure, these forms allowed for extraction of clinical comparison information over time, and the NP's outcome measurement practice was born. Summaries of the data trends soon found their way into administrative reports describing the practice and benefits associated with referrals to the NP. Over the years, the NP's sophistication in measuring and analyzing outcomes of practice improved; however, these early activities in her initial NP position were as satisfying and rewarding as subsequent, more detailed efforts—and describe this author's initial interest and efforts in outcome measurement.

It can be intimidating to contemplate establishing a formal process for measuring outcomes. However, it is increasingly becoming expected that providers such as NPs measure their outcomes as an objective indication of their quality, safety, and cost effectiveness. This chapter builds on the early chapters of this textbook by providing a practical framework that ambulatory care NPs can use in implementing outcome measurement in their practices. It will: (1) review the purpose and importance of measuring and documenting outcomes of individual NP practices, (2) briefly summarize some of the literature on NP outcomes, (3) describe the categories and examples of outcome measures relevant to ambulatory NPs, (4) discuss practical considerations for selecting outcomes and a measurement approach, (5) provide examples of how to approach outcome measurement in practice, and (6) discuss available resources relevant to primary care outcome measurement (see Table 7.1).

## IMPORTANCE/PURPOSE OF PRIMARY CARE OUTCOME MEASUREMENT

As noted in earlier chapters, there are many reasons for conducting outcome measurement in practice. Outcome research should ultimately improve the health of our patients. Further, there are many stakeholders interested in how and to what degree we improve the health of those we serve. These stakeholders include our current and potential patients, employers, colleagues, payors, policy makers, and others. They are interested in knowing how much NP care costs and saves, as well as what precisely NPs do in their patient encounters and the objective patient-centered benefits of that care. Ambulatory providers who receive fee-for-service payments from the Centers for Medicare & Medicaid Services are increasingly expected to participate in the Physician Quality Reporting System (PQRS). Not specific to physicians, PQRS reporting can result in incentive payments and/or payment adjustments. It is a major example of the increasing expectation for public reporting of data by health care systems, organizations, and providers in smaller practices. As practitioners of a relatively new role created in the mid-1960s, NPs must continue to document the outcomes of their care.

Evaluation of clinical outcomes is now an expectation of the NP role. The National Organization of Nurse Practitioner Faculties lists a number of competencies relative to outcome measurement in the 2012

Table 7.1  *Ambulatory Outcome Measures*

| Outcome Category | Outcome Examples |
|---|---|
| Physiologic status | Vital signs |
| | Physical examination findings |
| | Laboratory studies |
| Psychosocial status | Mentation |
| | Mood and affect |
| | Coping status |
| | Social function |
| Functional status | ADL function |
| | IADL function |
| Behavioral activities and knowledge | Performance of therapeutics |
| | Problem-solving ability |
| | Knowledge test scores |
| Symptom control | Pain |
| | Fatigue |
| | Dyspnea |
| | Nausea |
| | Incontinence |
| Patient perception | QOL |
| | Satisfaction with care |
| Resource utilization | Hospital readmission rates |
| | Emergency visits |
| | Unplanned office visits |
| | Health care costs |
| Performance measures | Availability of recommended resources |
| | Implementation of recommended practices |

ADL, (routine) activities of daily living; IADL, instrumental activities of daily living.

NP Core Competencies (National Organization of Nurse Practitioner Faculties, 2012). Examples of outcome-related competencies are evident throughout the domains, including using evidence to continuously improve the quality of care; evaluating the relationships among factors, such as cost, quality, and so on; and improving outcomes through application of clinical investigative skills.

## SUMMARY OF EXISTING PRIMARY CARE NP OUTCOME LITERATURE

The published research on NP outcomes has consistently supported the quality and cost effectiveness of NP practice. In 1974, a classic report of the Burlington Trial documented outcomes in mortality, as well as physical, emotional, and social function, concluding that NP and physician outcomes were comparable (Spitzer et al., 1974). The Congressional Budget Office reviewed studies on NP practice and outcomes in 1979, with the conclusion that the NPs' outcomes, diagnoses, and management were at least as good as those of physicians. In 1986, the Office of Technology Assessment came to the same conclusions. Later, meta-analyses of NP care had similar findings (Brown & Grimes, 1995; Horrocks, Anderson, & Salisbury, 2002; Laurant et al., 2004), as have additional review articles (Cunningham, 2004). Mundinger et al. (2000) and Lenz, Mundinger, Kane, Hopkins, and Lin (2004) described primary care outcomes of patients assigned to either physician or NP, finding equivalent outcomes for both sets of patients. Regarding cost effectiveness of NP care, studies have also consistently demonstrated that NPs provide quality care efficiently with reduced cost, compared with physicians (Burl, Bonner, & Rao, 1994; Chenowith, Martin, Penkowski, & Raymond, 2005; Office of Technology Assessment, 1981; Paez & Allen, 2006; Roblin et al., 2004). More recently, Newhouse et al. (2011) conducted a systematic review of the published literature (1990–2008) on NPs and other advanced practice nurses (APNs), confirming that the evidence continues to support high-quality outcomes associated with NP care.

## MEASURES RELEVANT TO AMBULATORY CARE PRACTICE

The outcomes selected by a given NP will depend on factors such as the type of practice, areas of interest, and available resources. Even in a focused subspecialty-type practice, there are several options to measure. Outcomes can be categorized in many ways. One categorization would classify outcomes as best demonstrating one of the following: physiologic status, psychosocial status, functional status, behavioral activities, and knowledge, symptom control, patient perception, or resource utilization. Within each category, there are likely measures relevant to any area of practice. Another common area of measurement that does not fit the definition of outcome but which must be considered relevant to contemporary ambulatory care involves performance measures.

Physiologic status involves those biomarkers that are usually readily available in the course of routine patient care. They include routinely collected vital signs, such as blood pressure, pulse, and temperature; physical exam findings, such as lung sounds and weight; and laboratory values, such as glucose and lipid levels. Abnormal findings in these physiologic markers are often the defining characteristics of health problems and the targets of care; thus, they provide a means of later following response to and outcomes of treatment. For instance, the outcomes of diabetes, hypertension, or hyperlipidemia management should include measurement of blood glucose/glycosylated hemoglobin, blood pressure, or lipids, respectively. A feature of physiologic measures, such as vital signs and laboratory findings, is that they are objective and quantified. Laboratory studies, in particular, are usually validated against some control procedure. The quality of vital signs and physical examination findings is dependent on the quality of the equipment and technique used in obtaining the measures.

Although psychosocial status includes measures often included in the history and which are qualitative in nature, psychosocial measures can be quantified through use of validated tools. Examples of psychosocial outcomes include mentation, mood and affect, attitude, coping status, and general social functioning. While psychosocial status outcomes often involve some degree of subjectivity, there are a number of validated and quantitative scales available, depending on the focus of concern. For instance, there are validated scales to measure depression and anxiety, confusion, and dementia. Depending on the outcome of interest, sources are often available to discuss measurement options. For example, the Mini-Mental State Examination is a common tool for cognitive function, well published and validated. Harvan and Cotter (2006) review and compare a range of dementia screening tools for use in clinical practice.

Specific functional status involves ability to achieve routine activities of daily living (ADL) and instrumental activities of daily living (IADL), and can be measured with global functional scales or measures more specific to select abilities such as mobility and communication.

A number of measures of functionality exist, including the Physical Activities of Daily Living and Instrumental Activities of Daily Living scales, as well as the 10-minute Screener for Geriatric Conditions. Others include the Functional Independence Measure Scale and the Barthel Scale.

Behavioral activities and knowledge include areas of both therapeutic competence and understanding of treatments. Therapeutic competence involves the ability to perform the skills necessary to carry out prescribed or recommended treatments, as well as the ability to solve problems related to therapeutic guidance. Understanding is related to basic knowledge regarding recommended diet, medications, and treatments without a behavioral component. Knowledge tests have been developed and described in the literature for select conditions. Measurement of behavioral activity competence is more complex to assess than knowledge, by comparison.

Symptom control is another area of outcomes where the history often includes the basic related details, but requires further quantification to serve as an outcome measurement. Examples of the symptoms that could be quantified as outcome measures include level of pain, fatigue, dyspnea, nausea, constipation, diarrhea, and incontinence. There are a number of validated scales to measure many symptoms, and pain scales are perhaps among the better known. One means of assessing specific symptoms would be to use a 10-centimeter visual analog scale (VAS), where the poles of the scale represent symptom extreme (complete absence of the symptom versus worst possible degree of the symptom), or having the symptom similarly rated using a numerical scale.

Patient perceptual category includes areas such as a patient's perceived quality of life (QOL) and expressed satisfaction with care. QOL refers to patients' satisfaction with their life circumstances and sense of well-being. It can further relate to a more narrowed focus of satisfaction with specific components of the patient's life, for instance, with how a specific symptom affects life quality. There are general and condition-specific QOL scales, and a VAS can also be used to measure perceived QOL. In contrast, satisfaction refers to satisfaction with the patient experience and care received. Patient perceptions also include a patient's determination of progress toward meeting goals. For instance, patients can identify their personal goals for treatment, then subsequently rate the degree to which they are able to accomplish the goal over time.

Resource utilization involves a range of outcomes, such as numbers of hospitalizations or readmissions, length of stay for any admission, the cost of care, and unplanned office or emergency visits. In many cases, it is difficult to accurately identify all hospitalizations or emergency visits, along with the cost for each, as dependent on the patient's recall. However, within a well-defined system such as a managed care organization, accountable care organization, or hospital-anchored system, pulling electronic or paper records of other visits, admissions, and associated costs are more easily accomplished. In addition to identifying any change in resource utilization associated with care, cost analysis of the actual care provides another outcome indicator.

Recommendations for performance, quality, and outcome assessment measures are available through a number of national initiatives and repositories, such as the National Quality Forum (NQF), the National Committee for Quality Assurance (NCQA), the National Quality Measures Clearinghouse (NQMC), and the AQA (formerly Ambulatory Care Quality Alliance). These entities are generally engaged in inter professional development, recommendation, and/or dissemination of quality measures for systems, organizations, and providers, so that it is critical to identify measures created for outpatient practice. An increasingly important source of outcome measures is available through the PQRS program.

Many recommended measures include a focus on performance, rather than the ultimate outcome. It is worthwhile considering the difference between performance measures and outcomes of care. Performance measures document what is performed or done, rather than the outcomes of that practice. Performance measures sometimes serve as surrogates for actual outcomes in various reporting programs. With the increasing availability of electronic health records, queries of coded procedures allow ready identification of completed clinical activities. Certainly, current "pay for performance" mandates are based primarily on documenting the resources available and the processes implemented, as opposed to actual outcomes, so that incentives are based on providers documenting activities such as making appropriate referrals, ordering and monitoring of suggested laboratory studies, and administration or ordering of recommended treatments (e.g., pneumonia vaccines for persons ≥65 years of age or older, or beta blockers for patients experiencing a myocardial infarction) rather than the associated outcomes that are subject to a number of intervening influences. Although clinical recommendations often imply that specific activities should result in improved outcomes, it is ideal to document the results of the performance measures, as well as the performance, to validate the desired result.

## SELECTING PRACTICAL OUTCOMES OF INTEREST

With the broad range of potential outcomes of primary care NP practice, the dilemma becomes determining what should and can be measured. It is advisable to start with an answerable question and then proceed to select the available measures and/or type of data that will contribute to the answer. Certainly one deciding factor should be the provider's own areas of interest and questions. Other considerations will include the context in which the care is delivered, the resources available to support outcome measurement, and anticipated patient variables.

The decision to measure outcomes of practice may be based on questions the NP has regarding how his or her practice outcomes compare to some benchmark or published report. In practices with an established performance improvement (PI) process, there may be baseline data that support the need for improvements and that trigger outcome measures. Just as PI activities typically focus on conditions of large volume, high cost, and high risk, these same three criteria are helpful in guiding decisions on where to expend energy in outcome measures.

The practice context is important, as practices vary in the range and quality of resources helpful to outcome measurement. The progress toward broad implementation of electronic health records in ambulatory practice offers great promise for increased ability to automate queries regarding specific outcomes or activities performed. Practices with a well-designed electronic health record have an advantage when it comes to identifying relevant patients and tracking and measuring outcomes and performance. When selecting outcome data to be collected from an electronic system, it is critical to ensure that data are accurately coded and entered. The use of narrative notations rather than pre-coded options limits the utility of pulling needed data once entered. It also remains critical that the language of the system accurately fits the data and the practice involved. Another organizational consideration involves a philosophical expectation or mission that could mandate select measures used for outcomes and collegial support for the effort. Because it is rare for a health-care provider to be the sole provider in an ambulatory clinic, it is often helpful for the team of providers to collaborate and select clinical topics and outcomes of interest. Moores, Breslin, and Burns (2002) describe the process of talking through problems with peers as a means of bringing the issue into focus as an answerable question.

Another type of resource specific to practices is the type of economic resources available for patient care. If a practice has a largely indigent population, the type of measures readily available may differ from one with a more affluent patient population, unless the practice has additional sources of funding to support patient care needs.

Patient-specific variables must be considered when planning outcome measurement. For instance, patients who tend to seek episodic care are not easily followed over time and short-term outcomes will be important rather than outcomes that are measured over time. For episodic visits, sometimes a performance measure may be helpful, such as the percentage of patients with a given diagnosis who receive or do not receive antibiotics, or the percentage of patients meeting specified criteria who receive appropriate immunization during visits. Of course, efforts to enhance continuity could be implemented and then long-term follow-up included as a measure itself.

In considering relevant outcome measures, ambulatory NPs must also consider what is recommended for select conditions; published clinical recommendations or guidelines provide an excellent source for outcome selection. These often identify a number of measures that could be used to track response to treatment, including specific validated tools. When focusing on a specific condition, it is often favorable to use condition-specific measures that will be more sensitive to change with treatment of that select condition whenever possible. For instance, while asthma affects psychosocial and functional outcomes, these may also be affected by a number of other comorbid conditions, so that these other conditions confound the response to care. By measuring specific asthma variables, outcomes are more easily attributed to treatment of that specific condition. There are scales to assess outcomes of treatment of conditions, such as arthritis, asthma, fibromyalgia, and benign prostatic hyperplasia, in addition to the relevant physiologic markers, such as pulmonary functions, blood glucose, and blood pressure. For varied conditions, generic outcomes could be used. For instance, generic functionality measures, or SF-36, are broadly used. Scales of QOL could be responsive to a number of health changes, as would pain scales.

When the topic of interest has been identified and feasible outcome measures identified based on the characteristics of the practice, patient population, and providers, a plan should be written to guide the continuing effort. While most NPs may be more comfortable with associating the outcome measurement process with continuous quality improvement (CQI) or PI than with more formal "research," outcome measurement is a form of exploratory research (Breslin, Burns, & Moores, 2002) and the methodological issues are important considerations. An important benefit of establishing a written plan early in the planning process is that the plan will help to identify any related costs as well as added resources needed.

In addition, even with CQI/PI projects, it is advisable to discuss the plans with a representative from the affiliated institutional review board or research board, to determine whether a formal application and approval are expected.

## CASE EXAMPLES

### The Shotgun Approach

The first case is an example of how using a "shotgun" approach to outcome measurement can "backfire." A newly hired NP inherited management of a disease management practice for patients with asthma and/or COPD, to find that her predecessor had created a very detailed plan for measuring the outcomes of the practice. At the baseline, initial visit, and again at 3, 6, 12, and 18 months, patients would be assessed with a focused history and physical, as well as by completing the following measures: the Center for Epidemiology Depression Scale, the State-Trait Depression and Anxiety Scale, the SF-36 Medical Outcomes Scale, the Modified Dyspnea Index, a record of peak flow usage, history of tobacco usage, medication list, a number of VASs (QOL, dyspnea), and a 6-minute walk with pulse oximetry, breath sounds, peak flow, and pulmonary functions before and after. In addition, the system's records were queried at these intervals for any emergency department visits and hospitalizations, as well as the costs and charges for each. Needless to say, even in a 1-hour visit, it was hard to conceive how anyone would accomplish all of the necessary outcome measures, if time were to be spent on patient problem solving, support, and education. The clinic NP provider had recently resigned and a temporary part-time NP was filling in, but perhaps not surprisingly, patients rarely returned after the second visit.

The NP manager and interim NP provider reviewed the processes and interviewed some of the practice's patients. Patient interviews ascertained that they saw little benefit in participating in all of the multi-item scales and found numerous depression, anxiety, medical outcomes, and dyspnea scales difficult to understand and confusing. Moreover, outcome measures had become the focus of the clinic, rather than the delivery of care.

Procedures were changed so that the focus would be patient-centered care delivery, and necessary outcomes would be embedded in the encounter record, with the number of outcomes significantly abbreviated. What did seem feasible was to record responses from dyspnea

VAS and other relevant symptom ratings (e.g., shortness of breath, cough, and interrupted sleep), peak flow averages, and tobacco use, as well as to quarterly system queries to document a cost analysis of resource utilization. Subsequently, the continuity of care immediately improved; patients remained in the clinic, and the outcomes improved as patients were being educated on their conditions. The physiologic measures showed improvement. The population's emergency department visits were cut in half, and the number of hospitalizations was decreased to approximately 15% of the historical data following enrollment to the clinic. On an ongoing basis, the clinic has been able to demonstrate positive outcomes and to serve as a model for other disease-managed clinics.

### Triangulation

An earlier chapter describes combining quantitative and qualitative efforts in outcome measurements to provide for triangulation. An NP involved in the pulmonary management described above monitored tobacco use in her patients. Instituting the "5A" approach (ask about patient's habits, advise of consequence of smoking, assess willingness to quit, assist with cessation plan development, and arrange for follow up) to smoking cessation and providing support based on her patient's level of readiness, she wanted to measure the outcomes of the process.

She asked all newly referred patients whether or not they smoked and, for those who did smoke, the number of cigarettes used per day. Thus, the measures used were tobacco use ("Yes/No") and number of cigarettes, collected from each patient at the first visit and again at 3, 6, and 12 months. At baseline and at 3 and 6 months, the percentage of patients who smoked was 45%, 43%, and 49%, respectively, and the number of packs per day for patients who smoked was 0.91, 0.65, and 0.60, respectively. Certainly, the decrease in amount of tobacco used per smoker was positive, but the anticipated outcome had included a decreasing percentage of smokers, not an increase.

The NP instituted a series of interviews with the patients to explore the tobacco use. For instance, she considered that prior to the first appointment, a number of patients might have "quit" smoking due to initial concern over their respiratory symptoms, but were unable to maintain abstinence. Instead, she found that the percentage of her patients who smoked was actually stable over time; however, some patients indicated that they had not been forthright in sharing whether they smoked during their initial visit, concerned that their care might be affected or that they would be lectured for the practice.

Only after they developed a comfort with the new provider, they were more likely to be open about their tobacco use.

The series of interviews also identified a number of other issues related to tobacco use for her patients. When she identified that her standard practice was not successful in helping her patients quit smoking, the NP used the findings to obtain external funding for an individualized tobacco-cessation program. The funded program provided a range of resources for patients during the smoking cessation process and did result in a decreased percentage of smokers. However, without the qualitative interviews, the necessary information would not have been identified to further improve practice and later outcomes.

## APPROACHES TO OVERCOMING POTENTIAL BARRIERS TO OUTCOME MEASUREMENT

There are many potential barriers to outcome measurement. These include lack of confidence, time, and support, as well as limited data analysis resources.

Primary care NPs are likely to struggle with where to start with outcome measurement and to be intimidated by the concept. Primary care is fraught with many competing demands and the need to remain current on the recommended approach to many conditions. This may leave little time for the individual NP to prepare himself or herself for practice in outcome measures and with the broad range of conditions encountered, to even decide what measures are important. Depending on the practice setting, there may not be a significant level of support for outcome measures or the emphasis may be on the basic performance measures rather than actual outcomes. Finally, given availability of outcome measures, many NPs will lack the initial knowledge of how to analyze the data.

Luckily, there are several resources that will facilitate the outcome measurement process. Resnick (2006) provides a four-step process to implementing outcomes research. While her discussion is directed toward implementation of projects that will develop new and generalizable knowledge rather than limited findings to one practice setting, the steps provide examples of how to go about the process as well as encouragement for NPs contemplating the process. The other resources cited earlier also provide guidance.

Key facilitators include the NP's desire to improve practice and to optimize the outcomes of care. In fact, an ideal way to launch outcome measurement may be through practice improvement projects. Practice, or performance, improvement (PI) is an area of growing interest by multiple professions. Physicians, in particular, have PI expectations as part of their maintenance of certification requirements. Thus, in multi-professional ambulatory practices, there is a growing tendency for PI to be implemented and often to involve team efforts—with all providers participating. NPs often are familiar with the PI process, regardless of which particular model they have used in their prior nursing practice. PI encompasses the principles important to overall outcome measurement; the target variables should be important to the practice, based on evidence, designed to measure improvement, and be practical to identify. A benefit of a PI focus is that there are a number of recognized PI models (PDCA, IMPROVE, and PDSA) that describe a step-by-step approach for measurement over time.

Another factor facilitating NP efforts in outcome measures is the clinical expertise that NPs bring to their practice. A sound knowledge of a clinical area supports understanding of expected outcomes of care, which should provide direction on how to proceed in measurement activities.

Finally, even when NPs practice in a setting without other providers with similar interests in outcome measurement, it can be very helpful for NPs to establish a collaborative process with providers in other settings who have similar needs. Through collaboration, the providers are able to work together to establish outcome processes and strategies for success. Alternatively, an external mentor can be sought to coach through the process. Finally, there are networks for practice-based research in which providers can participate to become involved in the research process.

## Answers to Chapter Discussion Questions

1. Physiologic: HbA1C; weight
   Behavioral/knowledge: Demonstrated self-injection technique; diabetes knowledge scores.
   Resource utilization: Emergency visits for hyper/hypoglycemia; pharmacotherapy costs.

2. NPs in collegial practices can find outcome measurement easier to accomplish when they are able to engage others within the practice, so that the overall requirements are less daunting. Another strategy involves taking advantage of the growing interest in practice improvement methods, selecting one of the recognized models, such as PDSA, to establish a focused project within the practice. Selecting variables that can be abstracted over time and relevant to an identifiable patient population from a well-designed electronic health record is helpful, simplifying the data-collection process.

3. Using the example of asthma guidelines (National Asthma Education Program Report 3: Guidelines for the Diagnosis and Management of Asthma), the following are recommended to monitor asthma periodically in clinical visit: responses to asthma assessment tools, such as the Asthma Control Test or the Asthma Therapy Assessment Questionnaire and spirometry, provide quantitative measures to follow over time as documentation of treatment outcomes.

4. Performance measures provide data on the completion of specific activities, depicting the degree to which recommended practices are accomplished. For diabetes, this could relate to documenting the percentage of patients for whom A1c is documented or the percentage of patients with diabetes for whom a retinal examination is documented. Performance measures differ from outcome measures, which would involve documenting the percentage of patients whose A1c was less than a selected level.

## WEB LINKS

The following organizations are excellent sources of current and developing measurement resources:

AQA (formerly Ambulatory Care Quality Alliance) ■ www.aqaalliance.org

National Committee for Quality Assurance (NCQA) ■ www.ncqa.org

National Quality Forum (NQF) ■ (www.qualityforum.org)

National Quality Measures Clearinghouse (NQMC) ■ www.qualitymeasures.ahrq.gov

Office of National Coordinator for Health Information Technology (HITECH) ■ www.healthit.hhs.gov

Physician Quality Reporting System ■ (www.cms.gov/medicare/quality-initiatives-patient-assessment-instruments/pqrs)

## REFERENCES

Breslin, E., Burns, M., & Moores, P. (2002). Challenges of outcomes research for nurse practitioners. *Journal of the American Academy of Nurse Practitioners, 14*, 138–143.

Brown, S., & Grimes, D. (1995). A meta-analysis of nurse practitioners and nurse midwives in primary care. *Nursing Research, 44*, 332–339.

Burl, J., Bonner, A., & Rao, M. (1994). Demonstration of the cost-effectiveness of a nurse practitioner/physician team in primary care teams. *HMO Practice, 8*, 156–157.

Chenowith, D., Martin, N., Penkowski, J., & Raymond, I. (2005). A benefit-cost analysis of a worksite nurse practitioner program. First impressions. *Journal of Occupational and Environmental Medicine, 47*, 1110–1116.

Congressional Budget Office. (1979). *Physician extenders: Their current and future role in medical care delivery.* Washington, DC: U.S. Government Printing Office.

Cunningham, R. (2004). Advanced practice nursing outcomes: A review of selected empirical literature. *Oncology Nursing Forum, 31*, 219–232.

Horrocks, S., Anderson, E., & Salisbury, C. (2002). Systematic review of whether nurse practitioners working in primary care can provide equivalent care to doctors. *British Medical Journal, 324*, 819–823.

Laurant, M., Reeves, D., Hermens, R., Braspenning, J., Grol, R., & Sibbald, B. (2004). Substitution of doctors by nurses in primary care. *Cochrane Database of Systematic Reviews, 2004*(1), Article CD001271. doi: 10.1002/14651858. CD001271.pub2.

Lenz, E. R., Mundinger, M. O., Kane, R. L., Hopkins, S. C., & Lin, S. X. (2004). Primary care outcomes in patients treated by nurse practitioners or physicians: Two-year follow-up. *Medical Care Research and Review, 61*, 332–351.

Moores, P., Breslin, E., & Burns, M. (2002). Structure and process of outcomes research for nurse practitioners. *Journal of the American Academy of Nurse Practitioners, 14*, 471–474.

Mundinger, M., Kane, R., Lenz, E., Totten, A., Tsai, W., Cleary, P., ... Shelanski, M. (2000). Primary care outcomes in patients treated by nurse practitioners or physicians: A randomized trial. *Journal of the American Medical Association, 283*, 59–68.

National Organization of Nurse Practitioner Faculties. (2012). Nurse practitioner core compeTencies, Amended 2012. Retrieved Sept 5, 2012, from http://nonpf.com/associations/10789/files/NPCoreCompetenciesFinal2012.pdf

Newhouse, R., Stanik-Hutt, J., White, K., et al. (2011). Advanced practice nurse outcomes, 1990–2008: A systematic review. *Nursing Economics, 29*(5) 1–22.

Office of Technology Assessment. (1981). *The cost and effectiveness of nurse practitioners.* Washington, DC: U.S. Government Printing Office.

Office of Technology Assessment. (1986). *Nurse practitioners, physician assistants, and certified nurse midwives: A policy analysis.* Washington, DC: U.S. Government Printing Office.

Paez, K., & Allen, J. (2006). Cost-effectiveness of nurse practitioner management of hypercholesterolemia following coronary revascularization. *Journal of the American Academy of Nurse Practitioners, 18*, 436–444.

Resnick, B. (2006). Outcomes research: You do have the time! *Journal of the American Academy of Nurse Practitioners, 18*, 505–509.

Roblin, D., Howard, D., Becker, E., et al. (2004). Use of midlevel practitioners to achieve labor cost savings in the primary care practice of an MCO. *Health Services Research, 39*, 607–626.

Spitzer, W., Sackett, D., Sibley, J., Roberts, R., Gent, M., Kergin, D., ... Olynich, A. (1974). The Burlington randomized trial of the nurse practitioner. *New England Journal of Medicine, 290*, 252–256.

# Chapter 8: Assessing Outcomes in Clinical Nurse Specialist Practice

JUDY E. DAVIDSON, MELISSA A. JOHNSON,
AND ANNE W. ALEXANDROV

## Chapter Objectives

1. List four different categories of outcomes measured as a product of clinical nurse specialist (CNS) work in hierarchical order of importance.
2. Describe an example of how to measure time-on activities, process measures, surrogate measures, and actual outcomes of CNS practice.
3. Describe how to integrate the CNS spheres of influence and categorical outcomes of a CNS project or activity.
4. Describe how outcomes from a project align with organizational goals, objectives, or pillars of performance.

## Chapter Discussion Questions

1. List four different categories of outcomes discussed in this chapter in hierarchical order of importance.
2. Using your own practice or experience during clinical rotations, describe one example of how you could personally measure time-on

activities, compliance with process measures, a surrogate measure of cost or quality, and an actual impact on patient or staff outcomes.

3. Select one project that you have been involved in or the plan for your capstone project, and make a table to include at least one measure for each of the four categories of outcomes listed in Question 1. Map these outcomes for each sphere of influence, as done in Exhibit 8.8.

4. For the project discussed in Question 3, describe how the outcomes align to organizational goals or objectives.

5. Describe the pros and cons of recording activities and tracking outcomes.

**C**linical nurse specialists (CNSs) work on an advanced level of practice in three spheres of influence: (1) patient/clients, (2) nurses and nursing practice, and (3) systems and organizations (National Association of Clinical Nurse Specialists [NACNS], 2004). As a result, CNSs contribute to promoting positive outcomes in a number of ways. Understanding the effect of CNS care on outcomes is important in today's health care system. Furthermore, the shift in the health care delivery system over the past several years to focus on outcomes management requires that CNSs be able to articulate and demonstrate their contributions to outcomes, both clinical and economic. The health reform legislation signed by President Obama in 2010 and the American Recovery and Reinvestment Act of 2009 require changes in health care organizations related to financing and the delivery of health care. Additionally, the emerging pay-for-performance paradigm is supported by payee (hospitals and individuals) in compliance with numerous process indicators, but is rapidly shifting toward the inclusion of potent outcome indicators to document health care quality (National Quality Forum, 2012). Many programs have resulted because of these events, such as accountable-care organizations, which rely heavily on interventions solely within the nursing scope of practice. In addition, increases in the numbers of people with insurance coverage will increase demands on the primary care system (Committee on the Robert Wood Johnson Foundation Initiative on the Future of Nursing at the Institute of Medicine, 2010). Much of the work of the CNS is focused around achieving quality outcomes while balancing cost-containment issues. In a cost-containment environment, communicating information about outcomes of CNS practice is paramount to the survival of the CNS as an advanced practice nurse (APN) (Davidson, 2011; Scott, 1999; Wojner, 2001). The purpose of this chapter is to describe a variety of strategies to select, measure, analyze, and promote outcomes using a hierarchical model familiar to operational leaders. Examples will be provided, including a case example and crosswalk, to visualize how outcome measures align to the CNS spheres of influence.

## FRAMEWORK FOR MEASURING CNS OUTOMES

In 1998, the NACNS published the *Statement on Clinical Nurse Specialist Practice and Education* (NACNS, 2004). Core competencies were revised and published by the NACNS in 2010 (National CNS Competency Task Force, 2010). Within these documents are descriptions of core CNS competencies and outcomes of practice. The competencies and outcomes are articulated in the spheres of influence that clearly differentiate the practice and outcomes of the CNS from other APNs. Although impact on the spheres of influence is important, it is critical to articulate the value of the CNS to nonclinicians in an understandable manner. Table 8.1 outlines categories of outcomes of CNS practice and roles across three spheres of influence, which are reflective of the CNS core competencies. Table 8.2 expands the outline of assessment of CNS practice to include the focus of practice, performance of subroles, and economic impact, in addition to the three spheres of influence. Using these categories can be helpful in identifying the impact of the CNS role and specific outcomes. Communicating outcomes of CNS work to the entire organization is an essential component to making a business case for retaining the CNS role during austere economic times (Amber, Carreon, Agan, Johnson, & Cahill, 2012; Davidson, 2010, 2011).

A number of studies have demonstrated the impact of CNS care on outcomes and have highlighted the importance of measuring the outcomes of CNS-led initiatives, program development, and patient care interventions (Cunningham, 2004; Dickerson, Wu, & Kennedy, 2006; Duffy, 2002; Forster et al., 2005; Fulton, 2006; Fulton & Baldwin, 2004; Hamilton & Hawley, 2006; Larsen, Neverett, & Larsen, 2001; Ley, 2001; McCabe, 2005; Prevost, 2002; Willoughby & Burroughs, 2001).

Table 8.1 *Categories of Outcomes of CNS Practice and Roles Across Three Spheres of Influence*

| Categories of Outcomes in Patient/Client Sphere | Categories of Outcomes in Nursing Personnel Sphere | Categories of Outcomes in Organization/Network Sphere |
|---|---|---|
| Programs of care are designed for specific populations (e.g., oncology, specific ethnic groups) | Knowledge and skill development needs of nursing personnel are profiled | Clinical problems are articulated within the context of the particular organization or network |
| Phenomena of concern with etiologies requiring nursing interventions are identified | **State-of-the-art knowledge and skills are reflected in registered nurse practice** | Patient care processes reflect continuous improvements that benefit the system |
| **Nursing therapeutics target specific etiologies** | The research base for innovations is articulated, understandable, and accessible | Policies are evidence-based and enhance the practice of nurse providers and multidisciplinary teams |
| **Nursing therapeutics, in combination with medical therapeutics, where appropriate, result in achievement of goals for prevention, alleviations, or reduction of symptoms, functional problems or risk behaviors** | **Nurses articulate nursing's unique contributions to patient care and expected nurse-sensitive outcomes** | **Innovative models of practice are developed, piloted, evaluated, and incorporated as appropriate across the continuum of care** |
| Health care plans are appropriate for meeting client needs within available resources | **Nurses solve patient care problems at the care delivery level** | Innovations in practice contribute to the achievement of quality, cost-effective outcomes for populations of patients |
| **Real and potential unintended consequences are errors are prevented** | **Desired patient outcomes are achieved through the synergistic effect of collaborative practice between nursing and other providers** | Stakeholders (nurses, other health care professionals, and management) share a common vision of practice outcomes |
| Nurse-sensitive outcomes are explicated | Nursing career enhancement programs are ongoing, accessible, innovative, and effective | Decision makers within the institution are informed regarding practice problems, factors contributing to the problems, and the significance of those problems with respect to outcomes and costs |

| | | Nursing care initiatives and programs are aligned with the organization's strategic imperatives, mission, and vision |
|---|---|---|
| Effective interventions are incorporated into guidelines for practice | Nursing personnel experience enhanced self-efficacy in patient care | |
| Interventions that do not meet evaluation standards are discontinued | Nursing personnel experience job satisfaction | |
| Collaboration with patient/client as well as physicians and other health care professionals occurs as appropriate | Competent nursing personnel are retained | |
| Innovative educational programs for patients, families, and groups are developed, implemented, and evaluated | Nursing personnel are engaged in learning | |
| Transitions across the continuum of care are smooth | Educational programs for nursing personnel focused on advancing the practice of nursing are developed, implemented, and evaluated | |
| Reports of new clinical phenomena and/or interventions are published | **The overall cost of care is reduced through judicious purchase and use of resources that enhance quality of patient care outcomes** | |

**Note:** Outcomes directly associated with CNS practice are **bolded**; other outcomes are reflective of sub-roles CNSs may use to indirectly influence practice outcomes.
**Source:** Adapted from NACNS (2004).

**Table 8.2 Summary of Assessments of CNSs Practice**

| Focus of Practice | Examples of Types of Assessments/Data | Examples of Sources of Evidence |
|---|---|---|
| Performance of subroles | Implementation of job expectation as advanced practice clinician, educator, consultant, and utilizer of research | Time-on activities logs/journals and summaries<br>Peer review and evaluations of staff nurses, and other health-care professional<br>Portfolio of products of practice |
| Client sphere | Morbidity, mortality data<br>Symptom experience<br>Functional status<br>Mental status<br>Stress level<br>Client satisfaction with care<br>Burden of care<br>Effective self-care behaviors/reduced risk behaviors<br>Avoidance of complications<br>Quality of life | Hospital databases<br>Instruments that specifically measure changes in patient problems and achievement of goals/outcomes of care from both nurse and client perspectives<br>Surrogate indices:<br>Morbidity, mortality, rehospitalization, discharge destination<br>Clinical data such as laboratory and x-ray reports<br>Chart audits, risk management information |
| Nursing Personnel Sphere | Recruitment and retention successes<br>Improved job satisfaction<br>Improvements in nursing personnel competency<br>Decreased cost of products and other resources used in patient care | Information from human resource department<br>Attendance at staff development meetings, chart audits<br>Financial data |
| Systems sphere | Length of stay, recidivism, use of post discharge health services<br>Achievement of benchmarks<br>Patient satisfaction<br>Workforce redesign/patient care | Systems databases including data from hospital, postdischarge services, physician offices<br>Benchmark data from internal data and comparison data provided by state and national sources<br>Satisfaction surveys<br>Nursing report cards |
| Economic impact | Revenue analysis<br>Cost-benefit analysis<br>Cost-effectiveness analysis | Fiscal databases reflecting cost savings, cost avoidance, and revenue generation. Relevant clinical indicators from the three spheres |

The following hierarchical model (Figure 8.1) is proposed (by these authors) for sorting outcomes by level of value to the organization and is derived from the system widely used to sort levels of evidence (Craig & Smyth, 2007; Melnyk, 2011; Schmidt & Brown, 2012). The levels are divided from weakest to strongest into (1) time-on activities, (2) process measures, (3) surrogate outcome measures, and (4) patient or staff outcomes. The pyramid portrays the fact that the least-valued measure is more easily produced and often used, whereas the strongest measures of patient or staff outcomes are hardest to obtain and least frequently reported. In the sections to follow, we will describe examples of each of these forms of outcome measures.

### Time-On Activities

#### Calendar

One easy strategy to track contributions without spending undue time is for every CNS to keep an electronic calendar populated with actual work done. At the end of the day, just before retiring, go back to the day's calendar and populate the "white space" with projects, rounds,

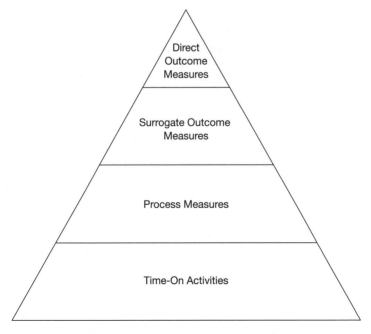

Figure 8.1 *Outcome Hierarchy Pyramid*

just-in-time education, and so forth. Populate meeting time with major decisions or outcomes. This will take 5 minutes or less if performed while the memory of the day is fresh. The data can then be used at the end of the month to populate an end-of-month productivity report.

### Productivity Report

Productivity reports describing CNS duties are a valuable tool to communicate CNS contributions to health care organization leadership. To increase visibility of the contributions CNSs make to the organization, record summaries of monthly productivity on a template with subheadings for each of the organization's pillars (Studer, 2008). Most organizations report a scorecard of metrics to the Board of Directors according to subheadings such as finance, quality, workforce development, and so forth. Instead of hiding activities under the subcategories of the CNS role functions that are known and understood mainly by the CNS community, use the organizational pillars as subheadings, and have each CNS complete the tool at the end of each month. This also helps CNSs to see how they directly contribute to the goals of the organization. Wherever possible, use cost figures or cost surrogates to estimate impact on finance. A predicted obstacle will be to move the team from qualitative descriptions of their work to quantitative objective outcomes reporting. The root of the problem is that most CNSs are not comfortable using estimates of cost reduction or savings, or literature-based cost estimates versus actual values. Because actual savings are difficult to capture, surrogates are acceptable and also save time in hunting for obscure organizational data. This normal business strategy will improve visibility and security. From our experience, moving from paragraph to concrete outcome descriptions took more than a year of practice (Davidson, 2011). In the case where a team is learning how to do this together, it is helpful to have the leader complete one of their own, leading by example. The leader's productivity report is distributed to the staff with a timely reminder to complete the end of month report. This sets clear expectations for the level of detail. Then the entire team's package can be attached to staff meeting minutes. In this manner, each member of the team can learn from peer examples. The leader of the team may call out especially positive examples and use the documents as a source of staff recognition. Exhibit 8.1 provides an example of how to structure a monthly productivity report. If each CNS submits one, the complete package can be forwarded up the chain of command each month for positive team exposure. The act of sending positive messaging about employees up the chain of command on

## Exhibit 8.1  *CNS Monthly Productivity Report*

**CNS Monthly Productivity Report**

Name_____                    Month_____, 2010

|  | Operational Accountabilities (put activities in this column that never go away, but you are making progress on) | Time-Limited Projects (put activities in this column that should be time-limited and eventually end) | Quantifiable Data ($ revenue or calculated avoidance, near miss saves related to either time-limited or operational accountabilities) |
|---|---|---|---|
| **Financial Performance** (Any activity which has direct revenue/ cost avoidance implications) |  |  |  |
| **Workforce Development** (Internal education/ development of practice tools) |  |  |  |
| **Medical Staff Development** (Education/ collaboration) |  |  |  |
| **Quality** |  |  |  |
| **Meeting Community Needs** (community involvement, public speaking, publications) |  |  |  |

a regular basis is called "managingup" and is promoted by Studer as a strong business tactic for organizational success (Studer, 2008).

### Preformatted Productivity Spreadsheet

This second example is offered for collating monthly performance data. Preformatted electronic spreadsheets provide a quick way to organize CNS activities. The following process was used by a team of CNSs to organize a simple method of tabulating time-on activities.

During a retreat, the group brainstormed the categories of activities for which each spent time. The total list was then numbered so each activity received a unique identifier. Then, of the total list, individualized lists were made to reflect activities pertinent to each person's scope of practice. The spreadsheets were then autopopulated with time spent on required meetings. At the end of the month, the CNS populated his or her own spreadsheet, which was then forwarded up the chain of command. The process was designed with the goal of spending less than 15 minutes per month tabulating time-on activities. The spreadsheet also provides the ability to capture time within the CNS spheres or within the organization pillars, which allows the data to be tailored to the target audience (Exhibit 8.2).

### Peer Review and CNS Visibility

Another strategy to increase CNS visibility and staff understanding of outcomes generated from activities within the CNS role is the peer evaluation process. One method to obtain peer review is to ensure first that the CNS job description is built according to the published role elements (National CNS Competency Task Force, 2010). The role-specific elements are then abstracted into a peer evaluation along with the standard organizational behaviors required by each employee. The supervisor may send out the peer evaluation electronically to physicians, operational leaders, and staff who work with the CNS on committees, projects, or in their area of practice (Exhibit 8.3). This accomplishes several goals. The recipient can see what the CNS is accountable for, as well as soliciting the input needed for evaluation. When sending out the peer evaluation, a leading message with at least two accomplishments can also be sent to manage up the CNS to others (Studer, 2008) and improve visibility of CNS outcomes (Exhibit 8.3). The peer evaluation can easily be sent as an electronic survey with the introductory email to automatically summarize the data according to subheading to cut and paste into the evaluation.

### Process Measures

### Rounding With a Purpose

It is known that educational offerings do little by themselves to change behavior (Bloom & Bloom, 2005) and, therefore, academic detailing in the form of bedside rounds is imperative to solidify practice change. Table 8.3 summarizes the effectiveness of different methods of

### Exhibit 8.2 *CNS-Specific Productivity Spreadsheet*

| Item/Activity | Time (hrs) | Units/Items | Pillar | Sphere | Role | Scope |
|---|---|---|---|---|---|---|
| Committee—CNS | 120 | 1 | | | | Facility-wide |
| Committee quality | 90 | 1 | | | | Facility-wide |
| Committee nurse practice council | 120 | 1 | | | | Facility-wide |
| Committee—Restraint | 90 | 1 | | | | Facility-wide |
| Committee—Restraint | 120 | 1 | | | | System-wide |
| Committee—Patient safety | 60 | 1 | | | | System-wide |
| Committee—Delirium | | 1 | | | | Facility-wide |
| Committee—Delirium | | 1 | | | | System-wide |
| Security subcommittee | 60 | 1 | | | | Facility-wide |
| Committee—AWS | | 1 | | | | Facility-wide |
| Committee—AWS | | 1 | | | | System-wide |
| Care management redesign | | | | | | System-wide |
| Patient satisfaction rounding— Assigned unit | | | | | | Unit specific |
| Rounding—Restraints | | | | | | Facility-wide |
| Rounding—Alcohol withdrawal | | | | | | Facility-wide |
| Rounding—Falls reduction | | | | | | Facility-wide |
| Rounding—Core measures | | | | | | Facility-wide |
| Evidence-based practice review | | | | | | System-wide |
| Conduct mortality and morbidities | | | | | | Facility-wide |
| Nasal bridle | | | | | | Facility-wide |
| Equipment demonstration | | | | | | Facility-wide |
| Student precepting | | | | | | Facility-wide |
| Occurrence report review | | | | | | Facility-wide |
| Auditing | | | | | | Facility-wide |
| Community service | | | | | | Community |
| Educating staff, managers | | | | | | System-wide |
| Rounding—Pain | | | | | | Facility-wide |
| Committee—System-wide | | | | | | System-wide |
| Computer screen development | | | | | | System-wide |

*Note:* This is a CNS-specific productivity report culled from a larger list of possible CNS activities. Standard meeting time is formatted to automatically populate. If viewed electronically, a drop-down list of pillars would appear for selection, as well as the drop-down list of spheres of influence. A drop-down list of CNS role requirements also appears. AWS = alcohol withdrawal syndrome; M&M = morbidity and mortality

**Exhibit 8.3** *Example Script for Peer Evaluation Request*

Nancy Nurse, CNS, is due for her yearly evaluation. We are hoping you will email feedback before June 7. Of note, Nancy has chaired the pressure ulcer committee over the last year with a resultant 30% reduction in hospital-acquired pressure ulcers. This reduction is estimated to have saved the organization over $250,000.00 in fines and lost revenue. Nancy has also spearheaded a program to improve compliance with the IHI Bladder Bundle. The Bladder Bundle Team has achieved an overall improvement in protocol compliance from 25% to 96%. There have been no hospital-acquired UTIs reported in the quarter following the launch of the pilot. We congratulate Nancy and the team on this success.

Nancy's evaluation has these subheadings.

Please comment on any in the form of a return email:

**Influencing Direct Care**

**Consultation**

**Systems Leadership**

**Collaboration**

**Coaching**

**Research**

**Ethical decision making**

Problem solving and making improvements

Compliance and organizational alignment

Workplace integrity and accountability

Communicating with others

Working with others

Creating a favorable impression

Serving others

Dependability

Resource utilization

*Note:* Bold items are subheadings specific to CNS core competencies. Normal text subheadings are specific to required organizational behaviors and will change facility to facility.

Table 8.3 *Expected Impact of Activity on Change in Practice*

| Method | High (30%–35%) | Moderate | Low (3%–5%) | None | Total Number of Studies |
|---|---|---|---|---|---|
| Didactic (classroom) | 0% | 15% | 35% | 50% | 20 |
| Information only (e.g., mailings) | 0% | 15% | 23% | 61% | 13 |
| Clinical practice guidelines | 0% | 60% | 40% | 0% | 5 |
| Opinion leaders | 0% | 33% | 44% | 22% | 9 |
| Interactive education | 38% | 46% | 15% | 0% | 13 |
| Audits with feedback | 26% | 47% | 17% | 9% | 23 |
| Reminders/prompts | 35% | 45% | 20% | 0% | 26 |
| Academic detailing (1 to 1) | 40% | 53% | 7% | 0% | 15 |

education in changing practice (Bloom & Bloom, 2005). There are several forms of rounds that CNSs make during the course of a day. They may round on vulnerable staff, new employees, staff floating outside their normal work environment, or staff working with patients who have unusual diagnoses or complex care. Another form of round is targeted rounds to followup on new projects, programs, or services. A third form might take the form of multidisciplinary rounds or discharge planning rounds. Last, the CNS might be responsible for certain quality metrics, such as restraints, falls, pressure ulcers, or hospital-acquired pneumonia and plans to round on patients with those issues to ensure that standards of care are being met and that the processes designed in meetings actually meet patients' needs without undue burden on staff. In all of these situations, rounds should be performed with a purpose (Studer, 2008) and conducted using tools to gather data and input from staff. The data from these rounds may also be used for monthly productivity reports.

### Rounding Tools

The CNS role was originally developed to foster evidence-based practice at the bedside, and this key function remains a critical aspect of the job. Although direct outcomes cannot always be measured, compliance with evidence-based process measures, which have been demonstrated to improve outcomes, can be captured prospectively enabling an opportunity for just-in-time education and practice improvement. CNS-led rounds provide an opportunity to showcase expert assessment and diagnostic skills, while encouraging application of evidence-based nursing interventions in real time.

Johnson et al. (2011) captured the types of evidence-based recommendations made during CNS-led rounds. The rounds were targeted at preventing ventilator-associated pneumonia (VAP), venous thromboembolism, and hospital-acquired infections, as well as use of progressive mobility and improved glycemic management. The number and types of recommendations and the frequency with which the recommendations were carried out could be captured. Johnson et al. found that CNS recommendations were carried out 63% of the time, and over the course of 1 year, CNS-led rounds lead to 345 evidence-based interventions. Exhibits 8.4 and 8.5 are examples of tools tailored for data collection from different types of rounds.

Another application of CNS process measurement targets key outcome indicators that change over time. For example, catheter-associated urinary tract infections (CAUTIs) occur infrequently and it may take many months to a year to see if an intervention has been effective. However, the Centers for Disease Control and Prevention has clear guidelines for the prevention of CAUTIs (Gould et al., 2009), and because CAUTIs are tied to pay-for-performance, this untoward outcome is ripe for CNS management. Figure 8.2 is an example of process data collected for the reduction of CAUTIs. Bar graphs are especially useful in displaying before and after data for a set of required process elements.

### Example of Process Measurement and Rounding Impact

The emergence of disease-specific management certification by The Joint Commission (TJC), tied to Centers for Medicare & Medicaid (CMS) pay-for-performance core measures and evidence-based guidelines, provides yet another opportunity for CNS project leadership. Among these TJC services, attainment of primary or comprehensive stroke center certification has become an expectation of many health care systems, and the majority of U.S. hospitals have achieved this recognition. However, although stroke centers were originally developed to increase the number of patients that could be treated with intravenous tissue plasminogen activator (tPA; Alteplase), U.S. treatment rates remain significantly lower than other countries around the world.

**Exhibit 8.4** *Outcome Measure: Data Collection Tool for Outcomes From Rounds*

---

### FOLLOW-UP ITEMS FROM ICU MULTIPROFESSIONAL ROUNDS

- Order for occupational therapy/physical therapy for evaluation and treatment
- Order for speech therapy/swallow evaluation and treatment
- Order for intermittent pneumatic compression device
- Order for venous thromboembolism medication
- Complete medication reconciliation form
- Complete vaccination/methicillin-resistant *Staphylococcus aureus* screening
- Discuss feeding tube placement/nutrition needs
- Discuss weaning from mechanical ventilation or tracheostomy
- Arrange patient/family conference
- Implement the ventilator associated pneumonia (VAP) bundle elements

  - Every 4 hour oral care/subglotal suctioning
  - If VAP endotracheal tube present, connect to low continuous suction
  - Venous thromboembolism prophylaxis
  - Head of bed up 30 degrees
  - Daily sedation wake-up/assessment of readiness for weaning and extubation

- Implement appropriate pressure ulcer precautions
  - Placed pressure ulcer order set in chart
  - Order special bed/surface _____

- Review need for central line/Foley catheter
- Consider discontinuation of central line/Foley catheter
- Spiritual care/social work consult
- Consider palliative/pain service consultation
- Recommend medication changes (i.e., PO vs. IV) _____
- Consider transfer out of intensive care unit
- Other _____
- Other _____

**Exhibit 8.5 Process Measure: Rounding Tool**

ICU Multiprofessional Rounds _____     Date: _____     Coordinator _____

| Room # | PT/OT/ST | Family conference | Transfer | VAP/Oral care/HOB/ Sed.Hol./GI proph./Vent wean? | VTE Proph | Medications:PO vs IV Duplicate therapy, antibiotics vs cultures, home medications? | Infection control | Diet | Skin | Lines | Foley | Glyc mgt | Other |
|---|---|---|---|---|---|---|---|---|---|---|---|---|---|
| | | | | | | | | | | | | | |
| | | | | | | | | | | | | | |
| | | | | | | | | | | | | | |
| | | | | | | | | | | | | | |
| | | | | | | | | | | | | | |

*Abbreviations:* PT, physical therapy; OT, occupational therapy; ST, speech therapy; VAP, ventilator-associated pneumonia; HOB, head of bed; Sed. Hol., sedation holiday; GI proph, gastrointestinal prophylaxis; VTE proph, venous thromboembolism prophylaxis; Vent, ventilator; Glyc mgt, glycemic management.

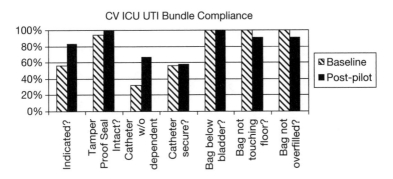

Figure 8.2 *Process Measure: Compliance With CAUTI Bundle*

Alexandrov and colleagues (2009) developed the first postgraduate academic APN (CNS and nurse practitioner) acute neurovascular fellowship program to prepare expert evidence-based APNs capable of driving improvement in intravenous tPA treatment rates for acute ischemic stroke. These investigators analyzed their first cohort of graduates for change in tPA treatment rates, documenting an absolute 7% increase in tPA treatment by the end of fellowship year 1, and an absolute 8.3% increase (95% CI = 6.4–10.2; $P < .001$) in tPA treatment by the end of year 3. Most importantly, rates for symptomatic intracerebral hemorrhage for patients identified and treated by these expert APNs were well beneath the U.S. Food and Drug Administration approved rate of 6.4%, at only 4.4% (Alexandrov et al., 2011). Despite only two (11%) CNSs in the cohort having prescriptive authority, there was no difference by type of APN in tPA treatment rate change, with CNS fellows primarily capable of driving the improvement in treatment rate through expert knowledge, skills, and an ability to positively influence physician stroke team members. Because treatment with intravenous tPA is associated with a 30% improvement in neurologic disability and functional status by 3 months, capturing an increase in tPA treatment rates is a potent example of the use of a process measure to capture the significant contribution of CNSs.

### Surrogate Outcomes

#### Surrogate Outcome Measures

Cost avoidance and reduction in adverse outcomes can be difficult to capture. Surrogate values are a valuable tool in these circumstances and have been used in medical and allied health literature (Dasta et al., 2010; Fraser, Riker, Prato, & Wilkins, 2001; Stahl et al., 2009). Costs of a specific test or treatment can be obtained through administrative accounting data providing an actual cost per case figure that is a better indicator than billing data. When a test or treatment is eliminated from care, the cost of the item plus the cost of staff time spent doing the test or treatment is calculated. Estimates of staff time are described below.

When using a surrogate figure that was published in the literature for an episode of care (e.g., pressure ulcer or VAP), currency of the published figure is evaluated and then adjusted for inflation. If the figure was published in 2010, the inflation factor can be obtained from the department of finance and added to the published cost to bring the cost up to date. The inflation rate methodology is specific to the organization due to geographic variation in inflation.

### Calculating Cost in Staff Time

One of the most desirable outcomes to measure is reduction in wasted time spent on unnecessary activities. For example, streamlined medication passes, decreasing the number of prompts in computerized documentation, or reduced time spent in hunting and gathering supplies could constitute cost savings. If a project has resulted in decreasing wasted process steps in the delivery of care, the hours of saved time can easily be converted into a surrogate figure for dollars saved. To do this, have your supervisor inform the department of finance that you are working on a project that requires this analysis. The data you will be requesting for the calculation is often considered sensitive and will not be granted unless there is verification that you are using it for a business need. If the change in practice will affect only one department, ask for the average nursing salary for that department. If the change will eventually affect all departments, ask for the organizational average salary. Average salary may differ widely based upon seniority. Also ask for the overhead rate that constitutes the percent over wage that is spent by the organization on provision of benefits. Then, measure the amount of time the wasted process step takes in minutes by conducting a time and motion study. Perform several observations and average the result. Create a spreadsheet using the following variables:

- Minutes of time saved by eliminating this activity.
- Average staff hourly wage.
- Overhead rate = (express percent in decimal: e.g., 30% = 0.3).

- Number of times this activity is done in a day.
- Number of patients receiving this activity in a day.
- Number of times a day the patients receive this activity.
- Number of days the activity is expected to occur in a year.

Embed formulas within the spreadsheet as shown in Exhibit 8.6 to calculate cost savings. In the example used in Exhibit 8.6, the deleted activity that took 15 minutes to perform and was routinely performed twice a day on 15 patients every day of the year by a nurse whose salary was $55.00/hour with an organizational overhead rate of 30% resulted in an estimated annual cost savings of $195,731.25.

Because salary figures are often sensitive, obtain approval prior to distributing the formula to those outside of the organizational leadership team. For every nonvalue-added activity that is deleted from a

**Exhibit 8.6** *Outcome Measure: Yearly Cost Savings*

|  | A | C | E |
|---|---|---|---|
|  | Variable |  | Formula Embedded in Column C |
| 4 | Average staff hourly wage in dollars | $55.00 |  |
| 5 | Overhead rate (express percent in decimal: e.g., 30% = .3) | 0.3 |  |
| 6 | **Total labor/hour** | **$71.50** | (C4*C5)+C4 |
| 8 | Minutes saved per activity expressed as portion of hour (15 minutes = .25) | 25% |  |
| 9 | **Dollars saved/activity** | **$17.88** | C6*C8 |
| 11 | # Patients receiving activity/day | 15 |  |
| 12 | # Times/day patients receive activity | 2 |  |
| 13 | Total activity times | 30 | C11*C12 |
| 15 | **Dollars saved per day** | **$536.25** | C13*C9 |
| 17 | # Days the activity is expected to occur/year | 365 |  |
| 19 | **Annual savings** | **$195,731.25** | C17*C15 |
| 20 | Formula |  | ((C4*C5)+C4)*C8*(C11*C12)*C17 |

nurse's workload, the CNS can promote managing the newly found free time, which is formally referred to as capacity in a way that is desirable to operational leaders. For example, if patients have not been satisfied with discharge education, the report on the project to save time in hunting and gathering could conclude with, "This xx minutes of care/day (xx/yr) saved in hunting and gathering could easily correct the problem we currently have with patient education if we manage the transition correctly."

## EXAMPLE OF SURROGATE DATA USE

The following project is explored as an example of the use of surrogates to capture avoidance of cost and adverse outcomes. Gutierrez and Cahill (2011) introduced a nasal gastric tube securement device in their organization and measured reduction in restraints, nursing time, and radiation exposure. Restraint days were measured, pre- and post implementation, and were reduced from 6.21 to 4.32 days, resulting in 53 restraint days avoided ($P < .001$). Cost savings from this are calculated to be $12,800, assuming 3 RN hours, 1 charge nurse hour, 1 manager hour, and .5 CNS hours per restraint day.

$$([\$41 \times 3] + [\$43 \times 1] + [\$47 \times 1] + [\$55 \times 0.5]) \times 53 = 12,746.50$$

Prior to the new securement device, these patients with nasal gastric tubes had an average of 5.75 abdominal radiographs done, which was reduced to 1.29 after introducing the new product. This resulted in a cost savings of $33,000 as well as a 28,080 millirad reduction in radiation. Because this project was performed over a 3-month period in one hospital, and there was no reason to assume there would be seasonal variation to the number of patients requiring a nasal securement device, the figures could be multiplied by four to obtain and report the estimated yearly savings. The values used in this example were very conservative because the calculation did not account for overhead costs, which is approximately 30% higher than the salary figure.

## CALCULATING COST OF NURSING TIME IN EDUCATION

The time nurses spend in educational programs is costly to the organization. When planning a change in practice, education is often planned as a first step in the change, but the cost of education time is often seen as a burden within any project. As a general principle, the value you anticipate to bring to the change needs to outweigh the burden of the cost of the education. For this reason, limit the didactic education to only what is necessary. Calculate time spent in the classroom using the average wage of the nurse, overhead cost, number of minutes, number of nurses who will be educated, and cost of instructor. Remember to add in replacement figures if the nurse will need to be replaced on the job (back-filled) to attend the class. If the back-fill is anticipated to accrue overtime, account for the overtime by using a replacement factor of 1.5 × the hourly wage.

Because classroom education is so expensive, an alternative that can decrease project burden is to teach 1:1 or in small groups at the bedside while conducting rounds. With careful scheduling and a train-the-trainer approach, many projects can be taught in this manner without adding educational costs while also enhancing valuable CNS exposure to nursing staff at the bedside.

## OUTCOMES

In some instances, direct outcomes of CNS interventions can be measured. This is the highest level of CNS outcome data, but it is also the most difficult to obtain. One nurse-sensitive indicator where data may be readily available is patient perception of pain control. Figure 8.3 is an example of outcome level data from a CNS intervention for pain (Cahill, Worthington, & Sisk, 2010).

Another strategy for demonstrating CNS contributions is measurement of outcomes produced by CNS-lead groups. The CNS is often involved in hospital-wide initiatives targeted at nurse-sensitive indicators, such as falls. Figure 8.4 illustrates the trend of fall rates in a hospital with a CNS-lead falls committee. Whenever available, a graph of this nature should be included with text report of achieved outcomes.

Linking process measures to outcomes tracked and reported up the chain of command by the Department of Quality is another strategy to link outcomes with CNS performance. For instance, in the process example described earlier, the CNS conducted rounds focused on compliance with the CAUTI bundle, providing feedback to staff when errors of omission occurred. The Department of Quality reports UTIs to the Infection Control Committee. Submitting the bundle compliance data highlighting improvement in compliance to the Department of Quality for inclusion in the report of UTIs to the Infection Control Committee leverages use of existing resources with CNS visibility at a high level within the organization.

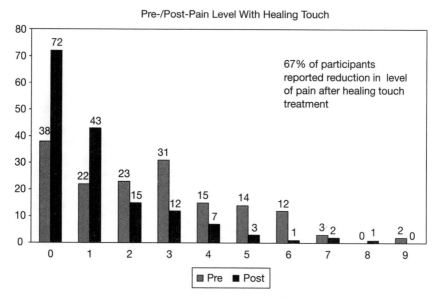

Figure 8.3  *Outcome Measure: Pain*

*Note:* Sixty-seven percent of participants reported reduction in level of pain after healing touch treatment.

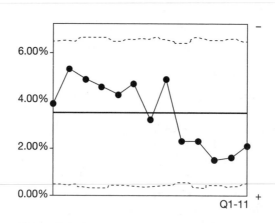

Figure 8.4  *Outcome Measure: Fall Reduction*

## PULLING IT ALL TOGETHER

### End of Year Report

End of the year reports can be used proactively by the CNS to collate process, surrogate, and outcome data. Usually time-on data are not included in this level of report. Exhibit 8.7 demonstrates an example of how to organize report data. Time the construction of an end of year summary so that it can be aggregated to reflect the work of the entire team and be available at the end of each fiscal year. This also becomes a good time to review committee charters and CNS participation within key committees and projects. In Exhibit 8.7, the organization's pillars are in bold. Change these if your organization's pillars are different. Typical CNS activities are listed under each subheading. At the end of the year, each CNS in the system would submit his/her personal contributions that could be collated and summarized in aggregate. The chief nursing officer could then complete the report with activities not performed by CNSs. The original version provides an overall picture of how the CNSs contribute to organizational goals. The end product will be balanced with contributions by others, but it can be predicted that the bulk of the activity to move the profession forward and enact change to improve important nurse-sensitive outcomes have been affected by the work of a CNS. This template is easily modifiable into an electronic survey that would automatically summarize the data.

## PROJECT CASE EXAMPLE AND CROSSWALK

The following project is explored because it was constructed to measure and report a variety of outcomes of a CNS-driven change in practice. Nolan, Burkard, Clark, Davidson, and Agan (2010) developed a new system for conducting mortality and morbidity (M&M) reviews for nurses in an attempt to reduce VAP. Nurses who were directly involved in providing care to each patient with a case of VAP were invited to the review and paid to attend. The primary outcome measure for the project was VAP. However, during the project several other key measures of success were evaluated and reported, such as percent compliance with elements (process measures) of the Institute for Healthcare Improvement VAP bundle. This investigator also used an unbiased observer to measure nurse accountability by recording how many times the staff used "I" versus "You" statements to reflect accountability for the omissions in care. Satisfaction with the

Exhibit 8.7 *End of Year Report Template*

---

### DEPARTMENT OF NURSING END OF YEAR REPORT

**Finance:** (Put any quantifiable data here including but not limited to reduction in cost of care estimates, cost abatement, avoided fines, avoided reimbursement denials; cite sources for literature-based surrogates at bottom of page):

**Quality:** Committee reports (List all committees where CNSs serve as chair, co-chair, liaison, or have significant impact)

- Nurse practice council
- Council of scientific inquiry
- Patient satisfaction
- Pain
- Restraint
- Pressure ulcer
- Falls
- Nursing satisfaction
- Pharmacy and therapeutics
- Institutional review board
- Care line committees

Performance improvement/evidence-based practice change projects Research (List titles, investigators):

Professional projects (Include team leaders' names):

**Workforce Development:** (List all activities surrounding educating or supporting staff: number of rounds conducted, number of staff affected, courses taught, educational programs developed, relate to outcomes whenever possible):

**Medical Staff Development:** (List interdisciplinary projects CNSs conduct in collaboration with physicians in this section. List programs that CNSs develop for medical education):

**Community Benefit**

- Lectures to the community (title, speaker)
- Community projects
- Professional presentations (title, speaker, venue)
- Publications (citation)

program was measured qualitatively with open-ended comments as well as quantitatively using Likert scale scoring, and included measures of CNS effect within the nursing personnel sphere. Cost of M&Ms was also measured to reflect an organizational outcome. Lastly, a surrogate measure for the cost of an episode of VAP was used and multiplied by the number of VAP cases that would have resulted without the M&M intervention. VAP rates were compared in a pretest/posttest fashion using similar months to account for seasonal variation. Results from the project included overwhelmingly positive nursing satisfaction, improved accountability ($x^2 = 24.041$, $P < .001$), protocol compliance improvement from 90.1% to 95.2%, and improved VAP rates. The final cost analysis yielded $100,000 prevention in costs associated with VAP per year, even when accounting for the cost of paying nurses to attend M&M reviews. Exhibit 8.8 demonstrates a crosswalk between the outcomes measured in this project and the hierarchical model presented in this chapter plus the spheres of influence.

## CONCLUSIONS

CNS outcomes can be measured in a variety of ways. CNS outcome visibility is enhanced when tools and terms understood by operational leaders are used. Time-on activities can be captured from well-kept calendars, committee minutes, and project summaries to be converted into productivity reports and end of year reports. Peer evaluations, when constructed and distributed to include examples of CNS outcomes promote visibility of the individual CNS. All projects can be designed to measure success. Rounds may be performed with intention to measure and improve protocol adherence following changes in practice. Surrogate measures and financial data can be used to create formulas to estimate outcomes affected by streamlining efficiencies or preventing episodes of illness. Finally, direct measurement of improvement in clinical outcomes can be reported. As highlighted in the NACNS's vision for the future of the CNS, outcome evaluation and measurement is a recommended area of core content specific to CNS practice (Goudreau et al., 2007). Assessing the outcomes of the CNS role to achieve important patient, provider, and health system goals can help to maximize the potential and long-term sustainability of the CNS role (Bryant-Lukosius et al., 2010). Continuing the focus on demonstrating the outcomes of CNS practice will help to ensure recognition of the value and impact of the role.

Exhibit 8.8 *Crosswalk of Project Outcomes to Outcome Hierarchy Pyramid and Spheres of Influence*

| Nursing Morbidity and Mortality Project | | | | | | | |
|---|---|---|---|---|---|---|---|
| Outcome Measure | Patient/ Client | Nursing Personnel | Organizational/ Network | Time-On | Process | Surrogate Outcome | Outcome |
| VAP bundle protocol adherence | | X | | | X | | |
| Evidence of nursing account-ability in the form of "I" versus "You" statements | | X | | | | X | |
| Qualititative measures of staff satisfaction | | X | | | | | X |
| Quantitative measures of staff satisfaction | | X | | | | | X |
| VAP | X | | | | | | X |
| Cost savings to the organization | | | X | | | X | |

## Answers to Chapter Discussion Questions

1. Time-on activities (least important), process measures, surrogate measures, outcome measures (most important).
2. Each individual will have a different answer to this question. Time-on activities may include tracking time spent on activities through the use of a calendar or spreadsheet. Process measures normally include compliance with new changes in practice. Surrogate

measures use published costs of care and estimations of events prevented through improved practices to calculate cost reduction. Actual outcome measures may include those focused on patients (e.g., length of stay, mortality, adverse events, readmissions) or staff (e.g., retention, satisfaction, comprehension, change in practice following education).

3. Each individual will create a unique table. If the learner has not yet done a project or planned a capstone, he/she should create a fictitious example based upon the last time he/she was expected to change practice as a nurse in response to a performance improvement project in the area of practice.

4. Answers will be individualized based upon the organization. Organizational objectives and goals normally center around publicly reported metrics and regulatory or accreditation standards, expanded services, and centers of excellence. The general themes of objectives are often clustered under pillars of performance such as finance, quality, workforce development, medical staff engagement, community involvement.

5. Cons include time spent to record and track activities, time, and effort to develop tracking tools. Literature-based surrogates are not available for all measures of interest. Extracting actual outcomes from organizational databases can be cumbersome, time consuming, or restricted. Pros include visibility, promotion/positive imaging of the CNS role, employment security, and justification of additional CNS positions. Tracking outcomes from change may also decrease resistance to change and help to solidify change when positive outcomes are shared with those affected by the change.

## ACKNOWLEDGMENTS

We would like to acknowledge the work of Nancy Dayhoff, EdD, RN, CNS, and Brenda Lyon, DNS, CNS, FAAN, who served as the authors for the chapter on assessing outcomes in CNS practice for the 2009 and 2000 editions of this book.

We would also like to acknowledge the following nurses whose projects have been showcased in this chapter as examples of outcome reporting: Rhonda Amber, MS, RN-BC, CMSRN, CNS; Donna Cahill, MS, RN-BC, CNS, CEN, CHTP; Nancy Carreon, MS, RN; Felipe Gutierrez, MS, RN, FNP; Scot Nolan, DNP, RN, CNS, PhN, CCRN, CNRN.

We would also like to acknowledge Donna Agan, Ed,D for her continued support and advancement of the outcome reporting tools used by these nurses.

## REFERENCES

Alexandrov, A. W., Baca, T., Albright, K. C., DiBiase, S., Alexandrov, A. V. for the NET SMART Faculty and Fellows. (2011). Post-graduate academic neurovascular fellowship for advanced practice nurses and physician assistants significantly increases tPA treatment rates: Results from the first graduating class of the NET SMART program. *Stroke, 43*(3), e352–353.

Alexandrov, A. W., Brethour, M., Cudlip, F., Swatzell, V., Biby, S., Reiner, D.,...Yang, J. (2009). Post-graduate fellowship education and training for nurses: The NET SMART experience. *Critical Care Nursing Clinics of North America, 21*(4), 435–449.

Amber, R., Carreon, N., Agan, D., Johnson, M., & Cahill, D. (2012). Quantification of clinical nurse specialist outcomes: Clinical nurse specialist rounds. *Clinical Nurse Specialist, 26*(2), E1–E49.

Bloom, B. S., & Bloom, B. S. (2005). Effects of continuing medical education on improving physician clinical care and patient health: A review of systematic reviews. *International Journal of Technology Assessment in Health Care, 21*(3), 380–385.

Bryant-Lukosius, D., Carter, N., Kilpatrick, K., Martin-Misener, R., Donald, F., Kaasalainen, S.,...DiCenso, A. (2010). The clinical nurse specialist role in Canada. *Nursing leadership, 23*, 140–66.

Cahill, D., Worthington, T., & Sisk, D. (2010). *Evaluating nurses' response and knowledge of the complimentary modality Healing Touch: Creating an environment of health/healing and improved pain management.* Paper presented at the 33rd Annual ACNL Conference: California Dreamin'—Nurse Leaders Honoring the Past and Envisioning the Future, Sacramento, CA.

Committee on the Robert Wood Johnson Foundation Initiative on the Future of Nursing at the Institute of Medicine. (2011). *The future of nursing: Leading change, advancing health.* Washington, DC: National Academies Press.

Craig, J. V., & Smyth, R. L. (2007). *The evidence-based practice manual for nurses* (2nd ed.). Edinburgh, Scotland: Churchill Livingstone Elsevier.

Cunningham, R. S. (2004). Advanced practice nursing outcomes: A review of selected empirical literature. *Oncology Nursing Forum, 31*, 219–230.

Dasta, J. F., Kane-Gill, S. L., Pencina, M., Shehabi, Y., Bokesch, P., Wiesmandle, W., & Riker, R. R. (2010). A cost-minimization analysis of dexmedetomdine compared with midazolam for long-term sedation in the intensive care unit. *Critical Care Medicine, 38*(2), 497–503.

Davidson, J. E. (2010). *Creation of a role for the DNP prepared nurse in hospital leadership.* Paper presented at the Doctor of Nursing Practice Conference, San Diego, CA.

Davidson, J. E. (2011). Measuring CNS outcomes. *Doctor of Nursing Practice Conference.* Retrieved July 19, 2012, from http://www.doctorsofnursing-practice.org/studentprojects.php

Dickerson, S. S., Wu, Y. B., Kennedy, M. C. (2006). A CNS-facilitated ICD support group: A clinical project evaluation. *Clinical Nurse Specialist, 20,* 146–153.

Duffy, J. R. (2002). The clinical leadership role of the CNS in the identification of nursing-sensitive and multidisciplinary quality indicator sets. *Clinical Nurse Specialist, 16,* 70–76.

Forster, A. J., Clark, H. D., Menard, A., et al. (2005). Effect of a nurse team coordinator on outcomes for hospitalized medical patients. *American Journal of Medicine, 118,* 1148–1153.

Fraser, G. L., Riker, R. R., Prato, S., & Wilkins (2001). The frequency and cost of patient-initiated device removal in the ICU. *Pharmacotherapy, 21*(1), 1–6.

Fulton, J. S. (2006). Disseminating outcomes of clinical nurse specialist practice. *Clinical Nurse Specialist, 20,* 264–265

Fulton, J. S., & Baldwin, K. (2004). An annotated bibliography reflecting CNS practice and outcomes. *Clinical Nurse Specialist, 18,* 21–39.

Goudreau, K., Baldwin, K., Clark, A., Fulton, J., Lyon, B., Murray, T., et al. for the National Association of Clinical Nurse Specialists (2007). *A vision of the future of the clinical nurse specialist.* Retrieved August 20, 2012, from http://www.nacns.org/docs/AVisionCNS.pdf

Gould, C. V., Umscheid, C. A., Agarwal, R. K., Kuntz, G., Pegues, D. A., Healthcare Infection Control Practices Advisory Committee (HICPAC). (2009). *Guideline for prevention of catheter-associated urinary tract infections.* Atlanta, GA: Centers for Disease Control and Prevention.

Gutierrez, F., & Cahill, D. (2011). *Nasal bridle: Decrease in restraints, nursing time, and X-ray exposure.* Paper presented at 20th Annual AMSN Conference, Boston, MA.

Hamilton, R., & Hawley, W. (2006). Quality of life outcomes related to anemia management of patients with chronic renal failure. *Clinical Nurse Specialist, 20,* 139–143.

Johnson, M., Amber, R., Azuma, N., Cahill, D., Nolan, S., & Davidson, J. (2011). Clinical nurse specialist multidisciplinary rounds as a strategy to translate evidence-based practice to the bedside. *Clinical Nurse Specialist: The Journal for Advanced Practice Nursing, 25*(2), 80.

Larsen, L. S., Neverett, S. G., & Larsen, R. F. (2001). Clinical nurse specialist as facilitator of interdisciplinary collaborative program for adult sickle cell population. *Clinical Nurse Specialist, 15,* 15–22.

Ley, S. J. (2001). Quality care outcomes in cardiac surgery: The role of evidence based practice. *AACN Clinical Issues, 12,* 606–617.

McCabe, P. J. (2005). Spheres of clinical nurse specialist practice influence evidence-based care for patients with atrial fibrillation. *Clinical Nurse Specialist, 19,* 308–317.

Melnyk, B. M. (2011). *Evidence-based practice in nursing & healthcare: A guide to best practice* (2nd ed.). Philadelphia, PA: Wolters Kluwer/Lippincott Williams & Wilkins.

National Association of Clinical Nurse Specialists. (2004). *Statement on clinical nurse specialist practice and education.* Glenview, IL: Author.

National CNS Competency Task Force. (2010). *NaCNS core competencies.* Retrieved from http://www.nacns.org/docs/CNSCoreCompetenciesBroch.pdf

National Quality Forum. (2012) Measures, reports & tools. Retrieved August 25, 2012 from http://www.qualityforum.org/Measures_Reports_Tools.aspx

Newhouse, R. P., Weiner, J. P., Stanik-Hutt, J., White, K. M., Johantgen, M., Steinwachs, D., . . . Bass, E. (2011). Advanced practice outcomes 1990–2008: A systematic review. *Nursing Economics, 29,* 230–250.

Nolan, S. W., Burkard, J. F., Clark, M. J., Davidson, J. E., & Agan, D. L. (2010). Effect of morbidity and mortality peer review on nurse accountability and ventilator-associated pneumonia rates. *Journal of Nursing Administration, 40*(9), 374–383.

Prevost, S. S. (2002). Clinical nurse specialist outcomes: vision, voice and value. *Clinical Nurse Specialist, 16,* 119–124.

Schmidt, N., & Brown, J. (2012). *Evidence-based practice for nurses: Appraisal and application of research* (2nd ed.). Sudbury, MA: Jones & Bartlett Learning.

Stahl, K., Palileo, A., Schulman, C. I., Wilson, K., Augenstein, J., Kiffin, C., & McKenney, M. (2009). Enhancing patient safety in the trauma/surgical ICU. *Journal of Trauma Injury, Infection, and Critical Care, 67*(3), 430–435.

Studer, Q. (2008). *Results that last: Hardwiring behaviors that will take your company to the top.* Hoboken, NJ: Wiley.

Willoughby, D., & Burroughs, D. A. (2001). CNS-managed diabetes foot-care clinic: A descriptive survey of characteristics and foot-care behaviors of the patient population. *Clinical Nurse Specialist, 15,* 52–57

Wojner, A. W. (2001). *Outcomes management: Application to clinical practice.* St. Louis, MO: Mosby.

# Chapter 9: Outcomes Measurement in Nurse-Midwifery Practice

SUZAN ULRICH, RHONDA ARTHUR, AND JULIE MARFELL

## Chapter Objectives

1. Present an overview of the historical implementation and importance of outcome measurement in nurse-midwifery practice and discuss the role that outcome measurement has in improving modern health care delivery in the arena of maternal and child health.
2. Summarize published examples of nurse-midwifery outcome studies.
3. Outline the use of the American College of Nurse-Midwives Benchmarking Project for use in outcome measurement and quality improvement.
4. Present the Uniform Data Set as a tool for collection of outcome measures and research.

## Chapter Discussion Questions

1. Briefly describe three reasons why outcome measurement is an essential practice in nurse-midwifery practice.
2. List the four areas that the American College of Nurse-Midwives (ACNM) Benchmarking project used to evaluate quality nurse-midwifery care.

3. Describe how the ACNM Benchmarking Project could be used for nurse-midwifery quality improvement.
4. What is the Optimality Index?
5. Name and define at least three classifications of outcome measurements for nurse-midwifery practice.

## HISTORICAL PERSPECTIVE

Outcome evaluation of nurse-midwifery practice in the United States is as old as the profession. Mary Breckenridge brought nurse-midwifery to America in 1925 and created the Frontier Nursing Service (FNS). FNS was a demonstration project that provided health care to the rural poor in southeastern Kentucky. Mrs. Breckenridge took the advice of one of her consultants, Dr. McCormack, the Health Commissioner for the Commonwealth of Kentucky, who said she would be unable to determine the effects of the FNS without a complete assessment of the health status of the community. Her first step in establishing the FNS was to ride over 700 square miles to obtain health histories of all the area families so that the impact of the nurse-midwives on horseback could be measured (Breckinridge, 1981).

Meticulous records were kept at the FNS. The Metropolitan Life Insurance Corporation was asked to analyze the data of the first 1000 births attended by the nurse-midwives at FNS. The results were incredible. Dr. Louis Dublin reported

> The study shows conclusively that the type of service rendered by the Frontier nurses safeguards the life of mother and babe. If such service were available to the women of the country generally, there would be a saving of 10,000 mothers' lives a year in the United States. There would be 30,000 less stillbirths and 30,000 more children alive at the end of the first month of life. (Breckinridge, 1981)

Measuring nurse-midwifery outcomes started with the first nurse-midwifery service in the United States and has been an integral component of establishing nurse-midwifery as a profession in the United States.

The success of the nurse-midwifery care provided in the home by Frontier nurses from 1925 to 1975 was reported in 1975 on the 50th anniversary of the FNS (Browne & Isaacs, 1976). The study of the first 10,000 births at FNS by the Metropolitan Life Insurance Company found 11 maternal deaths, two of which were not obstetrics related. This was much lower than the national maternal mortality rate of 36.3 per 10,000 live births for the midpoint years 1939 to 1941. There were fewer premature births, stillbirths, and neonatal deaths for FNS than the rest of the country.

Continuing throughout the history of nurse-midwifery in the United States, outcomes have been studied. Initially, they were scrutinized to determine the safety and feasibility of midwifery care. A classic study was conducted in Madera County, CA, in the early 1960s to determine if nurse-midwives could be utilized to assist physicians in providing maternity care in a rural underserved area and to measure the outcomes of this new model of care (Montgomery, 1969). At the time, nurse-midwifery was not recognized or licensed in the state of California, so this project utilized nurse-midwives but labeled them Nurse Obstetric Assistants (NOAs). A before-and-after comparison was done that showed the NOAs could provide the needed care, and the birth outcomes improved dramatically. The number of women who received prenatal care in the first trimester doubled. The percentage of women receiving more than six prenatal visits increased almost 10%. Prematurity rates declined by 5% and the neonatal mortality rate went from 23.9 per 1,000 live births to 10.3 per 1,000 live births. This project highlighted the successful utilization of nurse-midwives, and a report of the project was presented to the California Medical Association (CMA) with the hope that they would endorse legislation to allow NOAs to practice in California. However, the CMA did not endorse NOAs, and nurse-midwives were not recognized in California until 1974 (ACNM, 2012).

It is interesting to note that a follow-up study of the Madera County project compared the birth outcomes before, during, and after the use of NOAs (Levy, Wilkinson, & Marine, 1971). In the 3 years following the termination of the NOAs, 9% more women received no prenatal care. Women who did receive prenatal care received fewer visits. The rate of premature infants rose significantly from 6.6% to 9.8%. Neonatal mortality almost tripled going from 10.3 per 1,000 live births when care was provided by the nurse-midwives to 32.1 per 1,000 live births afterward. The authors concluded that the use of nurse-midwives should be encouraged because the maternity outcomes improved during the interim period when they provided care.

Later, studies demonstrated that midwifery outcomes were excellent and there were added benefits of cost effectiveness and patient satisfaction. Reid and Morris (1979) evaluated the implementation of nurse-midwifery care for the underserved in Georgia in the 1970s and included analysis of cost effectiveness. There was a substantial increase in the number of women who received early prenatal care, and a reduction in the number of women giving birth with little or no prenatal care for the 3 years after the implementation of the midwifery services compared with the 2 years before. Birth outcomes showed improvement in neonatal mortality, longer gestations, and higher birth weights. Infant mortality rates dropped significantly in the rural counties studied, while there were no differences in the comparison counties. The authors found the cost of prenatal care and hospital care decreased over the course of the project and they were cautiously optimistic, while recommending that future research should include prospective analysis of health expenditures for midwifery care. Anderson and Anderson (1999) found home births cost 68% less than hospital births.

Outcome measurement was also undertaken to determine whether birth centers, which were specifically designed for the practice of the hallmarks of midwifery, were a safe alternative to hospital birth. The landmark prospective study of birth outcomes for over 11,000 women from 84 birth centers was published in the *New England Journal of Medicine* in 1989 (Rooks, Weatherby, Ernst, Stapleton, Rosen, & Rosenfield). The birth center clients were screened as low risk for maternity complications, hence an out of hospital setting was appropriate for their care. There were fewer premature births for women giving birth in the birth center than for all women who gave birth in the United States. The cesarean section rate was 4.4%, which contributed to lower costs for maternity care. The intrapartum transfer rate was 15.8% with 2.3% being emergent transports. The infant outcomes for birth center mothers were comparable to those of women with low-risk pregnancies having hospital births. Patient satisfaction was high with 98.8% of the women who gave birth at the birth centers saying they would recommend a birth center, and 94% would return to the birth center for their next birth. The percentage of satisfaction was slightly lower for the women who were transferred to the hospital during labor with 96.9% recommending it, and 83.3% willing to use it again. The authors concluded that "Few innovations in health services promise lower cost, greater availability, and higher degree of satisfaction with a comparable degree of safety" (p. 1810).

Recent attention has been paid to how the midwifery model of care actually improves pregnancy and birth outcomes, which lowers health care costs for maternity services. The Cochrane Review found that maternity care lead by midwives was beneficial for women (Hatem, Sandall, Devane, Soltani, & Gates, 2009). Women randomized to midwifery-led maternity units had fewer antepartum hospitalizations, fetal losses, instrumental deliveries, and episiotomies. They had more spontaneous vaginal births and early breastfeeding initiation. The women were cared for during labor by a midwife they knew, and they felt a sense of control. The authors concluded that for women without significant medical or obstetrical problems, "Midwifery-led care confers benefits and shows no adverse outcomes" (p. 13).

## CURRENT EXPANSION OF OUTCOME MEASUREMENT

### *Benchmarking*

ACNM is the professional organization for nurse-midwives with the goal of improving the health and well-being of mothers and infants. The ACNM defines eight standards for the practice of midwifery. One standard specifically addresses the need for evaluation of nurse-midwifery outcomes using a program of quality management that includes data collection, problem identification and resolution, as well as peer review.

To assist midwives to measure the quality of care, ACNM developed a Benchmarking Project in 1997 (Collins-Fulea, Mohr, & Tillett, 2005). This program specifically examined four areas of quality midwifery care. The first area examined functional status that included the physical and emotional well-being of the mother. The second area was cost of care, including both direct and indirect costs. The third area was patient satisfaction, and the fourth area consisted of clinical outcomes. The first benchmarking data were obtained in 2004 from 45 practices attending over 23,000 births. Results were reported so each midwifery service could see how they performed compared with the other services for each indicator. They could contact midwifery services with high performance to learn best practices that could then be modified and incorporated into their own practice for quality improvement. The ACNM Benchmarking Project has continued and expanded. Results from 2011 included data from 203 practices with almost 900 nurse-midwives attending over 69,000 vaginal births (ACNM, 2011).

## UNIFORM DATA SET

The American Association of Birth Centers (AABC) developed the Uniform Data Set (UDS; an online data registry) that collects comprehensive data on both the process and the outcomes of the nurse-midwifery model of care. It is intended that the data set be used to simultaneously collect data from all providers in hospital, birth center, and home birth settings. The UDS is stored on a password-protected secured site and is HIPAA compliant. The UDS also provides the provider with comprehensive statistic reports that include required reports for birth center accreditation, benchmarking reports for the ACNM Benchmarking Project, registration logs, delivery logs, incomplete reports, and custom reports (American Association of Birth Centers, 2007).

Stapleton conducted a validation study of the 189-item UDS (2011). Five birth center practices had a random audit of 2% of their records. Data from the health record were compared with data entered into the UDS. There was a high level of consistency between the health records and the UDS with 97.1% of the variables matching. This study shows the reliability of the UDS and encourages its use for research and quality assurance. Using such large data sets will greatly facilitate health policy changes.

Data from the UDS was used in a study by Stapleton, Osborne, and Illuzzi (2013) of 15,574 women planning to give birth in 79 birth centers across the United States. The transfer rate from birth center to hospital was 12% with the majority being non-emergent. Only 6% of the births were by cesarean section with 93% of the women having a vaginal birth. There were no maternal deaths and the fetal and neonatal mortality rate was the same as other studies of births to women with low-risk pregnancies. This study mirrors the results of the National Birth Center Study (Rooks et al., 1989) showing the positive and durable results of birth center care.

## PURPOSE OF OUTCOMES MEASUREMENT IN NURSE-MIDWIFERY PRACTICE

The most compelling rationale for outcomes measurement is that it assists in efforts to improve the quality of health care for patients. A recent report by the ACNM (2008) highlights that high-quality care, which includes high levels of client satisfaction and lower cost, is provided by CNM's with equal to or better outcomes than those of obstetricians or gynecologists.

Enhanced cost effectiveness is another reason for evaluating outcomes. In cost-effectiveness studies, alternative methods of obtaining the same goal are compared. Clients with similar conditions may be treated with alternative approaches, often with significantly different costs but with very similar outcomes. Studies that document the cost effectiveness of nurse-midwifery practice while maintaining clinical outcomes have long been documented (Cherry & Foster, 1982; Lubic, 1981; Oakley et al., 1996; Reid & Morris, 1979; Stewart & Clark, 1982). Jackson et al. (2003) discuss collaborative care with CNM versus traditional physician-based care and the decrease in length of stay and decreased emergency department visits documented for women in collaborative care. The safety outcomes of the neonate in this study were similar across both groups.

Alternatively, clients of CNMs and physicians with similar conditions may be treated with different approaches and one group may experience superior outcomes. An example of this is that physicians more often perform episiotomies, while the CNM might try different approaches, such as perineal massage, warm packs, or positioning, to reduce the need for episiotomy and reducing overall perineal trauma during childbirth (Hastings-Tolsma, Vincent, Emeis, & Francisco, 2007; Robinson, Noritz, Cohen, & Liberman, 2000). Another example of comparing different approaches to maternity care is the use of the Optimality Index-US (OI-US) which measures optimal maternity care (Cragin & Kennedy, 2006). Optimal is defined as obtaining the best outcomes with the least amount of intervention while taking into consideration the woman's physical and emotional status. Cragin and Kennedy (2006) studied 375 women in labor with moderate pregnancy risk status. Midwives provided care for 196 women, and 179 women were cared for by a physician. The mean OI-US was significantly higher for the midwifery care group. The care provided by the midwives included more mobility, oral hydration, nonpharmacologic pain relief, and spontaneous vaginal births than the care provided by the physicians. Yet both groups experienced good perinatal outcomes, thus showing that less interventive care during labor for women with moderate risk factors produces positive outcomes. Finally, outcomes measurement gives evidence and support to the practice of midwifery. Examples of how quality outcomes can influence and increase appreciation and accessibility of nurse-midwifery practice in the United States include the 2004 Virginia Governor's Task Force on Health-Care Reform recommendations for the development and funding of pilot birth centers in rural areas. The purpose of these sites is to demonstrate the effectiveness of midwifery care and increase access to high-quality pregnancy-related care. The recommendations call for the pilot sites collection and annual reporting of data using the American Association of Birth Centers Uniform Data Set (Governor's Health Reform Commission, 2007).

The federal government is also intrigued by the positive outcomes of midwifery care and wants to determine whether the midwifery model of care can be a solution to the problem of a high cost with poor outcome maternity care system. The Center for Medicare & Medicaid Innovation has developed Strong Start for Mothers and Newborns (Center for Medicare & Medicaid Innovation, 2012). This initiative is seeking to fund projects related to group prenatal care, birth centers, and maternity homes, all of which are based on the midwifery model of care.

Research is the basis of all clinical practice, a guiding principle shared by all disciplines. It is this requirement for evidence-based practice that is another rationale for outcome measurement in nurse-midwifery practice. While outcome measurement is not synonymous with research, the two methodologies provide empirical support for evidence-based changes in clinical practice.

## CLASSIFICATION OF OUTCOMES MEASUREMENT FOR NURSE-MIDWIFERY PRACTICE

There are several approaches to the classification of outcomes within nurse-midwifery practice. Each method provides data for evidence-based clinical practice. The following outcome classifications will be discussed: physiological, perceptual, psychosocial, cognitive, functional, and fiscal.

Physiological outcomes are those that have to do with the impact of CNM interventions on the process of birth. The division of physiological outcomes is somewhat arbitrary because all nurses utilize a holistic approach to health care, recognizing the interrelatedness of perceptual and psychosocial outcomes. Physiological outcomes can be further divided into groups of expected birth outcomes as well as adverse outcomes. It may be more helpful in outcome studies to focus on expected birth outcomes and to designate adverse events as variances from the usual and expected outcomes. Both classifications are of interest to CNMs because this information provides direction for clinical care improvement. Examples of physiological outcomes in midwifery practice include blood glucose levels, iron deficiency anemia, fetal heart rate, maternal breathing patterns, and use of relaxation techniques in labor.

Perceptual outcomes are defined in terms of patient satisfaction. This may include satisfaction with CNMs as providers, with the facilities, with the care received, or with the clinical outcomes. It is important to understand that perception refers to the situation as the client views it or understands it. While it may not be entirely congruent with the provider's reality, it does not matter. What does matter is that this is the client's perception of reality. Perceptual outcomes are crucial to the marketing and public acceptance of nurse-midwifery service.

Psychosocial outcomes are those that have to do with such things as the client's affective state, self-image, self-esteem, and interpersonal relationships. Examples of psychosocial outcomes that would be of clinical interest to nurse-midwives include maternal infant bonding, presence of social support, confidence in the ability to care for the infant, comfort with a pregnant body image, and sense of self-actualization associated with childbirth.

Cognitive outcomes include the knowledge and skills that the client will need to safely and effectively care for herself and/or an infant. These would include the knowledge of prenatal nutrition, the signs and symptoms of postpartum infection, and breastfeeding skills.

Functional outcomes have to do with the maintenance or improvement of physical functioning. While there are standardized measures of functional outcomes, such as various activities of daily living or independent activities of daily living scores, most CNM clients are women involved in a healthy childbearing process. There are standardized tools that measure functional outcomes in the postpartum woman; for example, the Childbirth Impact Profile (Tulman, Fawcett, Groblewski, & Silverman, 1990) and the Inventory of Functional Status after Childbirth (Tulman & Fawcett, 1988). Examples of functional outcomes include the ability to care for the infant and readiness to return to a job outside the home.

Fiscal outcomes involve those having to do with the cost of care. Because health care is a business it is essential that nurse-midwives understand the fiscal aspects of maternity care. Fiscal measures include such things as cost per case, hospitalization costs and length of stay, incremental costs of specialized nursing care during labor, reimbursement by payer, and laboratory costs. There are two approaches to the measurement of fiscal outcomes: cost data and charge data.

### Charge Data Analysis

Some institutions utilize charges as a proxy measurement for costs. Charges are defined as the charges appearing on the client's bill. Charges are somewhat arbitrary and do include some profit or mark-up amount added to the cost of producing a service or product. Just as a department store adds a mark-up to the charge for clothing or appliances, so does a health care system add a profit amount to the cost of producing a service? Charges are the same for each client for each procedure and do not reflect policy or group discounts. Because contractual payers often receive a provider discount, it is important that charges be studied before the discounts are applied for the purpose of outcomes measurement. Charges can be collected from both the client billing records and from the provider professional service records.

### Cost Analysis

Other institutions have a cost accounting system that will permit the measurement of actual costs of client care, that is, the cost of the service being produced. Cost is a complex concept and can be further reduced to a consideration of direct costs (supplies, salaries, and rent) and indirect costs (employee benefits, costs allocated by other departments, for example, a portion of the building maintenance). Some costs are defined as fixed, that is, they do not change with an increase in client volume. An example of a fixed cost would be heat and light costs. Other costs are variable, meaning that they change with client volume. Laundry and housekeeping costs are examples of variable costs.

What is important in fiscal outcome measurement is that CNMs understand what is included in the costs or charges to make appropriate comparisons. Another consideration is that charges in a clinical practice may be bundled. This means that there is a prospective fee determined by an organization for a particular set of services. For example, hospital charges associated with a normal vaginal delivery may be set at $4,000. This is one all-inclusive fee and there will not be additional charges reflected on the client billing record. This approach does make it difficult to determine variation in fiscal outcomes. If there are no other cost data available when charges are bundled, it is difficult to assess the impact of practice changes on costs.

A decision must be made as to the appropriate interval or timing of charge or cost outcome data collection for nurse-midwifery clients. The purpose of the study will determine the period of measurement. If charges are to represent the entire period of pregnancy, one method to consider is to define the period from the date of determination of pregnancy until 2 months after birth to capture the full scope of the charges for the mother. When collecting fiscal data related to infant outcomes, similar decisions regarding the appropriate measurement interval must be made. Because many infants do not remain within the CNM system but move to pediatrician care, this is an important decision.

## DEVELOPING CLIENT OUTCOME MEASURES

Developing client outcomes measures is not difficult. It is something that was a part of undergraduate nursing education and included as a step in the nursing process: assessment, analysis, outcome identification, planning, implementation, and outcome evaluation. The CNM builds on that foundation and uses the knowledge and skill base of nurse-midwifery practice to identify and write outcomes supported by evidence-based practice guidelines for clients during the perinatal period. Two basic questions start this process:

1. What results are expected as a result of the implementation of evidence-based guidelines?
2. When will the results likely be achieved by the client and/or family?

When evaluating practice, it is essential to be cognizant of some fundamental principles in outcome analysis. These principles are listed below:

1. Outcomes must be measurable. ACNM outcome that states that "client satisfaction will improve" is not measurable. It is necessary to be explicit about the indicators that will be used to measure satisfaction. The CNM in this case must specify the tool to be used to measure client satisfaction. For example, "Scores on the Picker patient satisfaction tool will increase after CNM care" is a specific measurable outcome.
2. The outcome must relate to the care process or intervention. Spontaneous pushing during labor can reasonably be expected to relate to the postpartum perineal condition.
3. The outcome should be realistic for both the client and the CNM. While improving client nutrition is a desirable outcome, there will be some clients who have no interest in the outcome and no amount

of education and teaching material will impact their knowledge of nutrition and alter intake. It is important, however, to study negative outcomes as well as positive outcomes. There is much to be learned in both directions.

4. Outcomes are measured within an accessible time span. If a CNM wishes to study maternal infant bonding comparing attachment indications at 1 week of age to those of 1 year of age for the same subjects, there will be major difficulties in maintaining the subjects in the study. This is not to negate the value of the study, but to help the CNM to anticipate the inherent challenges in such a design.

5. The risk status of the subject population is described. Risk is defined as "the presence or absence of selected factors associated with non-optimal outcomes" (Selwyn, 1990). While the typical population of clients of CNMs is described as low to moderate risk, there are clinical differences among midwifery practices as to what constitutes low risk. Many studies utilize the risk factors that would preclude admission to the midwifery service as descriptors of the status of the population. This might include such things as: hypertension requiring medication during pregnancy, serious cardiac disease, chronic renal or lung disease, or known multiple gestation. While there is debate in the literature regarding the accuracy of obstetric risk assessment instruments, it is necessary that the risk profile is described in order that appropriate comparisons can be made.

6. All data collection has a cost. Often novices at outcomes studies ask, "How many subjects are needed?" The only answer is, "It depends." It depends on the size of the population available, the sensitivity of the instrument used to measure outcomes, and the resources available to commit to data collection. More is usually better, but it is necessary to be realistic about the cost of data collection. Some outcomes may be collected for all clients within the midwifery service. At other times sampling techniques may be used after preliminary analysis of a pilot that would yield sufficient data to conduct a power analysis. Such an analysis is a means of establishing that the study was conducted on a large enough sample to find an effect or relationship among variables if indeed it does exist.

Here are some examples of individual client outcomes measures written for a nurse-midwifery practice:

1. For a client at the first prenatal visit: Client will verbalize an understanding of 2,200 calorie diet, the food pyramid, dietary needs in

pregnancy, such as iron and calcium, and complete a 3-day intake diary by her next visit.

2. For a client at the 8-month visit: Client will demonstrate knowledge of signs and symptoms of onset of labor and verbalize when to call the CNM.
3. For a client at her first postpartum visit: Breastfeeding at least 8 to 12 times per day 1 week after delivery.

Note that all of these outcomes are written for an individual client. It is also important to recognize the importance of individual outcomes as well as the aggregate outcomes. CNMs are concerned with outcome evaluation on both an individual client basis and in aggregate groups. This process helps the CNM to rapidly identify deviations from expected outcomes and to adjust individual client care appropriately.

Outcome measurements on aggregate groups are defined as issues related to a specific, identified population. Outcomes for the aggregate group would be those that are appropriate for all clients within the nurse-midwifery service. These outcomes might include the following:

1. Verbalize signs and symptoms of postpartum endometritis before discharge from birthing center.
2. Demonstrate safety in: taking infant temperature, bathing infant, and positioning infant in crib within 24 hours of birth.
3. Adhere to recommended schedule for follow-up postpartum visits.
4. Presence and extent of perineal laceration.

It is often helpful to utilize a formal approach for identifying clinical outcomes.

It is assumed that the subject of the outcome is the client or an aspect of the client: a blood value, the position of the infant, and blood loss. The client behavior is the observable activity or measurement that the client will demonstrate at some future time. Things such as drink, walk, report, or achievement of specific vital signs or lab values are examples of client behaviors. The criterion of performance sets the parameters for the behavior identified in the outcome (Murray & Atkinson, 2000). In clinical practice, the CNM may want the hemoglobin not to drop below 10.5 g/dL and weight gain not to exceed 35 lb. The time frame is a realistic estimate of when the client can reasonably be expected to achieve the outcome. Some outcomes are specific to the first trimester (taking supplements that include folic acid, avoiding medications that are possible teratogens), and others begin at the first stage of labor (use of different techniques for relaxation, maintenance of hydration). Finally, a condition may be added if necessary. The CNM might specify the condition under which the behavior specified in the outcome is to occur. Examples of this might include with the assistance of client's mother, after 1 month of iron supplements, or using a food pyramid picture.

In clinical practice, when thinking of identifying client outcomes, it is important to emphasize that outcomes must be individualized for a particular client. Outcomes that are mutually established with clients are much more likely to be achieved than those that are solely determined by a CNM. There is also a cultural component to outcomes. What is desirable within one culture may be inappropriate in others. For example, in some cultures a grandmother plays a significant role in the care of the infant and the new mother. The CNM needs to incorporate the grandmother as a significant other in the care process, including outcome measurement.

## SCHEDULED MEASUREMENTS OF OUTCOMES

Essential to planning any evaluation is determining the measurement of the outcome. This is a major clinical consideration requiring the knowledge of nurse-midwifery practice. One schema used by CNMs is to consider time intervals. The following time periods during pregnancy may be used to evaluate specific objectives related to maternal fetal outcomes: prenatal care (trimesters or weeks), intrapartum care that may be further divided into stages of labor, and postpartum care (first 2 hours, first 12 hours).

Another way to define time intervals might be to consider interim and discharge outcomes. At the completion of the childbirth process, there are some outcomes that signify the completion of the care process for that episode of care. The client may be independent in infant care, may have established a strong maternal–child bond, and may have established new health and wellness patterns reflective of being a family. At this time, usually within 6 to 8 weeks postpartum, the CNM may discharge the client from the care relationship. While some women choose to continue to remain in the practice of CNMs for primary care, the focus shifts from maternity care to well-woman care. Thus, there is the completion of one phase of care. Outcomes may then be classified as interim outcomes, which were those occurring during the care process, and discharge outcomes, those occurring at the completion of the care process. If discharge outcomes are not achieved, it may be an indication that there is a need for additional care. For example, if a mother appears to be experiencing postpartum depression, the CNM may consider a referral to a mental health professional.

## VARIANCE FROM EXPECTED OUTCOMES

Variances occur when an expected outcome is not met at all, met later than expected, or even met ahead of the time defined for measurement (Murray & Atkinson, 2000). A rather standard classification system for variances has evolved in recent years. The system attempts to classify variances according to their cause. System variances are those that result from variations in the system, perhaps scheduling glitches or computer downtime (Murray & Atkinson, 2000). A patient may not have kept a scheduled appointment because the information was incorrectly entered into the computer and the client did not understand the date of her next appointment, resulting in a missed visit. If the clinical outcome being measured is rate of kept appointments, this will result in a variance.

Another type of variance is provider variance. One CNM provider may choose not to do certain lab procedures, feeling that for this particular client it is duplicative or unnecessary. This may result in a variance in lab charges due to provider variance.

The third kind of variance is client variance. One client may be physically active, within normal weight range, and accustomed to engaging in strenuous cardiovascular exercise three times per week. This client may experience fewer discomforts of pregnancy, less weight gain, a shorter labor, and a faster recovery than defined in clinical outcomes. This is also an example of a positive variance if weight gain and labor length still fall within normal ranges. It is important to understand that not all variances are negative. Variances can mean that the client exceeded the usual outcomes. It is equally important for CNMs to study both positive and negative outcomes to effectively change their clinical practice.

## TOOLS FOR OUTCOME DATA COLLECTION

Before selecting and purchasing a data collection tool or designing a new data collection tool that might be duplicative or have limited use, it is important to first understand what tools and programs are available and their intended uses and applications. Currently, there are several tools available to assist CNMs in the collection of outcome data, including the Uniform Data Set developed by the American Association of Birth Centers. The UDS is under revision and work is underway to integrate it with Electronic Medical Record.

Additional software programs are available both commercially and through the Centers for Disease Control and Prevention (CDC). These include word processing, epidemiological analysis, and data management programs.

## SOURCES OF OUTCOME DATA

Because outcome studies all involve some costs, it is useful to understand some of the existing sources of outcome data available for healthcare information. These sources may decrease effort and costs when assessing outcome data. These are some sources; not all health care systems will have all of these tools.

1. Routinely collected administrative data. This typically includes vital statistics (births, deaths), payer source, Medicare/Medicaid, claims data, which includes principle diagnosis and procedure codes, complications, comorbidities, and records of adverse events. There may also be a case mix index (CMI), which is a measure of the resources used to treat a clinical population (Adams, 1996). CMI is useful as a tool to make comparisons among populations when there is not another tool to use to adjust for severity of illness. The clients of CNMs could be assumed to typically have a low CMI relative to other hospitalized patients.
2. Birth logs. Outcome data may also be gathered from birth logs. Hospitals and birth centers routinely keep concise data that usually include information such as place of birth, maternal age, gravity/parity, date of first prenatal visit, number of prenatal visits, total weight gain, significant prenatal events, significant intrapartum events, and infant data. Historically, birth logs have been kept in handwritten logs on birthing units.
3. Data sets. Data may also be gathered from existing data sets. Data may be collected from data sets, such as the UDS or the ACNM's Data Set. Many of these sets include comprehensive care and outcome data.
4. Discharge summary. Upon discharge, hospitals complete a discharge summary that consists of data extracted from the chart. This

may include such data elements as Social Security number, medical record number, name, admission and discharge dates, length of
stay, disposition (home, nursing home, and sub-acute facility), total
charges, employment status, and race. A cautionary note is that
when race is included in this data set, it may be incomplete and
unreliable due to diversity within racial categories, the number of
people with bi-racial identities, and differences in self-assignment
to potential categories (Alvidrez, Azocar, & Miranda, 1996; Foster &
Martinez, 1995).

5. Obstetric discharge summary. Obstetric units will typically have
a department-specific form that will include additional data. This
form includes such data elements as intrapartum procedures, postpartum procedures, data related to lacerations, infection, or phle-
bitis. These data may be entered into a computerized database that
permits easy access and retrieval.

6. Program-specific data collection. Each health care system may collect
data related to specific programs. For CNMs this may include newborn
screens for hearing loss, medications used during hospitalization, tests
ordered, car seats distributed, teen births, and early discharge.

7. Disease registration. Some institutions participate in registries for
various diseases. Programs of interest to CNMs might include sexually transmitted diseases, HIV/AIDS, or birth defects. Some of the
registries are required by state law and reporting by providers is
mandated.

8. Critical pathways or evidence-based clinical practice guidelines.
These are a form of an interdisciplinary plan of care and are used in
many systems. Some perinatal clinical pathways are initiated at the
first client visit and outline a plan of care concluding at discharge
from the midwifery service. Most pathways contain outcomes that
are evaluated at specified times.

One caution when collecting outcome data is the need to protect
the confidentiality of the clinical record data. Most institutions maintain rigorous control over who may access data and for what purposes.
If a CNM is considering an outcome study that has the potential to be
published, the approval of a human subject's protection committee or
institutional review board is necessary. This must be done before the
initiation of such a study. Typically, the use of data for quality improvement studies does not require such approval but then the CNM must
understand that no publication of results is possible. When in doubt,
it is recommended to seek consultation with the chairperson of the
human subject protection committee at the institution.

## REVIEW OF NURSE-MIDWIFERY OUTCOME STUDIES

Discussion of several selected studies will illustrate approaches to outcome measurement within nurse-midwifery clinical practice. While the studies are largely from a research perspective rather than a quality improvement focus, the measurement principles are the same.

The National Birth Center Study (NBCS; Rooks et al., 1989) was a landmark investigation of 18,000 women who enrolled at 84 birth centers across the United States. A full report of the study included descriptions of the birth center clients, birth center care providers, and birth center care. The study measured clinical outcomes of birth centers and compared them with outcomes of low-risk hospital births. Client satisfaction and satisfaction with charges were also measured. Findings from this study led the researchers to conclude that there is no evidence that hospitals are a safer place than birthing centers for low-risk births. While a complete summary is beyond the scope of this chapter, the three articles that provide the complete report are essential reading for CNMs.

A second study (Paine & Tinker Dawkins, 1992) compared two types of bearing down techniques as they related to fetal and maternal outcomes of arterial umbilical cord blood pH and length of the second stage of labor. In this group, the care process was either using the Valsalva maneuver or spontaneous pushing. Although the subject size was small, the authors concluded that the bearing down method does not have a negative effect on either the mother or the infant.

In another study, Oakley et al. (1996) compared the outcomes of women cared for by obstetricians and CNMs in a hospital-based setting. The authors reported that fiscal outcomes, specifically hospital charges and professional service fees, were significantly less for women in the nurse-midwife group. The lesser charges are especially interesting because the charge for obstetrician services and CNM services were the same in this institution. There was one bundled charge for all perinatal care so the differences that existed between providers reflected charges beyond the usual and customary practice. Oakley also reported differences in clinical outcomes of infant–mother separation, extent of perineal laceration, and the number of maternal complications, with CNM providers being significantly lower on each outcome.

A study of macrosomic infant (birth weight greater than 4,000 g) outcomes (Nixon, Avery, & Savik, 1998) asked specific research questions: Is there a difference in Apgar scores, birth morbidity, and shoulder dystocias between infants with birth weights of 2,500 to 3999 g,

4,000 to 4.499 g, and greater than 4,500 g? They also studied route of delivery, maternal position at birth, and antenatal variables that might predict poor infant outcomes. Shoulder dystocia occurred more frequently in large infants but ICU admission rates did not. Apgar scores at 1 and 5 minutes were significantly higher for infants weighing greater than 4,500 g. The Apgar differences were not clinically significant. The authors concluded that nurse-midwifery management of the labor of these mothers, in consultation with physicians, produced outcomes similar to those reported in the medical literature.

A study (Sampselle & Hines, 1999) examined the perineal outcomes of 39 women who had spontaneous vaginal births. Chart data were examined for documentation of extent of episiotomy and/or laceration sustained. Findings indicated that women who used spontaneous pushing were more likely to have intact perineum and less likely to have episiotomies and second- or third-degree lacerations. Although the results of this study are consistent with previous findings in the literature, the authors cite the need for conclusive evidence to be gathered in randomized clinical trials.

One comparison study (Jackson et al., 2003) looked at outcomes, safety, and resource utilization differences between traditional physician-based care and a collaborative (CNM/obstetricians) management birth center. This study included 2,957 low-income pregnant women and their infants who presented for prenatal care at several sites. Data from this study revealed that complications in both groups were similar, while the collaborative care group had a greater number of spontaneous vaginal deliveries and less epidural anesthesia use. The study authors concluded that for low-risk women, both types of care result in safe outcomes for mothers, but there were fewer operative deliveries and less medical resources used in the collaborative care groups.

A recent comparison study (Cragin & Kennedy, 2006) looked at midwifery and medical care practices and measured optimal perinatal outcomes in 375 moderate-risk women. This pilot study used a new instrument (the OI-US) to compare nurse-midwife and physician care among women who had moderate risk for poor pregnancy outcomes. The instrument consisted of scoring 40 care processes and outcomes across pregnancy, parturition, neonatal condition, and postpartum maternal condition, with higher average OI scores indicating more optimal balance between interventions and outcomes for a given health status. These data were collected from patient records. The authors of this study found that like groups of moderate-risk women cared for by nurse-midwives experienced less use of technology and equal or better health outcomes than women cared for by physicians and had equally positive neonatal outcomes. The researchers acknowledge a limitation of this study was the use of a relatively small convenience sample and recommend additional similar studies using this tool with similar populations of women.

Hastings-Tolsma et al. (2007) examined factors related to perineal trauma in childbirth. This retrospective analysis used recorded birth data from the Nurse Midwifery Clinical Data Set from 510 singleton pregnancies with uncomplicated prenatal courses. Data revealed that for all women, laceration was more likely in lithotomy position for birth. Factors found to be protective of the perineum during birth included perineal massage, warm compress use, manual support, and birthing in the left lateral position. The authors concluded that side lying position for birth and perineal support and compress use are important interventions for decreasing perineal trauma during childbirth.

A study published in 2012 by Neal and Lowe presented a partograph to assist with labor assessment in low-risk nulliparous women. The evidence-based tool was designed to correctly identify abnormal labor progression and provide an ongoing evaluation of interventions. The goal is to decrease the cesarean section rate in low-risk nulliparous women.

## CONCLUSION

In 2009, CNMs attended 8.1% of all births and 11.4% of vaginal births (Declercq, 2012). This was a significant rise from 20 years prior, when CNM-attended births were noted to represent 0.6% of all births (Martin et al., 2007). As the number of births attended by nurse-midwives increases, it is important to assess outcomes to justify fiscal, quality, and safety goals for the care of women and babies. Nurse-midwives are poised to improve the quality of health care and to act as change agents in the policy arena related to maternal care. This chapter has reviewed outcomes for nurse-midwifery practice. Some suggested outcome classifications in nurse-midwifery practice, including examples of specific client and aggregate data and outcomes studies regarding nurse-midwifery practice, were presented. The definition of health care outcomes and the process of evaluating these in relation to nurse-midwifery practice have also been discussed.

Nurse-midwives should use the frameworks presented in this chapter to begin analyzing their practices and evaluating their own practice outcomes based on measurements used in previous studies. Evidence-based practice guidelines and protocols need to be evaluated and updated to reflect current clinical practice. Data demonstrating the safety, quality, and fiscal attributes provided by nurse-midwives need to be widely available for health care providers and consumers to evaluate when making decisions about maternal care. This information will increase the quality and safety of maternity care provided to women and babies and increases the availability of nurse-midwifery services.

## Answers to Chapter Discussion Questions

1. ▪ Outcome measurement improves the quality of clinical care for patients by defining effective practice protocols. Practices and protocols that are evaluated and found to have best outcomes can be replicated, thus improving care for mothers and babies.
   ▪ Outcome measurement enhances cost effectiveness. Through the use of cost-effectiveness studies, alternative methods of obtaining the same goal are compared. Practices and protocols with satisfactory outcomes and lower cost can be identified and implemented.
   ▪ Outcome measurement gives evidence and support for the practice of midwifery. Examples of quality outcomes can influence and increase appreciation and accessibility of nurse-midwifery practice in United States.
2. ▪ Functional status includes the physical and emotional well-being of the mother.
   ▪ Cost of care including both direct and indirect costs.
   ▪ Patient satisfaction.
   ▪ Clinical outcomes.
3. ▪ Data were collected on four specific areas: functional status that includes the physical and emotional well-being of the mother, cost of care including both direct and indirect costs, patient satisfaction, and clinical outcomes. Results of the data collection were compiled and nurse-midwifery services could see how they ranked compared with other practices for each indicator. Individual practices could then contact higher ranking services to learn best practices, which they could incorporate into their own practices.
4. ▪ The optimality measures optimal maternity care. Optimal is defined as obtaining the best outcomes with the least amount

of intervention, while taking into consideration the woman's physical and emotional status.

5. ■ Physiological outcomes are those that have to do with the impact of CNM interventions on the process of birth.

■ Perceptual outcomes are defined in terms of patient satisfaction. This may include satisfaction with CNMs as providers, with the facilities, with the care received, or with the clinical outcomes. Perception refers to the situation as the client views it or understands it.

■ Psychosocial outcomes are those that have to do with such things as the client's affective state, self-image, self-esteem, and interpersonal relationships.

■ Cognitive outcomes include the knowledge and skills that the client will need to safely and effectively care for herself and/or an infant.

■ Functional outcomes have to do with the maintenance or improvement of physical functioning. Fiscal outcomes involve those having to do with the cost of care (cost per case, hospitalization costs and length of stay, incremental costs of specialized nursing care during labor, reimbursement by payer, and laboratory costs). The two approaches to the measurement of fiscal outcomes are cost data and charge data.

## WEB LINKS

AABC homepage. AABC is a multi-disciplinary membership organization that comprises individuals and institutions who support the birth center concept. The Uniform Data Set registry is located at the site http://www.birthcenters.org.

ACNM homepage. The ACNM is the professional organization that represents Certified Nurse-Midwives (CNMs) and Certified-Midwives (CMs). The site reports on the latest updates on nurse-midwifery practice and has links to professional resources, including results of the ACNM Benchmarking Project (http://www.midwife.org).

Childbirth Connections evolved from the Maternity Center Association founded in 1918. It is a national nonprofit organization committed to transforming maternity care through evidence-based practice and consumer education. Results from the *Listening to Mothers* national survey

can be found on this website (http://www.childbirthconnection.org/
home.asp?Visitor=Professional).

*Journal of Midwifery & Women's Health*. The peer reviewed journal of the
American College of Nurse-Midwives presents evidence-based practice
research in the areas of maternity care, gynecology, primary care for
women and newborns, public health, health care policy, and global health
(http://onlinelibrary.wiley.com/journal/10.1111/(ISSN)1542-2011).

## REFERENCES

Adams, T. P. (1996). Case mix index: Nursing's new management tool. *Nursing
Management, 27*(9), 31–32.

Alvidrez, J., Azocar, F., & Miranda, J. (1996). Demystifying the concept of
ethnicity for psychotherapy researchers. *Journal of Consulting and Clinical
Psychology, 64*(5), 903–908.

American Association of Birth Centers. (2007). *American association of birth centers.* Retrieved June 23, 2008, from http:///www.birthcenters.org/

American College of Nurse-Midwives (ACNM). (2012). *California state fact
sheet.* Retrieved from http://www.midwife.org/index.asp?bid=&cat=11&b
utton=Search&rec=177

American College of Nurse Midwives. (2008). *Nurse-midwifery in 2008:
Evidence-based practice. A summary of research on midwifery practice in the
United States.* Retrieved July 7, 2008 from http://www.midwife.org/
siteFiles/news/nurse_midwifery_in_2008.pdf

American College of Nurse Midwives. (2011). *CNM/CN attended births.* Retrieved
from http://www.midwife.org/CNM/CM-attended-Birth-Statistics

Anderson, R. E., & Anderson, D. A. (1999). The cost effectiveness of home
birth. *Journal of Nurse Midwifery, 44,* 30–35.

Breckinridge, M. (1981). *Wide neighborhoods: A story of the frontier nursing service.* Lexington, KY: The University Press of Kentucky.

Browne, H. E., & Isaacs, G. (1976). The frontier nursing service: The primary
care nurse in the community hospital. *American Journal of Obstetrics and
Gynecology, 124*(1), 14–17.

Center for Medicare and Medicaid Innovation. (2012). *Strong start for mothers and newborns.* Retrieved from http://innovations.cms.gov/initiatives/
strong-start/index.html

Cherry, J., & Foster, J. (1982). Comparison of hospital charges generated by certified nurse-midwives' and physicians' clients. *Journal of Nurse-Midwifery,
77*(1), 7–11.

Collins-Fulea, C., Mohr, J. J., & Tillett, J. (2005). Improving midwifery practice:
The American college of nurse-midwives' benchmarking project. *Journal of
Midwifery and Women's Heath, 50*(6), 461–471.

Cragin, L., & Kennedy, P. (2006). Linking obstetric and midwifery practice with optimal outcomes. *The Association of Women's Health, Obstetric and Neonatal Nurses, 35*(6), 779–785.

Declercq, E. (2012). Trends in midwife-attended births in the United States, 1982–2009. *Journal of Midwifery & Woman's Health, 57*, 321–326.

Foster, S. L., & Martinez, C. R. (1995). Ethnicity: Conceptual and methodological issues in child clinical research. *Journal of Clinical Child Psychology, 24*, 214–226.

Governor's Health Reform Commission. (2007, September). *Roadmap for Virginia's health: A report of the governor's health reform commission.* Retrieved June 27, 2008, from http://www.hhr.virginia.gov/Initiatives/ HealthReform/MeetingMats/FullCouncil/Health_ReformComm_Draft_ Report.pdf

Hastings-Tolsma, M., Vincent, D., Emesis, C., & Francisco, T. (2007). Getting through Birth in one piece: Protecting the perineum. *Maternal Child Nursing, May/June,* 158–164.

Hatem, M., Sandall, J., Devance, D., Soltani, H., & Gates, S. (2009). Midwife-led versus other models of care for childbearing women. *The Cochrane Library, 2009* (3), 1–109.

Jackson, D. J., Lang, J. M., Swartz, W. H., Ganiants, T. G., Fullerton, J., Ecker, J., et al. (2003). Outcomes, safety, and resource utilization in a collaborative care birth center program compared with traditional physician-based perinatal care. *American Journal of Public Health, 93*(6), 999–1006.

Levy, B. S., Wilkinson, F. S., & Marine, W. M. (1971). Reducing neonatal mortality rate with nurse-midwives. *American Journal of Obstetrics and Gynecology, 109*(1), 50–58.

Lubic, R. (1981). Evaluation of an out-of-hospital maternity center for low-risk maternity patients. In L. Aiken (Ed.), *Health policy and nursing practice.* New York, NY: McGraw Hill.

Martin, J. A., Hamilton, B. E., Sutton, P. D., Ventura, S. J., Menacker, F.,... Munson, M. L. (2007). Births: Final data for 2005. *National vital statistics reports 56*(6). Hyattsville, MD: Centers for Disease Control, National Center for Health Statistics.

Montgomery, T. W. (1969). A case for nurse-midwives. *American Journal of Obstetrics & Gynecology, 105,* 309–313.

Murray, M. E., & Atkinson, L. D. (2000). Understanding the nursing process in a changing care environment (6th ed.). New York, NY: McGraw Hill.

Neal, J. & Lowe, N (2012) Physiologic partograph improve birth safety and outcomes among low risk, nulliparous women with spontaneous labor onset. *Medical Hypotheses, 76*(2), p 319–326.

Nixon, S. A., Avery, M. D., & Savik, K. (1998). Outcomes of macrosomic infants in a nurse-midwifery service. *Journal of Nurse Midwifery, 43*(4), 280–286.

Oakley, D., Murray, M. E., Murtland, T., Hayashi, R., Anderson, H. F., Mayes, F., & Rooks, J. (1996). Comparisons of outcomes of maternity care by obstetricians and certified nurse midwives. *Obstetrics Obstetrics & Gynecology, 88*(5), 823–829.

Paine, L. L., & Tinker Dawkins, D. (1992). The effect of maternal bearing-down efforts on arterial umbilical cord pH and length of the second stage of labor. *Journal of Nurse-Midwifery, 37*(1), 61–63.

Reid, M., & Morris, J. (1979). Prenatal care and cost effectiveness: Changes in health expenditures and birth outcomes following the establishment of a nurse-midwife program. *Medical Care, 17*(5), 491–500.

Robinson, J., Norwitz, E., Cohen, A., & Lieberman, E. (2000). Predictors of episiotomy use at first spontaneous vaginal delivery. *Obstetrics and Gynecology, 96*(2), 214–218.

Rooks, J. P., Weatherby, N. L., Ernst, E. K. M., Stapleton, S., Rosen, D., & Rosenfield, A. (1989). Outcomes of care in birth centers: The national birth center study. *The New England Journal of Medicine, 321*, 1804–1811.

Sampselle, C., & Hines, S. L. (1999). Spontaneous pushing during birth: Relationship to perineal outcomes. *Journal of Nurse-Midwifery, 44*(1), 36–39.

Selwyn, B. J. (1990). The accuracy of obstetric risk assessment instruments for predicting mortality, low birth weight, and preterm birth. In J. Merkatz & J. Thompson (Eds.), *New perspectives on premature care*. New York, NY: Elsevier.

Stapleton, S. R. (2011). Validation of an online data registry for midwifery practices: A pilot. *Journal of Midwifery and Women's Health, 56*(5) 452–460.

Stapleton, S. R., Osborne, C., Illuzzi, J. (2013) Outcomes of care in birth centers: Demonstration of a durable model. *Journal of Midwifery and Women's Health, 58*(1), 3–14.

Stewart, R., & Clark, L. (1982). Nurse-midwifery practice in an in-hospital birthing center. *Journal of Nurse-Midwifery, 27,* 21–26.

Tulman, L., & Fawcett, J. (1988). Return of functional ability after childbirth. *Nursing Research, 37,* 77–81.

Tulman, L., Fawcett, J., Groblewski, L., & Silverman, L. (1990). Changes in functional status after childbirth. *Nursing Research, 39,* 70–75.

# Chapter 10: Outcomes Assessment in Nurse Anesthesia

MICHAEL J. KREMER AND MARGARET FAUT CALLAHAN

## Chapter Objectives

1. Describe the historical influences on outcomes assessment of nurse anesthesia practice.
2. List constraining variables that limit research opportunities in the area of nurse anesthesia outcomes.
3. Review the outcomes to date of linking pay to performance for surgical procedures.
4. Suggest next steps for cost-effectiveness analyses of nurse anesthesia care.
5. Examine the role of human patient simulation in knowledge transfer to the clinical area and risk reduction.
6. Discuss the risks for certified registered nurse anesthetists associated with participation in prospective, multicenter anesthesia outcomes studies.

## Chapter Discussion Questions

1. What was the impetus for the development of closed malpractice claims research in anesthesia?

2. Describe the relationship between human patient simulation and outcomes in anesthesia care.

3. Why did investigators posit that Surgical Care Improvement Project compliance should not be used to determine Medicare and Medicaid reimbursement rates?

4. Regarding adverse perioperative outcomes, how is the role of anesthesia versus that of surgery in contributing to the adverse outcome determined?

5. What enabling and constraining factors are related to the implementation of evidence-based practice?

## AN OVERVIEW OF OUTCOMES RESEARCH IN NURSE ANESTHESIA

Certified registered nurse anesthetists (CRNAs) have provided anesthesia care to patients in the United States for over 125 years. Some 44,000 CRNAs administer 32 million anesthetics annually in the United States (American Association of Nurse Anesthetists [AANA], 2012a).

Assessing outcomes of nurse anesthesia care is an essential component of CRNA practice. Participating in quality assessment activities is among the *Standards for Accreditation of Nurse Anesthesia Educational Programs* (2012) promulgated by the Council on Accreditation of Nurse Anesthesia Educational Programs (COA, 2012) and in the *Scope and Standards for Nurse Anesthesia Practice* (AANA, 2010a). Studies have compared outcomes of care provided by various mixes of anesthesia providers (Dulisse & Cromwell, 2010; Hogan, Seifert, Moore, & Simonson, 2010; Needleman & Minnick, 2009, 2010; Pine, Holt, & Lou, 2003; Simonson, Ahern, & Hendryx) and have demonstrated satisfactory clinical outcomes with anesthesia provided by CRNAs. However, there are no prospective multicenter studies on anesthesia outcomes.

Methodological challenges in anesthesia outcomes research include the various mixes of anesthesia providers and the complexity of health care settings where anesthesia services are delivered. CRNAs provide anesthesia services in hospital operating rooms, labor and delivery suites, and in numerous ancillary areas, including cardiac catheterization laboratories, endoscopy suites, and interventional radiology settings. CRNAs may be the sole anesthesia providers in rural and medically underserved areas as well as in forward-deployed military operations. Anesthesia in ambulatory surgery centers and office-based practices may be provided by a CRNA working collaboratively with a surgeon, dentist, or podiatrist. In some settings, an anesthesiologist may work collaboratively with two to four CRNAs administering concurrent anesthetics.

The earliest outcome research in nurse anesthesia was conducted by pioneering nurse anesthetist Alice Magaw. Miss Magaw, a nurse anesthetist at the Mayo Clinic, published a paper in the *Northwestern Lancet* in 1899 detailing over 3,000 ether and chloroform anesthetics she administered without a fatality (Bankert, 1989). These anesthetics were administered to patients undergoing operations ranging from general to orthopedic; ear, nose, and throat; gynecological; and urological surgeries. Note that endotracheal intubation was not common until the mid-twentieth century, and that Korotkoff did not identify the five sounds associated with blood pressure measurement until 1905.

It has been suggested that subsequent legal challenges to nurse anesthesia practice were defeated through the documentation of safe, quality care provided by Miss Magaw (Bankert, 1989). Like Nightingale (McDonald, 2001), this leader in the specialty of nurse anesthesia recognized that in addition to clinical excellence, maintenance of a clinical outcomes database and dissemination of research findings in peer-reviewed literature, were requisites of professionalism.

## STUDIES OF ANESTHESIA OUTCOMES

Municipal or state-level study commissions that examined anesthetic morbidity and mortality in the 1930s and 1940s were hampered by the unwillingness of anesthesia providers to share their data (Ruth, 1945). No concerted effort was made to track anesthetic outcomes until the 1950s.

The first large-scale study of anesthesia morbidity and mortality was conducted by Beecher and Todd (1954). Muscle relaxants were found to be significantly associated with anesthetic morbidity and mortality. Almost 60 years later, investigators have noted a high incidence of postoperative residual blockade in contemporary anesthesia practices, despite the advances in pharmacology, technology, and provider education (Murphy, 2012).

In the 1970s, a rapid increase in malpractice insurance premiums prompted a new research method for investigating anesthetic outcomes: analysis of closed malpractice claims. Pioneered by the National Association of Insurance Commissioners, this methodology was adopted by the American Society of Anesthesiologists (ASA) that has conducted the largest anesthesia closed claims study to date with nearly 9,000 cases reviewed (Brunner, 1984; Cheney, 2010; Metzner, Posner, Lam, & Domino, 2011). Over 50 publications in peer-reviewed journals have emanated from this study, often with the focus of lessons learned in specific practice-related areas such as equipment, airway management, and specialty practice areas. Recent publications include risk factors associated with ischemic optic neuropathy after spinal fusion surgery (Lee et al., 2012); cervical spinal cord, root and bony spine injuries (Hindman et al., 2011); injury and liability associated with cervical procedures for chronic pain (Ramthell et al., 2011); and malpractice claims associated with medication management for chronic pain (Fitzgibbon et al., 2010).

The American Association of Nurse Anesthetists Foundation (AANAF) has also conducted a closed claims study that is methodologically similar to the ASA study. Peer-reviewed papers related to this study have also focused on lessons learned in specific areas such as preinduction activities and the genesis of perioperative respiratory, peripheral nerve, and other injuries (Crawforth, 2002; Fritzlen, Kremer, & Biddle, 2003; Jordan, Kremer, Crawforth, & Shott, 2001; Kremer, Faut-Callahan, & Hicks, 2002; Larson & Jordan, 2001; MacRae, 2007; Moody & Kremer, 2001). Distinctions in outcomes among anesthesia providers have not been described in these studies.

Research findings from both the AANAF and ASA studies demonstrate that the process of care, rather than patient acuity or procedure complexity, is most frequently associated with outcomes that are not optimal (Caplan, Vistica, Posner, & Cheney, 1997; Cheney, 2010; Jordan et al., 2001; Kremer et al., 2002; Metzner, Posner, Lam, & Domino, 2011; Petty, Kremer, & Biddle, 2002). To foster improved decision making and reinforce principles of care to decrease the incidence of adverse outcomes, human patient simulation has been used as an instructional tool for clinicians and trainees.

The use of human patient simulation in the context of high-fidelity simulation labs provides trainees and practitioners with opportunities to develop crisis management skills in rarely occurring, potentially fatal scenarios (Blum et al., 2004; Cooper et al., 2008; Coopmans & Biddle, 2008; Lucisano & Talbot, 2012; Register, Graham-Garcia & Haas, 2003). Human patient simulation has also been used for nurse anesthesia faculty development (Hartland, Biddle, & Fallacaro, 2003) and critically evaluated as an educational tool by health care educators.

A recent paper noted that the best features and practices of simulation-based education in health care include

■ Feedback provided to learners.
■ Deliberate practice that occurs away from the bedside.
■ Integration of simulation into health sciences curriculum.
■ Measurement of outcomes that may be influenced by simulation.
■ Fidelity of simulation.
■ Acquisition and maintenance of skills, for example, management of difficult airways, placement of central venous catheters.
■ Mastery learning, for example, the ability to practice skills in the simulation lab before performing the same skills at the bedside.
■ Transfer of simulation-based learning to clinical practice.
■ Team training.
■ High-stakes testing.
■ Instructor training (McGaghie et al., 2010).

The impact and educational utility of simulation-based education in health care are likely to increase in the future. However, simulation labs currently vary significantly in terms of their infrastructure and available resources. The Society for Simulation in Healthcare (SSiH) has developed criteria for the certification of simulation instructors and accreditation standards for simulation labs. At this writing, six of over 300 simulation labs worldwide have fulfilled the criteria for SSiH accreditation. As available resources for simulation education become more consistent, additional research on knowledge transfer from the simulation lab to clinical practice is needed.

There is a developing body of research evidence showing that there is knowledge transfer from the simulation lab to clinical practice with beneficial effects on clinical outcomes. For example, clinicians who participate in simulation-based training on difficult airway management have decreased incidences of failed airway management scenarios. In addition to decreasing the potential morbidity and mortality associated with airway mishaps, operating room time and professional fees based on time are decreased when less clinical time is required to teach trainees these skills at the bedside. However, there remain critical challenges and gaps in research on the transfer of knowledge, skills, and abilities from the simulation lab to clinical practice (McGaghie et al., 2011). Nurse anesthesia educators have critically evaluated human patient simulation as an educational tool (Hotchkiss, Biddle, & Fallacaro, 2002).

Another use of human patient simulation that has been described is during the interview process for prospective nurse anesthesia students. Applicants are assigned to small groups and provided with a critical scenario in which they must work collaboratively (Penprase et al., 2012). This type of observed interaction and operationalization of critical care nursing skills may provide useful information that is predictive of the potential success of these applicants in a nurse anesthesia program.

As noted earlier, a methodological and design challenge for outcomes research is that anesthetic mortality occurs rarely today, with approximately one death in 200,000 cases (Jones, 2001; Lema, 2003; Li, Warner, Lang, Huang, & Sun, 2009). The Centers for Medicare & Medicaid Studies, the American Hospital Association, the ASA, the American College of Surgeons, and the Veterans Administration developed a strategy to reduce surgical morbidity over a 5-year period (Lema, 2003). The result of that collaboration is the Surgical Care Improvement Project (SCIP). The goal of SCIP was to reduce surgical complication by 25% by 2010. These data are publicly reported on the Centers for Medicare & Medicaid Services (CMS) Hospital Compare website, http://www.cms.gov/Medicare/Quality-Initiatives-Patient-Assessment-Instruments/HospitalQualityInits/HospitalCompare.html (CMS, 2012a). SCIP measures include the following:

- SCIP Inf-1: Prophylactic antibiotics are received within 1 hour before surgical incision.
- SCIP Inf-2: Prophylactic antibiotic selection for surgical patients.
- SCIP Inf-3: Prophylactic antibiotics discontinued within 24 hours after surgery end time.
- SCIP Inf-4: Cardiac surgery patients with controlled 6:00 a.m. postoperative glucose.
- SCIP Inf-6: Surgery patients with appropriate hair removal.
- SCIP Info-10: Surgery patients with perioperative temperature management.
- SCIP Card-2: Surgery patients on beta-blocker therapy before arrival who received a beta-blocker during the perioperative period.
- SCIP VTE-1: Surgery patients with recommended venous thromboembolism (VTE) prophylaxis ordered.
- SCIP VTE-2: Surgery patients who received appropriate VTE prophylaxis within 24 hours before surgery to 24 hours after surgery (Thiemann, 2012).

As of 2011, SCIP compliance has affected Medicare and Medicaid reimbursement rates. One recent study examined compliance with the SCIP surgical site infection (SSI) module, requiring prophylactic antibiotic administration 1 hour prior to surgical incision between 2009 and 2010 to determine whether compliance with SCIP correlated with SSI rates reported by the National Surgery Quality Improvement Program (NSQIP) data for the same period. The authors found no statistically significant association in patients whose care failed SCIP Inf-1 guidelines and the rates of SSI. These investigators posited that SCIP compliance should not be used to determine Medicare and Medicaid reimbursement rates because there was no observed correlation between failure of SCIP Inf-1 and SSI (Garcia, Fogel, Baker, Remine, & Jones, 2012). Other studies have demonstrated a modest association with process measures and patient outcomes (Thiemann, 2012).

CMS has developed the Ambulatory Surgical Center (ASC) Quality Reporting (ASCQR) Program, which is a pay-for-reporting, quality data program. Under this program, ASCs report quality of care data for standardized measures to "receive the full annual update to their ASC annual payment rate, beginning with calendar year 2014 payments." See http://www.cms.gov/Medicare/Quality-Initiatives-Patient-Assessment-Instruments/ASC-Quality-Reporting/index.html. These measures include:

- Patient burns.
- Patient falls.
- Wrong site/wrong side/wrong patient/wrong procedure/wrong implant.
- Hospital transfer/admission.
- Prophylactic antibiotics within 1 hour of procedure.
- Use of patient safety checklist, for example, WHO checklist (WHO, 2012). Facility volume data on selected procedures.
- Influenza vaccination coverage among health care providers (CMS, 2012b).

As members of multidisciplinary teams providing perioperative care in both inpatient and outpatient settings, CRNAs exert leadership daily, helping to ensure compliance with regulatory guidelines. Measures of compliance with these guidelines reflect the outcomes of direct patient care and leadership provided by CRNAs.

Regarding variables related to anesthesia care, it is difficult to classify anesthesia-specific events versus surgery-specific events. Outcomes such as epidural abscesses following neuraxial anesthesia or patient awareness under general anesthesia are more likely to be associated with anesthesia care. However, there is not a validated algorithm to identify outcomes directly related to anesthesia care (Thiemann, 2012).

As noted earlier, there are no ongoing prospective multicenter studies of anesthesia outcomes. Creation of a national health information network (NHIN) will facilitate national quality improvement activities. The NHIN is a set of standards, services, and policies that allow for secure web-supported health information exchange. The network will provide a foundation for exchange of health information across diverse entities. The intent of NHIN is to specify a simple, secure, scalable standards-based method for participants to send authenticated, encrypted health information directly to known and trusted recipients over the Internet at http://healthit.hhs.gov/portal/server.pt?open=512 &objID=1142&parentname=CommunityPage&parentid=4&mode=2 (National Health Information Network, 2012). A limitation associated with NHIN is that only 10.7% of U.S. hospitals utilize a comprehensive electronic medical record (Adler-Milstein, DesRoches, & Jha, 2011). Outcomes tracked in this manner can provide data that substantiate the reasonable cost and high quality of services provided by CRNAs and other advanced practice nurses (APNs).

Implementation of NHIN would also require standardized definitions across all vendors so that risk factors and outcomes will be coded identically across all hospitals. Lack of standardization compromises efforts to use electronic data for quality improvement and benchmarking. Information technology infrastructure must allow for data exchange within regional networks. Centralized data management and analysis are vital to benchmarking clinical practices and further demonstration of outcomes associated with care provided by APNs (Thiemann, 2012).

Performance measures are critical to the national effort to ensure that patients receive appropriate and high-quality care. Pay for performance (P4P), or value-based purchasing, has endeavored to link clinical outcomes with reimbursement. P4P also includes disincentives for negative consequences of care or increased costs for "never" events, for example, wrong-site surgery, operative or postoperative complications, medication errors (Agency for Health Research and Quality [AHRQ], 2012a).

Investigators used Medicare data to examine 30-day mortality among over 6 million patients who had acute myocardial infarction, congestive heart failure, or pneumonia, or who underwent coronary artery bypass grafting between 2003 and 2009. These researchers found no evidence that the largest hospital-based P4P program led to decreases in 30-day mortality among these patients and suggested that expectations for improved outcomes related to P4P should be modest (Jha, Joynt, Orav, & Epstein, 2012).

Over 40 million surgical and diagnostic procedures, most accompanied by anesthesia, are performed annually in the United States (Anesthesia Quality Institute, 2009). Meaningful and accurate outcome data for the types of surgeries and anesthetics, with or without anesthesia providers, could be collected in a longitudinal multicenter prospective study. The costs associated with such a study would be offset by reductions in unnecessary surgery, risky surgery, poor health care providers, perioperative deaths, and delayed discharge times (Lema, 2003). To date, no such study has been designed or implemented. Political, logistical, and economical constraints may account for the failure to implement such a study. Research findings reported by closed claims investigators provide information regarding the genesis of anesthetic morbidity and mortality, but do not provide epidemiologic data, for example, numerator and denominator, or anesthetic morbidity and mortality.

## OUTCOMES IN RURAL SETTINGS

Nurse anesthetists are the primary anesthesia providers in rural America, which enables health care facilities in these medically underserved settings to offer obstetrical, surgical, and trauma stabilization services. In some states, nurse anesthetists are the sole anesthesia providers in nearly 100% of rural hospitals (AANA, 2012b). Little outcomes research exists on anesthesia provided in rural America. Orkin (1998) noted that case mix and patient outcomes had not been studied relative to the rural anesthesia workforce. Absent full implementation of NHIQ of similar strategies, this information deficit persists.

Rural CRNAs provide a broad range of anesthesia-related services within and outside of the operating room. One study found significant differences in the employment settings of medically directed and non-medically directed CRNAs, the availability of certain anesthetic agents and monitoring devices, and the representation of surgical specialists based on the size of the rural community and hospital. However, this study did not examine anesthetic or surgical outcomes (Monti Seibert, Alexander, & Lupien, 2004).

An analysis of cesarean section outcomes showed no difference in complication rates when anesthesia was provided by a CRNA or a CRNA–physician team. Because solo CRNAs often provide anesthesia in rural settings, these findings help to quantify the outcomes of CRNA-provided in rural settings (Simonson et al., 2007).

A rare prospective study of anesthesia outcomes in a rural hospital described data collected over a 25 year period on patients who underwent cholecystectomies. These patients were statistically compared with matched controls from urban medical centers. All the anesthetics were administered by the same CRNA. There were no statistically significant differences in outcomes, including postoperative complications, between the two datasets (Callaghan, 1995).

Another study of rural anesthesia services involved surveying hospital administrators regarding their satisfaction with anesthesia services in rural Washington and Montana (Dunbar et al., 1998). Survey respondents indicated that they were satisfied with the anesthesia services provided. The authors noted that "all the administrators rated the care provided in their anesthesia departments as either good or very good" (Dunbar et al., 1998, p. 805). A replication of this study was conducted with rural Illinois hospital administrators, which also demonstrated that the majority of respondent administrators rated anesthesia care in their facilities as "good or very good" (Kremer & Stark, 2000). The perceptions of hospital administrators regarding anesthesia care in their facilities are important, because administrators have access to data such as morbidity and mortality reports as well as patient satisfaction surveys.

## OUTCOME MEASUREMENT IN NURSE ANESTHESIA

There have been national-level discussions on the need for outcomes research in nurse anesthesia for many years. One of the first initiatives to collect outcomes data that could be analyzed in aggregate was with AANA AQ Plus program initiated in 1989 (Kraus, 1994). AQ Plus collected data points including patient demographics, surgical procedures, anesthetic agents, and techniques used. The program did not have wide market penetration and the software was not suitable for aggregate data analysis. To date, there have not been products developed for practicing CRNAs to track their clinical outcomes. Efforts such as NHIQ may provide a repository of individual and aggregate clinician performance data.

Many nurse anesthesia educational programs utilize web-supported clinical case-tracking applications. This type of software captures data such as patient demographics, procedures performed, types of anesthetic agents administered, duration of the case, and so forth. The data can be entered using a smart phone and later uploaded to the website of the vendor. Data can be viewed on the website or downloaded to a spreadsheet application for analyses of individual or group performance. Perhaps practitioners will employ similar software for quality improvement activities, but there may be concern that such data would be legally discoverable in the event of litigation.

Automated anesthesia records are used in some practice settings. When this is the case, the system chosen may have the capability to capture data related to quality improvement and outcome assessment activities. The availability of digital information on multiple patients permits analysis of patient characteristics or intraoperative events as related to clinical outcomes. It is clear that meaningful outcomes analysis of rarely occurring events, such as anesthetic mortality, requires large datasets. For some outcomes, a single facility may not have sufficient patient volume to conduct rigorous outcome analyses. Prior to the development of the NHIQ initiative, some authors advocated outcomes data sharing among institutions to increase analytic power. Third-party payers are also interested in patient outcomes, as demonstrated by the P4P program. The availability of anesthesia outcomes data in digital format allows for its integration into other internal and external databases. When information anesthesia care is incorporated into the medical record, the role of anesthesia in overall patient outcomes can be assessed. Individual provider variations in clinical practice can also be studied (Dutton & Dukatz, 2011).

## FAILURE TO RESCUE

"Failure to rescue" describes failure to prevent clinically important deterioration, such as death or permanent disability from a complication of an underlying disease or a complication of medical care. Failure to rescue provides a measure of the degree to which providers responded to adverse occurrences that developed on their watch. It may be related to the quality of monitoring or to the efficacy of actions taken once early complications are recognized, or both (AHRQ, 2012b).

Initial studies of surgical morbidity and mortality correlated with other quality measures. Rates of failure to rescue have been utilized as outcome measures in studies that have compared the educational level and experience of nurses against patient outcomes (Aiken, Clarke, Silber, & Sloane, 2003).

The AHRQ technical report that developed the *AHRQ Patient Safety Indicators* (McDonald et al., 2002) reviewed the evidence supporting failure to rescue as a measure of the quality and safety of hospital care. Although failure to rescue was included in the final set of approved indicators, the expert panels that reviewed each potential indicator identified some unresolved concerns about its use. For example, patients with advanced disease processes may be especially difficult to rescue from complications such as sepsis and cardiac arrest. Patients with advanced illness may not desire "rescue" from such complications (AHRQ, 2012b).

Failure to rescue methodology has been used to study anesthesia outcomes related to the anesthesia providers involved (Pine, Holt, & Lou, 2003; Silber et al., 2000). These two papers analyzed a Pennsylvania Medicare dataset. The risk-adjusted mortality rates of Medicare patients who underwent carotid endarterectomy, cholecystectomy, herniorrhaphy, hysterectomy, knee replacement, laminectomy, mastectomy, or prostatectomy were compared for anesthesiologist-directed and nonanesthesiologist-directed cases and analyzed for a 3-year period. The result was a statistically insignificant difference in negative outcomes between anesthesiologist-directed and nonanesthesiologist-directed cases.

Clinicians and administrators have assessed the degree to which the "failure to rescue" indicator identifies true problems in the process of care at the individual or system level. Failure-to-rescue complications can be flagged through administrative data, and the clinical course of events then evaluated. Many factors influence whether a case is included in the measure, such as existing health problems, the presence of complex comorbidities, and variations in clinical documentation and coding practices (Talsma, Bahl, & Campbell, 2008). Therefore, studies that employ failure to rescue methodology need to rigorously assess multiple covariates and their potential association with a given outcome.

## NURSE ANESTHESIA OUTCOME MEASURES AND PROJECTS

Anesthesia outcomes research has focused on what Lohr (1988) described as "the five Ds: death, disease, disability, discomfort, and dissatisfaction." A shift toward outcomes studies focused on other aspects of health such as survival rates, states of physiological and psychological health, and satisfaction with care rendered was described by Lohr (1988).

The AANAF funds research and professional development for nurse anesthetists. Outcomes studies have been among the top priorities of the AANAF research agenda for some time. The AANAF mission is "advancing the science of anesthesia through education and research" (AANA, 2012c). Over the course of its 30-year history, AANAF has awarded more than $2.2 million to 2,275 students and CRNAs for scholarships, fellowships, research grants, and poster presentations. Current AANAF research priorities include health care policy research, practice, and clinically oriented research and education (AANA, 2012d).

The thrust of AANAF nurse anesthesia outcomes research has been the ongoing study of closed malpractice claims filed against nurse anesthetists (Jordan et al., 2001). The goal of this ongoing study has been to determine the causes of anesthesia-related patient injury or death, identify trends in adverse anesthetic outcomes, and compare research findings with current standards of practice. The results of this study have affected practice standards (MacRae, 2007). For example, current COA requirements for pediatric clinical experience were affected by data from the AANAF closed claims study.

Data for the AANAF closed claims study were collected with the permission of insurance carriers for CRNAs who need to obtain their own malpractice coverage, such as those nurse anesthetists who are not hospital-employed or group-employed. Ongoing data analysis has demonstrated results that mirror those of the ASA closed claims study: The most frequently represented patients in the database are lower acuity patients who underwent elective surgical procedures. Monetary awards were directly related to the severity of the adverse outcome. When anesthesia care was determined to be inappropriate, the severity of the injury and monetary award were higher (Jordan et al., 2001).

These research findings resulted in recommendations to study nurse anesthesia educational curricula and continuing education offerings. For example, the area of office-based surgery and related closed claims research findings influenced the development of AANA guidelines for office-based anesthesia (AANA, 2012e).

CRNAs are pursuing doctoral education in greater numbers, which bodes well for the future of the specialty and the generation of additional outcomes research. Funding initiatives for doctoral study and interviews with CRNA doctoral students and active researchers attest to the richness of discovery that is evident in this growing community of scholars.

A recent cost-effectiveness analysis (CEA) of anesthesia providers found that CRNAs are less costly to train than anesthesiologists and can perform the same set of anesthesia services, including relatively rare and difficult procedures such as open-heart surgeries, organ transplantations, and pediatric procedures. In concert with the Institute of

Medicine (IOM) report, the investigators noted that "as the demand for healthcare continues to grow, increasing the number of CRNAs and permitting them to practice in the most efficient delivery models, will be a key to containing costs while maintaining quality of care" (Hogan et al., 2010).

Malpractice insurance premium rates for CRNAs indirectly reflect outcomes of care provided by nurse anesthetists. Insurance rates for self-employed CRNAs have declined significantly since the 1980s (AANA, 2010b). In 2009, the average CRNA malpractice premium was 33% lower than it was in 1988, or 62% lower when adjusted for inflation. This decline in malpractice premium rate reflects the safe care provided by nurse anesthetists. The rate drop is impressive given inflation, our litigious society, and generally higher jury awards (AANA, 2010b).

## EVIDENCE-BASED PRACTICE (EBP)

New clinical information is generated more quickly than it can be assimilated by trainees and practicing clinicians. Nurse anesthesia students, faculty, and practitioners need the most current information regarding health care and anesthesia practice. This information need is acute for student registered nurse anesthetists, because they must rapidly learn complex specialty-related content and use this information to justify clinical actions to their faculty (Pellegrini, 2006). Using EBP concepts helps balance the demand for current information with the exponentially increasing supply of specialty-related research information.

EBP has been described as "the integration of individual clinical expertise with the best available external clinical evidence from systematic research" (Sackett, Rosenberg, Gray, Haynes, & Richardson, 2007). Health care professionals may believe that their practices have always reflected evidence-based underpinnings, but performance assessments indicate this is not the case (McGlynn et al., 2003). Current literature advocates increased adoption of EBP, but EBP implementation is inconsistent (Kavey, 2008).

The Institute of Medicine Committee on the Health Professions Education Summit suggested a paradigm shift for health professions education. The principal goal of this process was that "all health professionals will be educated to deliver patient-centric care as members of an interdisciplinary team, emphasizing evidence-based practice, quality improvement approaches, and informatics" (Greiner & Knebel, 2003).

The American Association of Colleges of Nursing, health educators, and foundations released competencies and action strategies for interprofessional education in 2011. The goal for operationalization of these competencies is transformation of the health care delivery system to provide collaborative, high quality, and cost-effective care to better serve every patient. The Core Competencies for Interprofessional Collaborative Practice identified four domains of core competencies needed to provide integrated, high-quality care to patients in the current health care delivery system. The panel recommended that future health professionals be able to:

- Assert values and ethics of interprofessional practice by placing the interests, dignity, and respect of patients at the center of health care delivery and embracing the cultural diversity and differences of health care teams.
- Leverage the unique roles and responsibilities of interprofessional partners to appropriately assess the health care needs of patients and populations served.
- Communicate with patients, families, communities, and other health professionals in support of a team approach to preventing disease and disability, maintaining health, and treating disease.
- Perform effectively in various team roles to deliver patient/population-centered care that is safe, timely, efficient, and equitable (AACN, 2011a).

Another report, "Team-Based Competencies, Building a Shared Foundation for Educational and Clinical Practice," was held in 2011 and included 80 leaders from diverse health professions who previewed the Interprofessional Education Collaborative (IPEC) core competencies. These leaders created action strategies to transform health professional education and health care delivery in the United States (AACN, 2011b). Utilization of these competencies in the context of interprofessional education and practice has great potential to positively impact health care, including care delivered by APNs, including CRNAs.

The paradigm shift that is occurring in health care includes the movement of health care delivery away from the traditional physician-dominated practice toward the concept of the physician as team leader, seeking the best evidence for patient care. Ideally, such physicians and teams will have the ability and expectation to continuously learn and change through utilization of evidence-based clinical support, informatics, and clinical data repositories. The potential scope of this initiative clearly includes all health professionals (Kavey, 2008).

Nurses may have the most experience in using EBP, with a record dating back to the time of Nightingale (McDonald, 2001). Nurses are the largest group of health care providers, numbering 3,100,000 (ANA, 2012). The projected job growth in nursing over the time frame of 2008 to 2018 is 581,500, reflecting a 22% growth in nursing employment. The current vacancy rate for CRNA positions is low, but expected retirements from 2014 and beyond will greatly increase the market demand for nurse anesthetists (AANA, 2012f).

A survey of 3,000 licensed nurses in the United States demonstrated that almost half of the respondents were unfamiliar with the term evidence-based medicine. More than half of these survey respondents had not identified a clinical problem that required research, and 43% "sometimes, rarely, or never" read nursing journals or texts (Pravikoff, Tanner, & Pierce, 2005).

Significant information literacy and access to adequate information technology are needed for implementation of EBP with tools such as best-practice databases, clinical practice guidelines, electronic medical records, and computerized physician order entry. Nurses report that access to evidence-based information can be "extremely difficult." Fewer than 50% of respondents to Pravikoff's (2005) survey reported available workstation access to the Internet. This may be offset by the increasing use of smart phones with functional web browsers. However, attitudes toward EBP are complex, with a majority of nurses identifying a colleague or supervisor as their primary information source, rather than any independent literature source.

One suggested educational direction is to include EBP as a core competency throughout all levels of nursing curricula. Related competencies should include formation of PICOT questions, where P = patient population, I = intervention or area of interest, C = comparison intervention or comparison group, O = outcome, and T = time frame. Students and practitioners need to be able to search for the best evidence, for example, specifically preappraised evidence and evidence-based clinical practice guidelines, and integrate the best evidence with their clinical expertise and patient preferences related to clinical decisions. Students also need to be able to assess outcomes based on EBP changes and participate in team EBP projects. Graduate students should be required to demonstrate facility with synthesizing a body of evidence to initiate and evaluate practice changes to improve the health of individuals, lead practice changes based on the best evidence for populations of patients, generate evidence through outcomes management, and mentor others in EBP (NLN, 2008).

It is difficult for practitioners and trainees to remain current with the relevant advances in their fields of interest. The major bibliographic databases cover less than half of the world's literature and are biased toward English-language publications. Textbooks, editorials, and reviews that have not been systematically prepared may be unreliable. Much evidence is unpublished, and yet unpublished data may have clinical significance. More easily accessible research papers tend to exaggerate the benefits of interventions (Cochrane Collaboration, 2008).

The *Cochrane Library* consists of a regularly updated collection of EBP databases including *The Cochrane Database of Systematic Reviews*. This database includes systematic reviews of health care interventions that are produced and disseminated by the Cochrane Collaboration. The *Cochrane Library* is published quarterly and is available in digital format and online. Abstracts of the reviews are available to browse and search without charge on this website (www.cochrane.org; Cochrane, 2012). Anesthesia-related *Cochrane Reviews* topics have included the bispectral index (Punjasawadwong, Bunchungmonogko, & Pongschiewboon, 2008).

A recent review described the implementation of EBP in anesthesiology and critical care. The authors found that outcomes research employing evidence-based approaches was seen in subspecialty areas such as pediatrics, obstetrics, and general anesthesia, as well as in critical care. The integration of individual expertise with data from externally conducted systematic research was described as a benefit of EBP. While EBP has its origins in the treatment- and diagnosis-related competencies of primary care, its tenets are applicable to nontherapeutic specialties such as anesthesia and critical care (Schulman, Schardt, & Erb, 2002).

## NURSE ANESTHESIA COMPETENCIES, CURRICULAR MODELS, AND EVIDENCE-BASED PRACTICE

Organizations seek to identify the core capabilities, or competencies, that have sustainable value and wide applicability to the customers that they serve. Professional nursing organizations that serve the interests of patients generally identify role-related competencies that describe their vision of the skills and abilities that the individual must possess (Callahan, 1988). For example, the *AANA Code of Ethics for the Certified Registered Nurse Anesthetists* (2010c) describes competence as including involvement with lifelong professional educational activities, participating in continuous quality improvement initiatives and maintaining licensure according to the statutory and regulatory requirements for recertification.

In education, AANA has adopted master's-level educational competencies required of the CRNA for entry into practice. These are the acquired knowledge, skills, and competencies in patient safety, perianesthetic management, critical thinking, communication, and the professional role identified by the Council on Accreditation of Nurse Anesthesia Educational Programs (January, 2012) SIII: Program of Study, Criterion C-20. One of the related criteria in this standard is critical thinking, which "is demonstrated by the ability of the graduate to provide nurse anesthesia care based on sound principles of research and evidence" (COA, 2012).

The movement of advanced practice nursing education to the practice doctorate level has mandated additional competencies to reflect this educational level. The COA's additional criteria for practice-oriented doctoral degrees (COA, 2012) reflects additional doctoral-level competencies. These competencies are reflected in the curricula of nurse anesthesia programs at the clinical doctorate level that are accredited by the COA.

Several of the identified competencies for CRNAs prepared at the practice doctorate level address EBP. For example, the competency area of biological systems, homeostasis, and pathogenesis advocates the use of "a systematic outcomes analysis approach in the translation of research evidence and data in the arts and sciences to demonstrate that these interventions will have the expected effects of nurse anesthesia practice" (COA, 2012).

In the competency area of health care improvement, CRNAs prepared with practice doctorates are expected to use "EBP to inform clinical decision making in nurse anesthesia." Regarding competencies in technology and informatics, a CRNA with a practice doctorate would use "information systems/technology to support and improve patient care and health-care systems; design, select, and use information technology to evaluate programs of care and health systems; and critically evaluate clinical and research databases used as clinical decision support resources" (COA, 2012).

Pellegrini (2006) noted that as nurse anesthesia curricula and clinical practice evolve, instructional methods will need to reflect EBP. The paradigm of using clinical judgment and expertise as the basis for clinical decision making will shift to a structure that incorporates the best available evidence to formulate clinical decisions, as described above, in the technology and informatics competency, along with clinical experience and expertise. Implementation of EBP principles into nurse anesthesia education will yield a well-informed student along with ensuring that students and faculty remain at the forefront of the latest evidence that is available in the literature (Pellegrini, 2006).

When one is presented with a clinical question, the EBP analysis is as follows:

1. Define the problem or question in terms of the patient or problem, the intervention or comparison interventions used to answer the question, and the findings of the research reviewed.
2. Outline the current steps in one's clinical practice to address the problem.
3. Use a ranking system to determine the quality of evidence available in the literature. This hierarchy, in descending order, consists of findings from systematic review of well-designed clinical studies (meta-analyses); results of one or more appropriately designed studies (randomized trials, cohort studies); results of large case series and case reports; editorial and opinion pieces; animal research; and in vitro research.
4. Identify the resources available to implement any proposed changes to practice to differentiate which evidence is applicable to the current clinical setting.
5. Assess the validity of the research presented with a consistent rubric to review clinical trials that includes these questions:
   a. Did the clinical trials studied include elements such as randomization of subjects, adequate sample size, and appropriate statistical analysis?
   b. Were the results relevant to clinical practice?
   c. Were the therapeutic interventions reported feasible for clinical practice?
   d. Were all research subjects accounted for at the end of the study (Pellegrini, 2006)?

The "pyramid of evidence" is central to EBP. This concept is depicted in Figure 10.1. Utilization of EBP in anesthesia practice is increasing. Longitudinal outcomes studies in practices where EBP is employed can determine if associations exist between the implementation of EBP and improved outcomes.

The AANA has recognized the importance of EBP and its importance to health care and society. The AANA "realized the need to establish a systematic evidence-based process to analyze and resolve issues of import to the profession and clinical practice as the body of knowledge affecting nurse anesthesia continued to grow." Based on

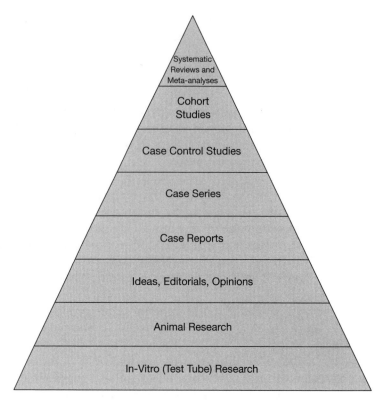

Figure 10.1 *The Evidence Pyramid*

the work of Sackett et al. (2007), the AANA adopted the definition of evidence-based nurse anesthesia practice as "integration and synthesis of the best research evidence with clinical expertise and patient values" in order to optimize the care of patients receiving anesthesia services (AANA, 2012g).

The member side of the AANA website (www.aana.com) lists these components of EBP:

- Patient preferences/values.
- Clinical expertise.
- Best research evidence.

Five steps of the evidence-based process are delineated:

*1.* Ask a clinical question.
*2.* Obtain the best research literature.

3. Critically appraise the evidence.
4. Integrate the evidence with clinical expertise and patient preferences.
5. Evaluate the outcomes of the decision (AANA, 2012g).

The AANA notes that as EBP is increasingly adopted, so are the available resources to translate evidence to practice. The AANA Professional Practice website (AANA, 2012g) provides information and resources to assist CRNAs and others who seek to learn more about EBP. The available resources include:

- EBP resources.
- EBP modules and tutorials.
- Guidelines and systematic reviews.
- Research terms and definitions.
- Types of evidence (AANA, 2012g).

This commitment to EBP at the level of the national professional organization is laudable. What is central to this discussion is the impact of promulgating EBP principles on the outcomes of care provided by CRNAs, which requires prospective longitudinal multicenter data collection and analysis.

## OUTCOMES ECONOMICS AND POLICY DEVELOPMENTS

A CEA of CRNA practice was conducted in 2010. The investigators found the CRNAs are less costly to train than anesthesiologists and have the potential for providing anesthesia care efficiently. The analysis noted that anesthesiologists and CRNAs can perform the same set of anesthesia services, including relatively rare and difficult procedures such as open-heart surgeries, organ transplantation, and pediatric procedures. In concert with the IOM report on the future of nursing recommendations to allow nurses to practice at the full scope of their education and training, this CEA has similar recommendations: "As the demand for healthcare continues to grow, increasing the number of CRNAs and permitting them to practice in the most efficient delivery models, will be a key to containing costs while maintaining quality care" (Hogan et al., 2010).

In 2001, the CMS allowed states to opt out of the requirement for reimbursement that a surgeon or anesthesiologist oversee anesthesia care provided by CRNAs. By 2005, 14 states opted out of this Medicare

Part A requirement. An analysis of Medicare data from 1999 to 2005 in the affected states found no evidence that opting out of the oversight requirement resulted in increased morbidity or mortality. Based on these findings, the authors recommended that CMS allow CRNAs in every state to work without the supervision of a surgeon or anesthesiologist (Dulisse & Cromwell, 2010; IOM, 2010).

As of this writing, 17 states have opted out of the federal supervision rule: Iowa, Nebraska, Idaho, Minnesota, New Hampshire, New Mexico, Kansas, North Dakota, Washington, Alaska, Oregon, Montana, South Dakota, Wisconsin, California, Colorado, and Kentucky. Some of these opt-outs have withstood legal challenges from the medical societies of their respective states. When opt-outs have been contested, the federal supervision rule was described as a measure to ensure patient safety. However, the supervision rule is a requirement that hospitals must meet in order to receive Medicare reimbursement for anesthesia services. This health care policy initiative helps to demonstrate the safety and quality of anesthesia care provided by CRNAs (AANA, 2012h).

## CONCLUSIONS

Outcomes research seeks understanding of the end results of certain health care practices and interventions. End results include effects that people experience and care about, such as improvement in functional status and quality of life, as well as morbidity and mortality. Linkage of care provided to the attained outcomes is a function of outcomes research, which can lead to improved care. Outcomes research has altered the culture of clinical practice and health care research by changing how we assess the end results of health care services. Outcomes research is the key to knowing the quality of care that can be achieved, and how providers can move to that level of care (AHRQ, 2012a).

Issues that face advanced practice nursing related to justification of the use of APNs and the measurement of the effects of APN services on patients and health care systems are similar but distinct from those faced by individual APNs evaluating the outcomes of their particular practices. There is clearly a need for well-designed longitudinal assessments of how APNs, including CRNAs, impact clinical outcomes. Since reimbursement decisions are driven by evidence of provider performance, APNs who lack valid, reliable data to substantiate their "impactfulness" will struggle for equitable reimbursement (Ingersoll, 2008).

To address the need for addition of APN-sensitive outcome indicators, development of electronic information systems that identify and track APN outcome data is required. This process requires national agreement on core outcome indicators germane to APNs and initiation of standards that support collection of APN-sensitive data. Health care organizations and third-party payers will be integral to the development of such systems (Ingersoll, 2008).

Outcomes measurement is interconnected with every other aspect of the APN role. Effective outcomes measurement and performance reviews related to outcomes criteria require APNs to work collaboratively with others, to plan and organize processes of care and assessment of quality in complex health services environments, and to allow scrutiny of their individual practices by others. In the end, the quality and value of care will improve along with recognition by the community of the impact of the APN on outcomes of care (Ingersoll, 2008).

Nurses and APNs, including CRNAs, continue to be interested and involved in the area of outcomes to ensure that patients are represented as more than a composite of physiologic variables or billing data. The use of outcomes measures has helped APNs to articulate their unique value and contributions to the well-being of patients. Many health care outcomes measures do not identify or quantify the contributions of nurses. In anesthesia care, the role of CRNAs in patient outcomes has been at times diminished as a result of the economic competition between CRNAs and their physician counterparts.

Given the worsening mismatch between population health care needs and available resources, APNs and CRNAs must continue to demonstrate their quality and cost effectiveness. Implementation of the Affordable Care Act will provide an unprecedented opportunity for CRNAs and APNs to demonstrate the value added to the health care delivery system by this cadre of safe, cost-effective providers.

Historically, quality of care has been described using variables such as morbidity, mortality, length of stay, readmission, and cost. Methods have not been readily available to define quality in terms of the effect of health care delivery on the health of patients (Ditmyer et al., 1998). Combined administrative and health-related databases can demonstrate outcome associated with nurse anesthesia practice.

Nurse anesthesia has made outcomes research an urgent priority. The benefits of this research in the policy arena are evident in the Hogan et al. (2010) and Dulisse and Cromwell (2010) papers. Development of methodologically sound outcomes research requires the preparation of more scholars within the specialty who have the expertise in research design and measurement. Fortunately, more CRNAs are rising to the challenge of doctoral education, with 3% of AANA members prepared at the doctoral level.

Continuing to strive for the accurate measurement of nurse anesthesia outcomes remains a goal of the nurse anesthesia specialty. Continued research, application of EBP principles, and operationalization of the recommendations of the IOM Future of Nursing Report will facilitate attainment of this goal.

### Answers to Chapter Discussion Questions

1. The impetus for the development of closed malpractice claims research was a significant rise in anesthesia malpractice premiums in the 1970s.
2. There are gaps in research on the transfer of knowledge, skills, and abilities acquired in human patient simulation. However, there is evidence that simulation-based training in skills such as difficult airway management improve performance as demonstrated by a decreased incidence of failed airway management for those clinicians who have completed simulation-based training in difficult airway management.
3. Investigators believe that SCIP compliance should not be used to determine Medicare and Medicaid reimbursement rates because there was no correlation between SCIP INF-1 (prophylactic antibiotics are received within 1 hour of surgical incision) and SSI.
4. Determining the contributions of anesthesia and surgery, respectively, to adverse perioperative outcomes is complex. For example, surgical aspects of spine surgery, such as positioning, the duration of surgery, and blood loss associated with the operation, can contribute to the development of postoperative ischemic optic neuropathy. However, factors under the control of the anesthetist, such as temperature regulation, ensuring that pressure points are padded, fluid management, and maintenance of hemodynamic stability, can also impact this problem.
5. The implementation of EBP is limited by the reliance of some clinicians on colleagues for information, rather than seeking information from peer-reviewed sources. Adoption of EBP is more likely with access of clinicians to Internet search engines, through the web browsers in their smart phones, and computer workstations in clinical areas.

## WEB LINKS

CMS Hospital Compare is a consumer-oriented website that provides information on how well hospitals provide recommended care to their patients. On this site, the consumer can see the recommended care that an adult should get if being treated for a heart attack, heart failure, pneumonia, or having surgery. The performance rates for this website generally reflect care provided to all U.S. adults with the exception of the 30-day Risk Adjusted Death and Readmission measures and the Hospital Outpatient Medical Imaging measures that only include data from Medicare beneficiaries. Website: http://www.cms.gov/Medicare/Quality-Initiatives-Patient-Assessment-Instruments/HospitalQualityInits/HospitalCompare.html

The Nationwide Health Information Network: This network is a set of standards, services, and policies that enable secure health information exchange over the Internet. The network will provide a foundation for the exchange of health information across diverse entities, within communities, and across the country. This critical part of the national health IT agenda will enable health information to follow the consumer, be available for clinical decision making, and support appropriate use of health care information beyond direct patient care so as to improve population health. Website: http://healthit.hhs.gov/portal/server.pt?open=512&objID=1142&parentname=CommunityPage&parentid=4&mode=2

CMS has developed the ASCQR Program, which is a pay-for-reporting, quality data program. Under this program, ASCs report quality of care data for standardized measures to "receive the full annual update to their ASC annual payment rate, beginning with calendar year 2014 payments." See: http://www.cms.gov/Medicare/Quality-Initiatives-Patient-Assessment-Instruments/ASC-Quality-Reporting/index.html.

## REFERENCES

AACN. (2011a). *Statement on interprofessional education.* Retrieved from http://www.aacn.nche.edu/news/articles/2011/ipec

AACN. (2011b). *Team-based competencies: Building a shared foundation for education and clinical practice.* Retrieved from http://www.aacn.nche.edu/news/articles/2011/ipec

Adler-Milstein, J., DesRoches, C., & Jha, A. (2011). Health exchange among U.S. hospitals. *The American Journal of Managed Care, 17*(11), 761–768.

Agency for Health Research and Quality. (2012a). *Agency for healthcare research and quality: Never events.* Retrieved from http://www.psnet.ahrq.gov/primer.aspx?primerID=3

Agency for Health Research and Quality. (2012b). *Agency for healthcare research and quality: Failure to rescue.* Retrieved from http://www.psnet.ahrq.gov/glossary.aspx?indexLetter=F

Aiken, L., Clarke, S., Silber, J., & Sloane, D. (2003). Hospital nurse staffing, education and patient mortality. *LDI Issue Brief, 9*(2), 1–4.

American Association of Nurse Anesthetists. (2010a). *Scope and standards for nurse anesthesia practice.* Park Ridge, IL: Author. Retrieved from http://www.aana.com/resources2/professionalpractice/Documents/PPM%20Scope%20and%20Standards.pdf

American Association of Nurse Anesthetists. (2010b). *Malpractice insurance premium rates for CRNAs.* Retrieved from http://www.aana.com/aboutus/Documents/quality_nap.pdf

American Association of Nurse Anesthetists. (2010c). *Code of ethics for nurse anesthetists.* Retrieved from http://www.aana.com/resources2/professionalpractice/Documents/PPM%20Code%20of%20Ethics.pdf

American Association of Nurse Anesthetists. (2012a). *Certified registered nurse anesthetists (CRNAs) at a glance.* Park Ridge, IL: Author.

American Association of Nurse Anesthetists. (2012b). *Certified registered nurse anesthetists' contributions to rural and medically underserved Americans.* Retrieved from http://www.aana.com/myaana/Advocacy/fedgovtaffairs/Documents/20120716-AANA_CommentLCD24473.pdf

American Association of Nurse Anesthetists. (2012c). *AANA Foundation mission statement.* Retrieved from http://www.aana.com/aanaaffiliates/aanafoundation/Pages/About-the-Foundation.aspx

American Association of Nurse Anesthetists. (2012d). *AANA Foundation FY 13 research priorities.* Retrieved from http://www.aana.com/aanaaffiliates/aanafoundation/Documents/AANA%20Foundation%20Research%20Agenda%202013.pdf

American Association of Nurse Anesthetists. (2012e). *AANA guidelines for office-based anesthesia.* Retrieved from http://www.aana.com/myaana/ProfessionalPractice/Documents/PPM%20Table%20of%20Contents.pdf

American Association of Nurse Anesthetists. (2012f). *AANA member survey slides.* Park Ridge, IL: Author.

American Association of Nurse Anesthetists. (2012g). *Evidence-based practice.* Retrieved from http://www.aana.com/resources2/professionalpractice/Pages/Evidence-Based-Practice.aspx

American Association of Nurse Anesthetists. (2012h). *AANA state governmental affairs update on opt-out states.* Park Ridge, IL: Author.

ANA. (2012). *Nursing workforce fact sheet.* Retrieved from http://nursingworld.org/NursingbytheNumbersFactSheet.aspx

Anesthesia Quality Institute. (2009). *Anesthesia quality institute. Surgeries performed annually in the U.S.* Retrieved from http://aqihq.org/Anesthesia%20in%20the%20US%202_19_10.pdf

Bankert, M. (1989). *Watchful care—A history of America's nurse anesthetists*. New York, NY: Continuum.

Beecher, H., & Todd, D. (1954). A study of deaths associated with anesthesia and surgery. *Annals of Surgery, 140*, 2–25.

Blum, R., Raemer, D., Carroll, J., et al. (2004). Crisis resource management training for an anaesthesia faculty: A new approach to continuing education. *Medical Education, 38*, 45–55.

Brunner, E. (1984). The National Association of Insurance Commissioners closed claims study. *International Anesthesiology Clinics, 22*, 17–30.

Callaghan, J. (1995). Twenty-five years of gallbladder surgery in a small rural hospital. *American Journal of Surgery, 169*, 313–315.

Callahan, L. (1988). Competence models: From theory to practical application. *American Association of Nurse Anesthetists, 56*, 5.

Caplan, R., Vistica, M., Posner, K., & Cheney, F. (1997). Adverse anesthetic outcomes arising from gas delivery equipment: A closed claims analysis. *Anesthesiology, 87*, 741–748.

Cheney, F. (2010). The American Society of Anesthesiologists closed claims project: The beginning. *Anesthesiology, 113*(4), 957–960.

CMS. (2012a). *Centers for Medicare and Medicaid Services Hospital Compare Website*. Retrieved from http://www.cms.gov/Medicare/Quality-Initiatives-Patient-Assessment-Instruments/HospitalQualityInits/HospitalCompare.html

CMS. (2012b). *Ambulatory Surgical Center (ASC) Quality Reporting (ASCQR) Program*. Retrieved from http://www.cms.gov/Medicare/Quality-Initiatives-Patient-Assessment-Instruments/ASC-Quality-Reporting/index.html

COA. (2012). *Standards for Accreditation of Nurse Anesthesia Educational Programs*. Park Ridge, IL: Council on Accreditation of Nurse Anesthesia Educational Programs.

Cochrane Collaboration. (2012). *Cochrane reviews*. Retrieved from http://www.cochrane.org

Cooper, J., Blum, R., Carroll J., et al. (2008). Differences in safety climate among hospital anesthesia departments and the effect of a realistic simulation-based training program. *Anesthesia and Analgesia, 106*, 574–584.

Coopmans, V., & Biddle, C. (2008). CRNA performance using a handheld, computerized decision-making aid during critical events in a simulated environment: A methodologic inquiry. *American Association of Nurse Anesthetists, 76*, 29–35.

Crawforth, K. (2002). The AANA Foundation Closed Malpractice Claims study: Obstetric anesthesia. *American Association of Nurse Anesthetists, 70*, 97–104.

Dulisse, B., & Cromwell, J. (2010). No harm found when nurse anesthetists work without supervision by physicians. *Health Affairs, 29*(8), 1469–1475.

Dunbar, P., Mayer, J., Fordyce, M., Lishner, D., et al. (1998). Availability of anesthesia personnel in rural Washington and Montana. *Anesthesiology, 88*, 800–808.

Dutton, R., & Dukatz, A. (2011). Quality improvement using automated data sources: The anesthesia quality institute. *Anesthesiology Clinics, 29*(3), 439–454.

Fitzgibbon, D., Ramthell, J., Michna, E., et al. (2010). Malpractice claims associated with medication management for chronic pain. *Anesthesiology, 112*(4), 948–956.

Fritzlen, T., Kremer, M., & Biddle, C. (2003). The AANA foundation closed malpractice claims study: Nerve injuries during anesthesia care. *American Association of Nurse Anesthetists, 71*, 347–352.

Garcia, N., Fogel, S., Baker, C., Remine, S., & Jones, J. (2012). Should compliance with the surgical care improvement project (SCIP) process measures determine Medicare and Medicaid reimbursement rates? *The American Surgeon, 78*(6), 653–656.

Greiner, A., & Knebel, E. (Eds.) (2003). *Health professions education: A bridge to quality.* Washington, DC: The National Academies Press. Retrieved from http://books.google.com/books/about/Health_Professions_Education .html?id=Ib6pckASxjkC

Hartland, W., Biddle, C., & Fallacaro, M. (2003). Accessing the living laboratory: Trigger films as an aid to developing, enabling and assessing anesthesia clinical instructors. *American Association of Nurse Anesthetists, 71*, 287–291.

Hindman, B., Palcek, J., Posner, K., et al. (2011). Cervical spinal cord, root and bony spine injuries. A closed claim analysis. *Anesthesiology, 114*(4), 729–731.

Hogan, P., Seifert, R., Moore, C., & Simonson, B. (2010). Cost effectiveness analysis of anesthesia providers. *Nursing Economics, 28*(3), 159–169.

Hotchkiss, M., Biddle, C., & Fallacaro, M. (2002). Assessing the authenticity of the human simulation experience in anesthesiology. *AANA Journal, 70*, 470–473.

Ingersoll, G. (2008). Outcomes evaluation and performance improvement: An integrative review of research on advanced practice nursing. In A. Hamric, J. Spross, & C. Hanson (Eds.), *Advanced practice nursing: An integrative approach* (p. 724). St. Louis, MO: Saunders Elsevier.

IOM. (2010). *The future of nursing: Leading change, advancing health.* Retrieved from http://www.iom.edu/Reports/2010/The-Future-of-Nursing-Leading-Change-Advancing-Health.aspx

Jha, A., Joynt, K., Orav, E., & Epstein, A. (2012). The long-term effect of premier pay for performance on patient outcomes. *The New England Journal of Medicine, 366*(17), 1606–1615.

Jones, R. (2001). Comparative mortality in anaesthesia. *British Journal of Anaesthesia, 87*, 813–815.

Jordan, L., Kremer, M., Crawforth, K., & Shott, S. (2001). Data-driven practice improvement: The AANA Foundation closed malpractice claims study. *AANA Journal, 69*, 301–311.

Kavey, R. (2008). IOM roundtable on evidence-based medicine, health professions sector statement. Retrieved from http://www.iom.edu/Object.file/

Master/44/388/Health%20Professionsa_Is%20Sector%20-%20formatted. pdf

Kraus, G. (1994). Quality assessment and improvement in the 1990s. In S. Foster & L. Jordan (Eds.), *Professional aspects of nurse anesthesia practice* (pp. 291–306). Philadelphia, PA: F.A. Davis.

Kremer, M., Faut-Callahan, M., & Hicks, F. (2002). A study of clinical decision making by certified registered nurse anesthetists. *American Association of Nurse Anesthetists, 70*, 391–397.

Kremer, M., & Stark, P. (2000). Rural realities revisited: Anesthesia care in rural Illinois. Poster presentation, AANA Annual Meeting, August 16.

Larson, S., & Jordan, L. (2001). Preventable adverse patient outcomes: A closed claims analysis of respiratory incidents. *AANA Journal, 69*, 386–392.

Lee, L., Roth, S., Todd, M., et al. (2012). Risk factors associated with ischemic optic neuropathy after spinal fusion surgery. *Anesthesiology, 116*(1), 15–24.

Lema, M. (2003). Safe anesthetic practice—fact, fantasy, or folly? *ASA Newsletter, 67*(6), 1.

Li, G., Warner, M., Lang, B, Huang, L., & Sun, L. (2009). Epidemiology of anesthesia-related mortality in the United states, 1999–2005. *Anesthesiology, 110*, 759–765.

Lohr, K. (1988). Outcomes management: Concepts and questions. *Inquiry, 25*(1), 37–50.

Lucisano, K., & Talbot, L. (2012). Simulation training for advanced airway management for anesthesia and other health care providers: A systematic review. *AANA Journal, 80*, 25–31.

MacRae, M. (2007). Closed claims studies in anesthesia: A literature review and implications for practice. *AANA Journal, 75*, 267–275.

McDonald, K., Romano, P., Geppert J., et al. (2002). *Measures of patient safety based on hospital administrative data—the patient safety indicators.* Rockville, MD: Agency for Healthcare Research and Quality. Publication No. 02–0038. Retrieved from http://www.ahrq.gov/clinic/evrptfiles.htm#psi

McDonald, L. (2001). Florence Nightingale and the early origins of evidence-based nursing. *Evidence-Based Nursing, 4*, 68–69.

McGaghie, W., Darycott, T., Dunn, W. Lopez, C., & Stefanidis, D. (2011). Evaluating the impact of simulation on translational patient outcomes. *Simulation in Healthcare, 6*, S42–S47.

McGaghie, W., Issenberg, S. Petrusa, E., & Scaelse, R. (2010). A critical review of simulation-based medical education research: 2003–2009. *Medical Education, 44*(1), 50–63.

McGlynn, E., Asch, S., Adams, J., et al. (2003). The quality of healthcare delivered to adults in the United States. *NEJM, 348*, 2635–2645.

Metzner, J., Posner, K., Lam, M., & Domino, K. (2011). Closed claims' analysis. *Best Practice & Research. Clinical Anaesthesiology, 25*(2), 263–276.

Monti Seibert, E., Alexander, J., & Lupien, A. (2004). Rural nurse anesthesia practice: A pilot study. *American Association of Nurse Anesthetists, 72*, 181–189.

Moody, M., & Kremer, M. (2001). Preinduction activities: A closed malpractice claims perspective. *AANA Journal, 69*, 461–465.

Murphy, G. (2012). Residual neuromuscular blockade: An important patient safety issue. Presentation at AANA Annual Meeting, 8/15/2012. Retrieved from http://www.aana.com/myaana/Meetings/Documents/Murphy_ Neuromusclar%20Blockade.pdf

National Health Information Network. (2012). *National health information network website.* Retrieved from http://healthit.hhs.gov/portal/server.pt?open =512&objID=1142&parentname=CommunityPage&parentid=4&mode=2

Needleman, J., & Minnick, A. (2009). Anesthesia provider model, hospital resources and maternal outcomes. *Health Services Research, 44*, 464–482.

NLN. (2008). *National League for Nursing: Transforming nursing education: Position statement.* Retrieved from http://www.nln.org/aboutnln/position-statements/transforming052005.pdf

Orkin, F. (1998). Rural realities. *Anesthesiology, 88*, 568–571.

Pellegrini, J. (2006). Using evidence-based practice in nurse anesthesia programs. *American Association of Nurse Anesthetists, 74*, 269–273.

Penprase, B., Mileto, L., Bittinger, A., et al. (2012). The use of high-fidelity simulation in the admissions process: One nurse anesthesia program's experience *AANA Journal, 80*, 43–48.

Petty, W., Kremer, M., & Biddle, C. (2002). A synthesis of the Australian Patient Safety Foundation Anesthesia Incident Monitoring Study, the American Society of Anesthesiologists Closed Claims Project and the American Association of Nurse Anesthetists Closed Claims Study. *AANA Journal, 70*(3), 193–204.

Pine, M., Holt, K., & Lou, Y. (2003). Surgical mortality and type of anesthesia provider. *AANA Journal, 70*, 193–202.

Pravikoff, D., Tanner, A., & Pierce, S. (2005). Readiness of U.S. nurses for evidence-based practice. *AJN, 105*, 45–51.

Punjasawadwong, Y., Bunchungmongkol, N., & Pongchiewboon, A. (2008). Bispectral index for improving anesthetic delivery and postoperative recovery. Retried from http://summaries.cochrane.org/CD003843/monitoring -the-bispectral-index-bis-to-improve-anaesthetic-delivery-and-patient-recovery-from-anesthesia

Ramthell, J., Michna, E., Fitzgibbon D., et al. (2011). Injury and liability associated with cervical procedures for chronic pain. *Anesthesiology, 114*(4), 918–926.

Register, M., Graham-Garcia, J., & Haas, R. (2003). The use of simulation to demonstrate hemodynamic responses to varying degrees of intrapulmonary shunt. *AANA Journal, 71*, 277–284.

Ruth, H. (1945). Anesthesia study commissions. *JAMA, 127*, 514–524.

Sackett, D., Rosenberg, W., Gray, J., Haynes, R., & Richardson, W. (2007, February). Evidence based medicine: What it is and what it isn't. *Clinical Orthopaedics and Related Research, 455*, 3–5.

Schulman, S., Schardt, C., Erb, T. (2002). Evidence-based medicine in anesthesiology. *Current Opinion in Anesthesiology, 15*(6), 661–668.

Silber, J., Kennedy, S., Even-Shoshan, O., et al. (2000). Anesthesiologist direction and patient outcomes. *Anesthesiology, 93*(1), 152–163.

Simonson, D., Ahern, N., & Hendryx, M. (2007). Anesthesia staffing and anesthetic complication during cesarean delivery: A retrospective analysis. *Nursing Research, 56*, 9–17.

Talsma, A., Bahl, V., & Campbell, D. (2008). Exploratory analyses of the "failure to rescue" measure: Evaluation through medical record review. *J Nurs Care Qual, 23*(3), 202–210.

Thiemann, L. (2012). Quality performance measurement and nurse anesthesia practice. Presentation at AANA Annual Meeting, 8/8/2012. Retrieved from http://www.aana.com/myaana/Meetings/Documents/Thiemann_Quality%20Performance%20Measurement.pdf

WHO. (2012). *World Health Organization surgical safety checklist.* Retrieved from http://www.who.int/patientsafety/safesurgery/ss_checklist/en/index.html

# Chapter 11: Measuring Outcomes of Doctor of Nursing Practice

*Marguerite J. Murphy and Kathy S. Magdic*

## Chapter Objectives

1. Examine the current research available related to Doctor of Nursing Practice (DNP) outcomes.
2. Explore rationale for the limited numbers of studies of DNP-related outcomes.
3. Identify areas for future research related to DNP outcomes.

## Chapter Discussion Questions

1. Based on the literature supporting the DNP as the entry level degree for advanced practice nurses (APNs) and the American Association of Colleges of Nurses's (AACN) *The Essentials of Doctoral Education for Advanced Nursing Practice*, what are some of the outcomes of DNP degree-prepared nurses that should be evaluated?
2. What factors have influenced the study of DNP outcomes to date?
3. Describe DNP outcomes that should be considered for future study?

*T*hough a practice doctorate degree in nursing has been offered for more than 20 years, an organized effort to examine and make recommendations for future development of a nursing practice doctorate occurred in 2002 when the American Association of Colleges of Nursing (AACN) convened a task force appointed for this reason (AACN, 2004). In 2004, the AACN proposed the development of practice-doctorate programs for APNs, the DNP (AACN, 2004). Rationale supporting the need for the DNP degree included quality and safety issues in health care addressed in the Institute of Medicine's (IOM) reports *Crossing the Quality Chasm: A New Health System for the 21st Century* (IOM, 2001) and *To Err is Human* (IOM, 1999), increasingly complex patient care, rapidly changing health care systems, and the shortage of nursing faculty (AACN, 2004). DNP graduates are impacting health and health care outcomes as they implement initiatives, apply evidence-based practice changes, and explore the impact of system and practice changes. This chapter presents an overview of the DNP and reviews the outcomes literature related to DNP practice.

## AN OVERVIEW OF THE DNP

The DNP curriculum is conceptualized as having two components: the DNP essentials and specialty competencies. The DNP essentials consist of eight foundational outcome competencies deemed essential for all DNP graduates and serve as a guide for standardization of all DNP degree programs (see Exhibit 11.1). Specialty competencies, developed by national specialty nursing organizations, are intended to prepare the DNP graduate for a particular specialty (AACN, 2006). For example, in 2006, the National Organization of Nurse Practitioner Faculties developed the Nurse Practitioner (NP) Practice Doctorate Competencies, which identified the entry level competencies for all NPs who complete the DNP. These are intended to be used in conjunction with the DNP essentials as a framework to develop DNP NP curricula (National Organization of Nurse Practitioner Faculties [NONPF], 2006, 2011).

Early supporters of AACN and the DNP degree cited increasingly diverse and vulnerable populations, rapidly evolving health care systems and increases complexity of care as needs for better prepared health care providers (Draye, Acker, & Zimmer, 2006; Marion et al., 2003; Mundinger, 2005). The literature identifies multiple attributes that the DNP degree would develop in APNs, thus better preparing

**Exhibit 11.1** *AACN Essentials of Doctoral Education for Advanced Nursing Practice*

| | |
|---|---|
| I. | Scientific underpinnings for practice |
| II. | Organizational and systems leadership for quality improvement and systems thinking |
| III. | Clinical scholarship and analytical methods for evidence-based practice |
| IV. | Information systems/technology and patient care technology for the improvement and transformation of health care |
| V. | Health care policy for advocacy in health care |
| VI. | Interprofessional collaboration for improving patient and population health outcomes |
| VII. | Clinical prevention and population health for improving the nation's health |
| VIII. | Advanced nursing practice |

*Source:* American Association of Colleges of Nurses. (2006). The Essentials of Doctoral Education for Advanced Nursing Practice.

them to become leaders in the ever-changing future health care environment (see Table 11.1). This early rationale and growing national acceptance for the DNP degree continue to serve as the impetus for recommending that APNs and nurse administrators are educated at the practice doctorate level.

A survey conducted by O'Dell (2012) requested data from 175 academic institutions with a DNP program and, based on responses from 123 institutions (70.3%), O'Dell projects there will be an estimated total number of 10,331 DNP graduates in 2012 and 59,872 by 2015 (2012). With the current and expected increase in number of DNP programs and DNP graduates, it is time to examine the outcomes associated with DNP-prepared APNs.

Although evidence exists in the literature regarding the positive impact that APNs have on health care outcomes, evidence reflecting the impact of DNP-prepared APNs is non existent. A literature search using CINHAL, OVID, ProMED, and commercial search engines, such as Google and Bing, revealed no research studies specific to the impact of DNP-prepared nurses on health care outcomes. Reasons for this include there are not enough DNP graduates to effectively study (Cronenwett et al., 2011), and the DNP graduates are scattered across varied practice foci decreasing the likelihood of finding a concentrated group of DNP nurses to include in an outcomes study. Unlike evidence from the landmark study by Aiken, Clark, Cheung, Slone, and Silber (2008) that found that care provided by bachelor of science in nursing

Table 11.1  *Projected Attributes of DNP-Prepared Advanced Practice Nurses*

| Attributes | Source(s) |
|---|---|
| Leadership in patient care and health care systems | Marion et al. (2003), Drayer et al. (2006), Montgomery and Poter-O'Grady (2010), Bellflower and Carter (2006) |
| Influence on health care policy | Bellflower and Carter (2006) |
| Improve quality care and safety issues | Marion et al. (2003), Mundinger (2005), Mundinger et al. (2000) |
| Improve clinical management | Draye et al. (2006), Marion et al. (2003), Mundinger (2005), Mundinger et al. (2000) |
| Improve interprofessional practice | Drayer et al. (2006) |
| Improve integration of evidence-based practice into health care | Bellflower and Carter (2006), Syler and Levin (2012) |
| Improve health promotion/risk reduction | Draye et al. (2006) |
| Improve coordination of care | Draye et al. (2006) |
| Use of technology for data collection and analysis of information | Draye et al. (2006), Montgomery and Poter-O'Grady, 2010 |
| Doctoral-prepared clinical educators | Marion et al. (2003) |

(BSN) graduates demonstrated better patient outcomes than care provided by non-BSN graduates, similar evidence does not yet exist for graduates with a DNP. Until such studies are undertaken, the impact of DNP-prepared nurses remains unknown.

## DNP OUTCOMES

### *Individual Personal and Professional Outcomes*

Anecdotal reports regarding the impact of obtaining a DNP degree on individual graduates' personal outcomes have been reported related to personal satisfaction with degree achievement and professional outcomes related to increased salaries, and movement into a more desirable, higher level professional position (Kung, 2012). The salary increase reported anecdotally is supported in the 2011 National Salary Survey for nurse practitioners and physician assistants, which indicated that DNP-prepared nurse practitioners make an average of $98,826 compared with an average of $90,250 made by master's-prepared nurse

practitioners (Pronsati, 2011). A recent survey of self-selected participants reinforced the findings that nurses entered DNP programs for
the primary purposes of personal satisfaction and job advancement or
job change (O'Dell, 2012).

### Trends in DNP Education

Currently, most data come from survey reports demonstrating increasing trends in numbers related to growth of DNP programs and DNP
graduates. For example, as of May 2012, the AACN (2012b) reported that
there are 184 DNP programs enrolling students at schools of nursing
across the country with an additional 101 DNP programs in the planning stages. DNP programs are available in 40 states plus the District
of Columbia with Florida, Massachusetts, Minnesota, New York,
Pennsylvania, and Texas listed as the states with the highest number
of programs, each with more than five. Between 2010 and 2011, the
number of enrolled students in DNP programs increased from 7,034 to
9,094 and the number of DNP graduates increased from 1,282 to 1,595
(AACN, 2012a). As mentioned above, O'Dell estimates that there will
be 10,331 DNP graduates in 2012 and 59,872 by 2015 (2012)

### DNP COMPETENCIES

Three years (2010–2012) of national survey data related to DNP outcomes were collected to answer the question: "Are graduates of DNP
programs utilizing these core competencies in practice?" (slide 29,
O'Dell, 2012). While the number of self-selected respondents was small
for each of the 3 years, 294, 359, and 248, respectively, there were some
interesting findings. The DNP degree was initially established for APNs
with a clinical focus; however, over time the degree has expanded to
include the practice of the nurse executive. Data from the O'Dell survey indicated that the largest majority of students are in programs of
clinical concentration, with above 60% of respondents indicating this
area of focus in each year for 2010, 2011, and 2012. Approximately 20%
of respondents reported leadership in the area of concentration for
these same years, making it the second highest area of concentration
of DNP program focus (2012). The survey also indicated the number
of DNP graduates accepting jobs as nursing faculty was increasing, a
finding that supports one of the initial incentives for the DNP degree—
to increase doctoral-prepared clinical faculty. Other findings indicated
that the largest majority of DNP graduates feel competent in the DNP

policy, evidence-based practice (EBP), leadership, and practice change essentials (O'Dell, 2012).

Professional contributions of DNP graduates include publications in journals and podium and poster presentations (O'Dell, 2012), and is an area that is being recognized and evaluated as a DNP outcome measure (Broome & Riner, 2012, Newland, 2012). A survey by Broome and Riner (2012) identified over 300 articles published in 59 journals from 2007 to 2012, where at least one author displayed DNP credentials. The number of publications increased steadily over the 5-year period with most of the publications being focused on practice. A review of the 300 articles to determine the focus or type of articles identified 147 data-based articles, which included nurses and/or staff focus ($n$ = 61) and patient focus ($n$ = 86). Other areas identified in this survey included clinical intervention or original research ($n$ = 115), evaluation of EBP guideline ($n$ = 16), clinical teaching ($n$ = 21), organization and systems improvement ($n$ = 23), and practice or educational survey ($n$ = 12). This survey also identified interdisciplinary authorship of medical doctors (MD) and doctors of philosophy (PhD). The increase in publications and presentations by DNP-prepared nurses indicate the increased leadership and scope of practice (slide 19, Broome & Riner, 2012) originally noted in AACN's call for the DNP degree. Table 11.2 provides samples of articles published in nursing journals in 2011 and 2012.

Table 11.2  *Sample of Articles Published in Nursing Journals Within the Last 3 Years With Primary Author With DNP Degree*

| Journal | Article Title |
| --- | --- |
| AANA Journal | Intrathecal Hydromorphone for Postoperative Analgesia After Cesarean Delivery: A Retrospective Study |
| Advances in Neonatal Care | Neonatal Nurse Practitioner Workforce Survey Executive Summary |
| International Journal of Nursing Practice | Understanding Overweight Adolescents' Beliefs Using the Theory of Planned Behaviour |
| Journal of Advanced Nursing | Paediatric Nurse Practitioner Managed Cardiology Clinics: Patient Satisfaction and Appointment Access |
| Journal of Association of Vascular Access | Evaluation Methods for the Assessment of Acute Care Nurse Practitioner Inserted Central Lines: Evidence-Based Strategies for Practice |
| Journal of Cardiovascular Nursing | Managing Heart Failure: A Critical Appraisal of the Literature |

*(continued)*

**Table 11.2** *continued*

| | |
|---|---|
| *Journal of Midwifery and Women's Health* | Treatment Options and Recommendations to Reduce Preterm Births in Women With Short Cervix |
| *Journal of Neuroscience Nursing* | Concussion and the Adolescent |
| *Journal of Nursing Administration* | Evidence Supporting Excellence |
| *Journal of Wound, Ostomy and Continence Nursing* | Post-Thrombotic Syndrome Patient Education Based on the Health Belief Model: Self-Reported Intention to Comply With Recommendations |
| *Nursing Education* | Using Social Media to Enhance Nursing Education |
| *Nurse Practitioner* | When Tension Headaches Become Chronic |
| *Oncology Nursing Forum* | Feasibility Pilot on Medication Adherence and Knowledge in Ambulatory Patients With Gastrointestinal Cancer |
| *World Views on Evidence-Based Nursing* | Using Clinical Pathways to Aid in the Diagnosis of Necrotizing Soft Tissue Infections Synthesis of Evidence |

## DNP STUDENT PROJECTS

Data are being reported about DNP programs and the DNP graduate, but there remains little data documenting the impact of the DNP graduate on outcomes related to the original established goals of improving nursing practice and patient outcomes, enhancing leadership skills to strengthen practice and health care delivery, and increasing faculty for practice instruction. At this point, there are no published studies comparing outcomes of DNP-prepared graduates to non-DNP-prepared graduates in similar roles. There are some data related to the profile of the DNPs' practice (O'Dell, 2012), but scarce data as to the outcomes of that DNP practice. So the question remains: Does the knowledge and skills gained by this doctoral degree translate into improved patient, systems, and educational outcomes?

In an attempt to discover areas where DNP graduates are focusing their efforts, an informal web search for DNP Capstone projects was performed. In addition, emails and phone calls were made to a number of schools with DNP programs requesting a list of titles and/ or abstracts. The search yielded 512 DNP capstone projects from over 51 schools; 243 were accompanied by abstracts. The remainder consisted of simple listings of DNP Capstone project titles. Capstone project titles and abstracts were reviewed to identify emerging trends of the foci for DNP Capstone projects. If an abstract was not available for review, the project title itself was reviewed. Some titles were detailed enough to clearly identify the focus of the project; however, some titles were either too vague or not explicit enough to clearly appreciate the intent of the project. Broad categories were established in an attempt to categorize elements of the projects with regard to population, setting, and problem. As expected, many of the projects spanned multiple categories. Exhibit 11.2 provides examples of titles of DNP Capstone projects from each of the schools sampled.

### Exhibit 11.2  *Examples of DNP Capstone Projects*

**Health Promotion**

Empowering Community Health: A Faith-Based Approach

Promoting Nutritional Awareness and Improving Dietary Habits: A Community-Based Approach

Clinical Decision Support System Improves Bone Mineral Density Screening Rates in 65-Year-Old Women

Developing Evidence-Based Evaluation Strategies for a Campus-Workplace Violence Prevention Program

Clinical Practice Guidelines: Screening for Anal Cancer in HIV-Infected Men Who Have Sex with Men

Cardiovascular Disease Awareness: Promoting Healthy Lifestyles in African American Females

Colorectal Cancer Screening in a Free Primary Care Program for the Uninsured

Teenage Pregnancy: An Impact of the Healthy Choices Abstinence Program

An Evidence-Based Toolkit to Prevent Meningococcal Meningitis in College Students

Provider Focused Process Improvement Project to Enhance Patient Participation in a Tobacco Smoking Cessation Program

Bully Victim Identification and Intervention Program for School Nurses

**Population/Diagnosis Focus**

Assessment of Male Partner Needs and Experiences During Labor and Birth

Neonatal Hypoglycemia and Prompted Interventions During the Pre-Transport Phase of Care

Childhood Obesity Prevention in the Context of Family Activity: Development of an Evaluation Tool for the PAK Family Activity Event

Evaluation of a Multidisciplinary Clinical Intervention on Childhood Obesity at Seattle Children's Hospital

Perceptions of Body Image, Body Satisfaction, and Knowledge of Obesity-Related Health Risks Among African American College Students

Improving Diabetes Self-Care Behaviors of Adolescents Through a School-Based Diabetes Care Initiative

*(continued)*

## Exhibit 11.2 *continued*

Missed Opportunities for the HPV Vaccine in Thirteen-Year-Old Girls Receiving Care at NeighborCare Health

A Transition Checklist for Adolescents with Sickle Cell Disease

Examining the Influence of Structured Diabetes Self-Management Education on Patient Outcomes in an Outpatient Setting

Dehydration in Terminal Disease: An Evidence-Based Protocol for Establishing Goals of Group Intervention of Life Enhancement of People in the Older Adult

The Predictive Value of Second Trimester Blood Pressures on the Development of Preeclampsia

Acute Pain Management: A Nursing Education Program for Improved Outcomes

ACES: A Quality Improvement Program to Improve Asthma Outcomes

The Effect of an Evidence-Based Support Intervention to Facilitate Treatment Preference Decision Making by Surrogates of Persons With Incapacitating Dementia

Translation of Autism Screening Research Into Practice

An Evaluation of a School-Based Asthma Program

Pressure Ulcer Prevention Protocol of Older Adults in a Nursing Home Setting

**Focus on Veterans**

Effectiveness of a Four-Item Screening Tool for Returning Operation Iraqi Freedom/Operation Enduring Freedom Veterans

Gap Analysis: Transition of Health-Care from the Department of Defense to the Department of Veterans Affairs

Cognitive Behavioral Therapy for the Treatment of Sleep Disturbances in Soldiers With Combat Associated Mild Traumatic Brain Injury

**Hospital Care**

The Evaluation of the Implementation of an Individualized Educational Program on the 30-Day Readmission Rate for Patients With Heart Failure in a Community Hospital

Application of the Iowa Model of EBP to Promote Quality Care in the Peri-Operative Management of Pacemakers and Implantable Cardioverter-Defibrillators

Evaluation of Cue vs. Schedule-Based Infant Feeding Protocols in the Neonatal Intensive Care Unit

Implementing an Evidence-Based Risk Assessment Model for Chemotherapy-Induced Neutropenia

Evaluation of an Evidence-Based, Nurse-Driven Checklist Designed to Prevent Hospital-Acquired Catheter-Associated Urinary Tract Infections in Intensive Care Units

Patient Rounding in the LTAC Setting: An Opportunity to Positively Impact Patient Call Light Use, Patient Satisfaction and Patient Safety

Evaluation of a New Program to Admit Heart Failure Patients to an Emergency Department Observation Unit

(continued)

## Exhibit 11.2  *Examples of DNP Capstone Projects*  (continued)

Blunt Cerebrovascular Injuries at the R. Adams Cowley Shock Trauma Center and the University of Maryland Medical Center: A Systems Analysis at a Tertiary Care Center

Implementation and Evaluation of an Evidence-Based Oral Care Guideline in a Mechanically Ventilated Patient Population

Improvement of Family Centered Care Practices in the Neonatal Intensive Care Unit

Evaluation of the Effectiveness of the Ruby Slipper Program in Reducing Falls on a Medical Surgical Unit

Implementation of Early Goal-Directed Therapy in Management of the Septic Patient

Inpatient Fall Prevention Program: Reducing Patient Falls Through Implementation of a Clinical Fall Prevention Team

Quality Improvement Intervention Using Split-Dose Protocol for Bowel Preparation for Colonoscopy

Transition Home for Patients With Heart Failure: A Pilot Program at a Critical Access Hospital

Exploring Coping Mechanisms of Palliative Care Patients in an Acute Care Setting

**Psychiatric-Mental Health**

Tele-Psychiatry: Pilot Training Program for Washington State Department of Corrections Psychiatric Prescribers

Enhancing Mental Health Services Utilization Among African Immigrants and Refugees in the Northwest

Heightened Mental Health Awareness on a Diverse, Urban Public University Campus Through a Medical Outreach Campaign

Developing a Treatment Guide for PTSD

Evaluation of Alcohol Management Practices in a Community Hospital

Educating Nurses About Postpartum Depression in the Acute Care Setting

Examining the Effectiveness of an Aggression Management Program in an Inpatient Psychiatric Setting

**Cultural and International Focus**

Implementation and Evaluation of a Model of Expanded Nursing Practice in Germany: A Pilot Program

Case Study from the Urban Village in Central Russia: Evaluating Barriers to Vaccine Administration and Vaccine Compliance

Improving Cardiovascular Health for Haitians in Dumay Using a Community Organization Approach

A Multi-Factorial Tailored Intervention to Improve Adherence in Uninsured and Underserved African Americans With Hypertension

Education of Incarcerated African American Males on Sexually Transmitted Diseases

*(continued)*

## Exhibit 11.2 *continued*

Can an Educational Intervention Lower Blood Sugar Levels in Latinos at Risk for Developing Diabetes Mellitus

Storytelling, a Cognitive Behavior Pain Management Strategy for American Indian and Alaska Natives

Evaluation of the Impact of Information on HPV, Cervical Cancer and PAP Smear Knowledge Among Costa Rican Women Enrolled in HPV Vaccination Trial

Policy Development to Improve Quality of Life Outcomes of Breast Cancer Survivors in a Northwest Tribal Community

Evaluation of Spanish Diabetes Group Visits at a Community Health Center

**Technology**

Use of the Electronic Health Record in the Measurement of Nurse Practitioner Performance

Tele-Visitation: A Strategy to Reduce Distress Among Isolated Blood and Bone Marrow Transplant Patients Post-Transplantation

Using Computerized Physician Order Entry (CPOE) to Improve Prescribing of Analgesics and Benzodiazepines to Persons 65 and Older

Feasibility of a Webinar for Coaching Patient with COPD on Endo-of-Life communication

The Use of Documentation Prompts as an Intervention Strategy for Primary Care Providers Managing Children in Out of Home Placement

Identification and Elimination of Barriers to the Use of a Technology-Based Patient/Family Education System

Crisis Team Training of Perinatal Health-Care Professionals Using Simulation Technology

Treatment Fidelity Evaluation of Tele-Health Stage-Based Motivational Interviewing Interventions

My Papp: An Android App to Educate about Pap Testing

The Use of Documentation Prompts as an Intervention Strategy for Primary Care Providers Managing Children in Out of Home Placement

Home But Not Alone: Telephone Support for the First-Time Breastfeeding Mother

Efficacy of an Electronic Integrative Protocol in Managing Alcohol Withdrawal Syndrome: A Quality and Safety Initiative

Development of Smartphone Application to Detect Hypertension in Children and Adolescents

**Health Policy**

Policy Development for Prenatal Care Assurance: A Strategic Approach to Improve Maternal and Infant Health Among AIAN Communities in Washington State

Methicillin-Resistant *Staphylococcus aureus* (MRSA) Infection Control Policy at First Place School: A Policy Development in Vulnerable Community

Public Policy Involvement and Behavioral Intentions Toward Health Policy Research Among Nurses With Professional Doctorates

(continued)

**Exhibit 11.2** *Examples of DNP Capstone Projects* *(continued)*

**Professional and Administrative Nursing**

Strategies to Improve Patient Flow in an Urgent Care Facility

Nurse Manager Leadership Development Program Evaluation

Transformational Leadership Behaviors of Successful Nurse Managers

Integration of Nurse Practitioner Practice into a Patient Centered Medical Home

Roadmap to Improved Trauma Outcomes: The ACNP Practice Model

The Use of Mentoring by a Nurse Executive to Affect Nurse Managers' Use of Transformational Leadership Behaviors

Does the DNP Change Clinical Practice

Developing a Farm Team: Succession Planning for Nurse Managers

Examining and Reducing Distractions and Interruptions During Medication Administration

**Education**

Acute Pain Management: A Nursing Education Program for Improved Outcomes

Disaster Preparedness and Response: Implication for Nurse Practitioner Education

Predictors of the First-Year Nursing Student at Risk of Early Departure

An Educational Intervention to Implement SBAR for Nurse Provider Telephone Communication

Acute Pain Management: A Nursing Education Program for Improved Outcomes

Evaluation of Nurses' Education Program on End of Life Care

**Practice Models**

MD-NP Collaborative Practice: Models, Barriers and Improvement Strategies

Use of Nurse Case Managers in Diabetic Care

Collaboration in an Outpatient Clinic Setting: Strengthening Care for Patients

Nurse Practitioner Led-Heart Failure Clinic

Development of an Online Learning Module Focusing on the Principles of EBP for Newly Hired Registered Nurses

Integrating Cardiology Acute Care Nurse Practitioners into a House Staff Model of Care: Development of Performance and Value-Added Outcome Measures

Promoting the Coordination of Care for Patients With a Diagnosis of Chronic Illness and Substance Abuse in a Managed Care Organization

The Development of a National, Multimodal, Multidiscipline Evidence-Based Clinical Practice Guideline for the Prevention and Management of PONV/PDNV in Adult Patients

## POPULATION AND SETTING FOCI OF DNP PROJECTS

While it was difficult to determine the specific population for all projects as some project titles did not specifically identify a population, it appeared that the population ranged from neonates to the older adult, with the majority of the projects focusing on adult males and females. African Americans were the predominant minority race specifically identified as the population of interest, followed Latinos, American Indian/Alaskan Natives, and Northwest Tribes. International projects included Germany, Nigeria, Central Russia, Costa Rica, and Haitians in Dumay. Interestingly, there was an interest in issues related to veterans. There were a high number of project titles focusing on nurses, APNs, and students. Many of the nurse-focused projects were directed toward education regarding practice change efforts or influence on attitudes. Settings for projects ranged from the community, long-term care, and retail health settings to hospitals and intensive care units.

## PROBLEM FOCI AND INTERVENTIONS OF DNP PROJECTS

As might be expected, chronic disease was a major focus, specifically, cardiovascular disease, valvular heart disease, heart failure, stroke, diabetes, hypertension, liver disease, chronic obstructive pulmonary disease (COPD), asthma, and end stage renal disease. Other disease-specific foci included various cancers, HIV, obesity (especially childhood obesity), transplant, dementia, attention-deficit disorder, and autism. Pain, end of life, hospice, and palliative care were noted as areas where health care needs were identified. Additional projects addressed women's health, psychiatric mental health, use of technology, informatics, telemedicine, and disaster preparedness.

Within these populations, settings, and diagnoses, projects were focused on health promotion strategies, development and evaluation of practice guidelines and quality improvement initiatives, practice models, models of care transition, interdisciplinary care, and health policy changes. Projects focusing on academic curriculum development, continuing education, and administrative topics, such as leadership and systems changes, were also included.

As previously stated, this was an informal review of DNP Capstone project titles and abstracts when available. Without the ability to review the entire project, it becomes difficult to truly appreciate the impact that the DNP degree has on outcomes. However, it is exciting to see the breadth of projects being conducted by DNPs.

## FUTURE RESEARCH-RELATED DNP OUTCOMES

The current focus on health care outcomes, compounded by the ongoing monitoring of educational outcomes, spotlights the need for research of DNP-related outcomes. But what will shape this research? The IOM in conjunction with the Robert Wood Johnson Foundation and the Josiah Macy Foundation is calling for APNs to be used to the fullest extent of the education to help meet the increasing health care needs in the United States (Cronenwett et al., 2011; IOM, 2010). In addition, the recent IOM report, *The Future of Nursing: Leading Change, Advancing Health*, calls for doubling the number of doctoral-prepared nurses (IOM, 2010). It is clear that the need for doctoral-prepared nurses will increase in the future; however, research is needed to document that DNP-prepared nurses can improve quality of care, provide leadership in policy reform, and reduce costs. Research that demonstrates a positive impact can be used to garner support of key decision makers, such as legislators, other health care providers, the community, third-party payers, and administrators (Newland, 2012).

## RECOMMENDATIONS FOR DNP OUTCOME STUDIES

### Policy

DNP graduates have primarily focused on local and regional policy initiatives (O'Dell, 2012); however, nursing has a history of leading policy changes at a national level, such as the Magnet process, which is affiliated with the American Association of Colleges of Nursing (Leavitt, 2009; American Nurses Credentialing Center, 2008). The DNP essentials and early supporters of the DNP degree cited leadership in policy reform to improve health care outcomes as a key role. Though nursing research has grown in the areas of education and clinical practice, the transition of research findings into public policy reform is necessary but lacking. Because analysis and synthesis of evidence is a cornerstone of DNP education and practice, this places the DNP in the role to serve as the advocate to champion policy change. It has been suggested that all nursing researchers should examine the policy implication of their research (Leavitt, 2009).

### Evidence-Based Practice

As the number of hospitals striving for and maintaining Magnet status increases and the implementation of EBP in health care delivery continues, there will be growing needs for leadership and mentors in this area (Melnyk, Fineout-Overholt, Gallaher-Ford, & Kaplan, 2012; Syler & Levin, 2012). The DNP-prepared nurse is the logical choice to help fill these roles. The impact of DNP-lead EBP changes needs to be documented in the areas of quality care, patient outcomes, cost reduction, and employee satisfaction (Melnyk et al., 2012). Research related to the impact of the implementation of EBP clinical guidelines on patient care outcomes is warranted in a multitude of settings and a variety of patients. The use of EBP is not limited to the clinical practice setting. Research is needed in academic arenas to determine the most effective teaching modalities, curriculum structure, and the impact that DNP-prepared faculty have on educating nurses of tomorrow.

### Quality and Safety Improvement

The Quality and Safety Education for Nurses expanded its recommended knowledge, skills, and attitudes (KSA) to the advanced practice nursing level, with the APN expected to take the leadership role in combining EBP, information technology, and outcome measures related to quality and safety measures (Cronenwett et al., 2009). These recommendations were supported in word or in spirit by the national organizations representing APNs. The quality and safety arena is open for research regarding outcomes related to DNP-prepared nurses to include the educational curriculum using the APN KSA as outcome measures for DNP students and graduates. The KSA can also be used to select quality and safety outcomes to be monitored and impacted by DNP-prepared nurses.

### Academic Education

As the number of DNP programs is being developed across the United States, it is important that research is done to demonstrate the quality and rigor necessary to adequately prepare DNP graduates. What are the essentials necessary to educate DNP graduates to be practice change leaders that require the incorporation of information systems, research review, and integration of change within systems (p. 112, Broom, 2012)? What faculty is necessary to guide the development of leaders at this level? What courses are needed to provide the foundational concepts and encourage application of the concepts to prepare for practice in the future health care? These are questions that need to be answered with research that is focused on outcomes to guide decisions in the academic arena. Additional research is needed with regard to the impact that DNP-prepared faculty have on the outcomes related to the education of nursing students, the impact of tenure versus non tenure track appointments for DNP-prepared faculty, the leadership of DNP-prepared faculty in academic settings, and the impacts of practice requirements of DNP–APNs who are full-time faculty.

## HEALTH CARE OUTCOMES IN SPECIALTY PRACTICE

Pulling from the DNP essentials to improve health care outcomes, doctoral-prepared nurses are expected to lead health care teams for the purpose of improving health care outcomes. National organizations representing nurse anesthetists and all seven of the nurse practitioner organizations' APNs have endorsed the doctoral preparation entry level requirement. The nurse midwifery organization and the clinical nurse specialist national organizations have maintained the master's entry, though the Society for Clinical Nurse Specialist Education has endorsed the DNP education for clinical nurse specialists and has begun development of curriculum guidelines to support this (Dennison, Payne, & Farrell, 2012). It is essential that the impact DNP-prepared nurses have on health care outcomes be demonstrated through research to support the decisions regarding the educational level necessary for entry into practices as an APN. Until this evidence is available, the educational debate will continue.

### Professional Outcomes

The DNP degree has been identified as having a positive impact on the empowerment of nurses to influence parity with other health care professionals and to impact health care (Dennison et al., 2012). The issue of achieving parity with other health care providers is also a rationale provided in the AACN's development of the DNP entry level proposal (AACN, 2004). Research to determine the degree to which parity and empowerment are being achieved in DNP-prepared nurses is necessary to demonstrate the level to which these goals are being accomplished.

## CONCLUSIONS

It is obvious through the review of the literature that while there is little research on outcomes related to DNP-prepared nurses, there is an increasing awareness of the need for this research as evidenced by many articles and editorials citing the need. Certainly there is research to support that APNs educated at a master's level are highly competent, providing care with equal if not better outcomes than physicians. However, future questions that need to be answered include: (1) How do outcomes achieved by DNP-prepared nurses compare with outcomes achieved by non-DNP-prepared nurses? and (2) Will the master's-prepared APN be as well prepared to provide care in the increasingly complex and diverse health care system as the DNP-prepared APN? Health care policy decisions, such as the Affordable Care Act, and future initiatives proposed by leaders in the field of health care, such as the Josiah Macy Jr. Foundation, the IOM and the Robert Wood Johnson Foundation, have and will continue to open the door for DNPs to shape the course of health care through projects developed to positively impact outcomes. This, in turn, should drive the need for research as to who is best prepared with the knowledge, skills, and abilities to demonstrate positive outcomes. Will it be the DNP-prepared nurse? The expectation is that it will be; however, research is needed to validate that assumption.

## Answers to Chapter Discussion Questions

1. The AACN essentials outline leadership, systems change, quality and safety improvement, integration of EBP, informatics, health care policy, interprofessional collaboration, population health, and specialty clinical care as outcomes that nurses with DNP degrees would positively impact. A review of the literature identifies support for the essentials as well as additional areas of outcomes that supporters of the DNP degree addressed, and include improved health promotion and risk reduction, improved coordination of care, and increase of doctoral-prepared nursing faculty.

2. Reasons for minimal research to date on DNP outcomes include not enough DNP graduates to effectively study, and that DNP graduates are scattered across varied practice foci decreasing the likelihood of finding a concentrated group of DNP nurses to include in an outcomes study. Anecdotal reports regarding the impact of obtaining a DNP degree on individual graduates' personal outcomes have been reported related to personal satisfaction with degree achievement and professional outcomes related to increased salaries and movement into a more desirable, higher level professional position.

Survey studies related to the number of DNP program, graduates, and overview of DNP curricula provide the primary source of data; however, surveys regarding impact on salary change and other professional outcomes are beginning to be found in the literature.
3. There are multiple factors that will impact the focus of future studies of DNP outcomes. Future decisions regarding health care policy, reimbursement sources, and increased focus on outcomes in health care and nursing education will require studies of DNP outcomes to support and document the impact of DNP-prepared nurses. The outcome studies should include but not be limited to outcomes related to policy reform; clinical practice—specifically care provided by DNP-prepared practitioners compared with MSN-prepared practitioners; development, implementation, and evaluation of EBP guidelines; quality and safety; and the impact of DNP-prepared nurse educators.

## WEB LINKS

American Academy of Colleges of Nurses: This site houses many of the essential documents related to the organized directive to call for the DNP as the entry level degree for APNs, including the initial Task Force report from 2004 and the DNP Essentials Document approved in 2006, which outlines the DNP core essentials. This site also maintains a list of all academic institutions with DNP programs, as well as Fact Sheets updated annually to reflect data trends related to DNP enrollment, numbers of graduates, and so on (website: http://www.aacn.nche.edu/dnp).

Doctors of Nursing Practice: This website was developed to serve as a virtual community for DNP-prepared nurses. The site houses abstracts of self-submitted DNP student projects as well as a collection of articles related to the development of the DNP degree. This organization hosts an annual conference that showcases presentations by DNP-prepared nurses. An annual survey is conducted regarding DNP outcomes and the summarized results are posted on this site: http://www.nonpf.com/displaycommon.cfm?an=1&subarticlenbr=27 (website: http://www.doctorsofnursingpractice.org/index.html).

National Organization of Nurse Practitioner Faculties, NP Curriculum Material: This site contains a link to DNP Scholarly Project Titles Exemplars from several universities (website: http://www.nonpf.com/displaycommon.cfm?an=1&subarticlenbr=27).

DNP Project Lists and Samples: The following websites provide lists of titles or samples of DNP Capstone projects completed by DNP graduates.

Past DNP Capstone Projects, University of Washington: http://nursing.uw.edu/academic-services/degree-programs/dnp/past-capstone-projects.html

Capstone Project Fulfillment Roster, University of Medicine and Dentistry of New Jersey: http://sn.umdnj.edu/academics/dnp/CompletedCapstoneList.pdf

Examples of DNP Projects, Rush University: http://www.rushu.rush.edu/servlet/BlobServer?blobcol=urlfile&blobtable=document&blobkey=id&blobwhere=1222091410478&blobheader=application%2Fpdf&blobnocache=true

Doctor of Nursing Practice Scholarly Projects, Vanderbilt University.
2012:http://www.nursing.vanderbilt.edu/dnp/pdf/dnp_scholarlprojects _2012.pdf
2011:http://www.nursing.vanderbilt.edu/dnp/pdf/dnp_scholarlprojects _2011.pdf
2010:http://www.nursing.vanderbilt.edu/dnp/pdf/dnp_scholarlprojects _2010.pdf

## REFERENCES

Aiken, L., Clarke, S. P., Cheung, R. B., Sloane, D. M., & Silber, J. H. (2003). Educational levels of hospital nurses and surgical patient mortality. *Journal of American Medical Association, 290*(12), 1617–1623. doi:10.1001/jama.290.12.1617

American Association of Colleges of Nursing. (2004). *AACN Position Statement on the Practice Doctorate in Nursing.* Retrieved from http://www.aacn.nche.edu/publications/position/DNPpositionstatement.pdf

American Association of Colleges of Nurses. (2006, October). *The Essentials of Doctoral Education for Advanced Nursing Practice.* Retrieved from http://www.aacn.nche.edu/publications/position/DNPEssentials.pdf

American Association of Colleges of Nurses. (2012a, March 22). *New AACN Data Show an Enrollment Surge in Baccalaureate and Graduate Programs Amid Calls for More Highly Educated Nurses.* Retrieved from http://www.aacn.nche.edu/news/articles/2012/enrollment-data

American Association of Colleges of Nurses. (2012b, May 29). *Fact Sheet: Doctor of Nursing Practice.* Retrieved from http://www.aacn.nche.edu/media-relations/fact-sheets/DNPFactSheet.pdf

American Nurses Credentialling Center. (2008). Magnet recognition program. Retrieved from http://www.nursecredentialing.org/Magnet.aspx.

Bellflower, B. & Carter, M. A. (2006). Primer on the practice doctorate for neonatal nurse practitioners. *Advances in Neonatal Care, 6*(6), 323–332. doi:10.1016/j.adnc.2006.08.001

Broom, M. E. (2012). Doubling the number of doctorally prepared nurses [Editorial]. *Nursing Outlook, 60,* 111–113. doi:10.1016/j.outlook.2012.04.001

Broom, M. E., & Riner, M. B. (2012, August). *Contributions of scholarly papers in literature: Dissemination practices of DNP graduates.* Podium presentation at Promoting Quality and Excellence in DNP Education, Chicago, IL.

Cronenwett, L., Dracup, K., Grey, M., McCauley, L., Meleis, A., & Salmon, M. (2011). The doctor of nursing practice: A national workforce perspective. *Nursing Outlook, 57,* 9–17. doi:10.1016/j.outlook.2011.11.003

Cronenwett, L., Sherwood, G., Pohl, J., Barnsteiner, J., Moore, S., Sullivan, D. T.,...Warren, J. (2009). Quality and safety education for advanced nursing practice. *Nursing Outlook, 57,* 338–348. doi:10.1016/j.outlook.2009.07.009

Dennison, R. D., Payne, C., & Farrell, K. (2012). The doctorate in nursing practice: moving advanced practice nursing even closer to excellence. *Nursing Clinics of North America, 47,* 225–240. doi:10.1016/j.cnur.2012.04.001

Draye, M. A., Acker, M., & Zimmer, P. A. (2006). The practice doctorate in nursing: Approaches to transform nurse practitioner education and practice. *Nursing Outlook, 54*(3), 123–139. doi:10.1016/j.outlook.2006.01.001

Institute of Medicine. (1999). *To Ere is Human: Building a Safer Health System.* Retrieved from http://www.nap.edu/catalog.php?record_id=9728#toc

Institute of Medicine. (2001). *Crossing the Quality Chasm: A New Health System for the 21ˢᵗ Century.* Retrieved from http://books.nap.edu/openbook. php?record_id=10027

Institute of Medicine. (2010). *Report Brief: The Future of Nursing: Leading Change, Advancing Health.* Retrieved from http://www.iom.edu/~/media/ Files/Report%20Files/2010/The-Future-of-Nursing/Future%20of%20 Nursing%202010%20Report%20Brief.pdf

Kung, M. (March, 2012). How the DNP changed me. *Advance for NPs & PAs.* Retrieved from http://community.advanceweb.com/blogs/np_7/default. aspx

Leavitt, J. K. (2009). Leaders in health policy: A critical role for nursing. *Nursing Outlook, 57*(2), 73–77.

Marion, L., Viens, D., O'Sullivan, A. L., Crabtree, K., Fontana, S., & Price, M. M. (2003). The practice doctorate in nursing: future or fringe? *Topics in Advanced Practice Nursing eJournal, 3*(2), 1–8. Retrieved from http://www. medscape.com/viewarticle/453247_print

Melnyk, M. B., Fineout-Overholt, E., Gallaher-Ford, L., & Kaplan, L. (2012). The state of evidence-based practice in the US nurses: critical implication for nurse leaders and educators. *The Journal of Nursing Administration, 42*(9), 410–417. doi:10.1097/NNA.0b013e3182664e0a

Montgomery, K. L., & Porter-O'Grady, T. (2010). Innovation and learning: Creating the DNP nurse leader. *Nurse Leader, 8*(4), 44–47. doi:10.1010/j. mnl.2010.05.001

Mundinger, M. O. (2005). Who's who in nursing: Bringing clarity to the doctor of nursing practice. *Nursing Outlook 53*(4), 173–176. doi:10.1016/j. outlook.2005.05.007

Mundinger, M. O., Cook, S. S., Lenz, E. R., Piacentini, K., Auerhahn, C., & Smith, J. (2000). Assuring quality and access in advanced practice nursing: A challenge to nurse educators. *Journal of Professional Nursing, 16*(6), 322–329. doi:10.1016/jpnu.2000.18177

National Organization of Nurse Practitioner Faculties. (2011, April). *Nurse Practitioner Core Competencies.* Retrieved from http://www.nonpf.org/ associations/10789/files/IntegratedNPCoreCompsFINALApril2011.pdf

National Organization of Nurse Practitioner Faculties & National Panel for NP Practice Doctorate Competencies. (2006). *Practice doctorate nurse practitioner entry level competencies.* Retrieved from http://www.nonpf.org/ associations/10789/files/DNP%20NP%20competenciesApril2006.pdf

Newland, J. A. (2011, April). The nurse practitioner salutes the DNP. [Editorial]. *The Nurse Practitioner, 5.* doi:10.1097/01.NPR.0000412897.94383/64

O'Dell, D. G. (2012, September 22). *The State of DNP Degree: Analysis of Three Years of National Survey Data.* Presentation at Fifth National DNP Conference, Saint Louis, MO. Retrieved from www.doctorsofnursingpractice.org/documents/ODellDNPOutcomesFinal.pptx.pdf

Pronsati, M. P. (2011). *National salary report 2011: Advance for NPs and PAs.* Retrieved from http://nurse-practitioners-and-physician assistants. advanceweb.com/Features/Articles/National-Salary-Report-2011.aspx

Syler, J., & Leving, R. F. (2012). Evidence-based practice: on the doctor of nursing practice (DNP). *Research and Theory for Nursing Practice: An International Journal, 26*(1) 6–9. doi:org/10.1891/1541–6577.26.1.6

# Chapter 12: Resources to Facilitate Advanced Practice Nursing Outcomes Research

DENISE BRYANT-LUKOSIUS, ALBA DICENSO,
SAADIA ISRAR, AND RENÉE CHARBONNEAU-SMITH

## Chapter Objectives

1. Describe the role and impact of a nationally funded chair in advanced practice nursing (APN) for building APN research capacity and expertise.
2. Provide an overview of the PEPPA Framework and how it has been applied to guide the successful design, implementation, and evaluation of APN roles.
3. Describe an APN Research Data Collection Toolkit for selecting APN-sensitive outcome measurement tools and other measurement instruments relevant to different stages of role development.

## Chapter Discussion Questions

1. What five features of complex health care interventions are consistent with common characteristics of APN roles?
2. What are common barriers to conducting meaningful APN role evaluations?

3. How can participatory action research (PAR) be used to inform the development and implementation of APN roles? Why is this process important?
4. Provide examples of APN role structures, processes, and outcomes. When should structure–process–outcome evaluations be conducted during role development?

B ased on UK Medical Research Council guidelines, advanced practice nursing (APN) roles meet the criteria of a complex health care intervention (Craig et al., 2008). They involve a number of interacting components including role competencies and related activities (clinical, education, research, leadership, consultation, and collaboration) that, when enacted in combination, are greater than the sum of their parts (Canadian Nurses Association [CNA], 2008). These role activities are often directed at a number of target groups (patients and families, nurses and other health care providers, organizations and health systems) to address difficult health care problems and to achieve a variety of outcomes relevant to each target group. As a health care intervention, APN roles also need to be highly flexible and responsive to the dynamic needs and contexts of the patient populations they serve and the environments and practice settings in which they work.

Like other complex health care interventions, high-quality and meaningful evaluations of APN roles require a sophisticated research skill set to determine the purpose of the evaluation and to apply the most appropriate methods for examining the role at different stages of development (Bryant-Lukosius, 2009). While numerous reviews document the effective outcomes of APN roles (e.g., Horrocks, Anderson, & Salisbury, 2002; Newhouse et al., 2011), the quality of individual APN studies included in the reviews is inconsistent. Advanced practice nurses frequently report that they lack the research knowledge, skills, and experience to evaluate the impact of their roles (Bryant-Lukosius, DiCenso, Browne, & Pinelli, 2004). A common limitation of APN role evaluations is the failure to use relevant theoretical frameworks and rigorous research methods in designing both the role and the evaluation plan. This contributes to poorly defined roles and evaluation designs that do not improve our understanding about the complexity of the role and relationships between role activities and outcomes, or how these roles did or did not achieve expected outcomes. Similarly, the lack of clearly defined APN roles and poor agreement among key stakeholders about expected role outcomes are barriers to the selection of APN-sensitive outcomes and the collection of baseline data for future comparative evaluations (Bryant-Lukosius et al., 2004).

This chapter reviews work being done in Canada to further APN outcomes research, by providing resources to address these five major barriers (i.e., lack of advanced practice nurse research expertise, guiding frameworks, role clarity, sensitive outcome measures, and baseline data) to evaluating these complex health care interventions. These resources include a nationally funded APN Research Chair to build research capacity and expertise; a conceptual framework and related toolkit for guiding the APN role design, implementation, and evaluation process; and an APN Research Data Collection Toolkit for selecting APN-sensitive outcome measurement tools and other measurement instruments relevant to different stages of role development. An overview of these research resources will be provided and their application to promote high-quality outcome assessments of APN roles will be examined.

## RESEARCH CHAIR IN APN

In 2000–2001, the Canadian Health Services Research Foundation (CHSRF), an organization established by the Canadian government, and the Canadian Institutes of Health Research (CIHR), the federal government's health research funding agency, partnered to create a number of nursing and health services chairs, each funded for 10 years. These chairs were created primarily to provide a mentoring and teaching resource for graduate and postgraduate students and junior faculty in health services and policy research. Unlike traditional research chairs, the focus of the CHSRF/CIHR chairs was on mentoring and education so as to build a capacity of new researchers who could independently contribute to applied health services and nursing research issues. Central to each chair's activities were partnerships with decision-making organizations to facilitate the conduct and dissemination of timely and policy-relevant research and to promote the use of research findings in health care planning and decision making.

One of these chairs was awarded to a co-author of this chapter (A.D.) and focused on APN. The goal of this chair program was to increase Canada's pool of nurse researchers with the ability to lead and conduct applied APN-related research that would meet the needs of clinicians, managers, and policy makers in the health sector. Chair activities designed to achieve this goal focused on (1) the education of nurse researchers at the graduate level, (2) linkage and exchange with decision makers to ensure policy relevance and the dissemination and uptake of research results, (3) mentoring of junior faculty and postdoctoral fellows to launch an APN-related research program, and (4) the conduct of research to inform the practice of APN across Canada.

Annually, through a competitive process, a maximum of three Canadian graduate students (both master's and PhD level) planning to conduct APN-related health services research were accepted into the Chair Program and awarded a $10,000 bursary. In addition to the university requirements for degree completion, the Chair Program required that all participating students (1) enroll in a graduate course on "Research Issues in the Introduction and Evaluation of APN Roles" specifically developed for APN Chair students and available via distance learning, (2) write an APN-related commentary for the journal *Evidence-Based Nursing*, (3) complete a 90-hour practicum in a policy setting and a 90-hour research internship with a senior research team, (4) identify an interdisciplinary thesis committee to oversee an APN-related health services research study, (5) partner with a decision maker to identify a policy-informing thesis topic, and (6) attend monthly meetings of Chair Program students via remote technology. Chair funding permitted graduate students from across the country to enroll in the APN-related graduate course by covering travel and accommodation costs for face-to-face classes at the beginning and end of the course, with teleconferencing and web-based communication for the remainder of the course.

## IMPACT OF THE CHAIR PROGRAM ON BUILDING APN RESEARCH CAPACITY AND EXPERTISE

Between 2001 and 2008, the Chair Program accepted 24 graduate students from five provinces across Canada (6 MSc, 16 PhD, and 2 Doctorate of Nursing Practice) who were enrolled in nine Canadian and American universities. Those who complete their PhDs were eligible to compete for a junior faculty position funded and supervised by the Chair Program with the goal to secure postdoctoral funding. Three junior faculty were funded through the Chair Program, all of whom were successful in subsequently competing for externally funded postdoctoral fellowship awards. Two additional postdoctoral fellows were supervised by the Chair. On completion of their research training, the postdoctoral fellows continued to participate in the Chair Program as

**Exhibit 12.1** *Sample Thesis Topics of APN Chair Program Students*

| |
|---|
| Nurse practitioner (NP)–physician collaboration collaborative service delivery models in long-term care |
| Facilitators and barriers to the implementation of an NP role in public health |
| Psychometric testing of the collaborative practice questionnaire: A measure of collaboration between NPs and physicians in primary care |
| Delineation of the clinical nurse specialist role in First Nations and Inuit communities |
| Practice patterns of CNSs working with First Nations and Inuit communities |
| Effectiveness of an APN role in secondary prevention of myocardial infarction |
| Development of an APN supportive care role in advanced prostate cancer |
| Participatory action research (PAR) with primary health care NPs: relevance of interprofessional collaboration to NP integration |
| Job satisfaction of primary care NPs |
| Development of an instrument to measure interprofessional collaboration |
| A case study of the implementation of the NP role in a regional health authority |
| Team perceptions of the effectiveness of the cardiology acute care NP role |

McMaster University-based senior faculty or as affiliate faculty from other Canadian universities. In addition to the graduate students, numerous advanced practice nurses from across Canada enrolled in the graduate course on "Research Issues in the Introduction and Evaluation of APN Roles." In total, 87 advanced practice nurses, graduate students, and health care administrators completed the course. The final assignment for this course was the preparation of a research proposal related to the development, implementation, or evaluation of an APN role. Exhibit 12.1 illustrates some of the student thesis topics of Chair Program graduate students.

Over the 10-year span of the APN Chair Program (2001–2011), its mandated effort to develop the research expertise of a large cadre of trainees had substantive impact on the capacity to conduct APN research in Canada. The program received over $3.5 million in additional research funding to complete 48 APN-focused studies. Research trainees and faculty presented their study findings and other scholarly work in 605 oral and 182 poster peer-reviewed presentations at national and international conferences and in 236 peer-reviewed publications and 21 book chapters. Through linkage and exchange activities among graduate students, advanced practice nurses, researchers, and health care administrators, the Chair Program fostered the development of other national APN research enterprises, supported national collaboration within research teams conducting APN research, and enabled the conduct of studies of national importance. For example, one clinical nurse specialist (CNS), who is also a co-author of this chapter (D.B.L.), transitioned through each research training opportunity provided by the Chair Program and went on to receive funding to establish a Canadian Centre of Excellence in Oncology APN. Similar to the APN Chair Program, this center provides research training, mentorship, and consultative services, and promotes the uptake of research findings through knowledge translation focused on advanced practice nurses in cancer control. More information about the center can be found at http://oapn.mcmaster.ca/.

Chair students and faculty from several provinces also collaborated to lead a landmark national study and interdisciplinary research team to examine the role of nurse practitioners (NPs) in long-term care settings. A second national study led by Chair faculty and graduate students established the foundation for the next generation of APN research in Canada (DiCenso & Bryant-Lukosius, 2010). In 2010, the results of this comprehensive study were summarized in a special issue of the *Canadian Journal of Nursing Leadership* that included 10 publications outlining evidence-based recommendations for the individual, organizational, and health system supports required to better integrate CNS and NP roles into the Canadian health care system. A major finding of this study was the need for further research about the outcomes and cost-effectiveness of APN roles within the context of the Canadian health care system. The special issue can be accessed freely online at http://www.longwoods.com/content/22264?utm_sou rce=Longwoods+Master+Mailing+List&utm_campaign=17b93e9e2d-NL_Vol23SP_Issue_TOC_Alert4_8_2011&utm_medium=email.

In July 2011, the 10-year funding for the Chair Program ended but its legacy continues with the establishment of the Canadian Centre for APN Research (CCAPNR) at McMaster University. As evidence of growing research capacity and the importance of succession planning to maintain research productivity and momentum, this center is led by senior and affiliate faculty from three provinces who are graduates of the Chair Program, with the former chair acting as its chief advisor. In contrast to the APN Chair Program, the primary focus of the center is on conducting research and on knowledge translation, with a continued but less prominent emphasis on the training and mentorship of APN researchers. To further the development of APN research expertise and to strengthen our understanding of these complex roles, CCAPNR has expanded its mandate to support collaborative, interdisciplinary research nationally and internationally. More information on CCAPNR can be found at http://fhs.mcmaster.ca/ccapnr/

Two additional resources arising from the Chair program are the PEPPA Framework and the APN Research Data Collection Toolkit. The PEPPA Framework was developed by a co-author of this chapter (D.B.L.) as a doctoral student in the APN Chair Program. PEPPA is an acronym for a participatory, evidence-informed, patient-centered process for APN role development, implementation, and evaluation (Bryant-Lukosius & DiCenso, 2004). As the Chair Program students planned and conducted their research, they used a number of existing data collection tools and developed a variety of instruments. Having become widely known across the country, the APN Chair Program was often approached by researchers and decision makers for information about the availability of APN-related research data collection tools. As a result, the Chair Program, with funding from a provincial decision maker partner, created the APN Research Data Collection Toolkit. Researchers conducting APN research may find both these resources, the PEPPA Framework and the APN Research Data Collection Toolkit, useful. The remainder of this chapter will describe these two resources.

## THE PEPPA FRAMEWORK

The PEPPA Framework was developed to provide APN researchers, health care providers, administrators, and policy makers with a guide to promoting the optimal development and deployment of APN roles. A critical feature of this framework is that strategies to support meaningful outcome evaluations of APN roles are incorporated throughout role planning and implementation. The underlying premise of the PEPPA Framework is that *the mandate of all APN roles is to maximize, maintain, or restore patient health through innovation in nursing practice and in the delivery of health services* (CNA, 2008; Davies & Hughes, 2002; Hamric, 2000; McGee & Castledine, 2003). This mandate is consistent with international views of advanced nursing practice. There is a heightened demand worldwide for advanced practice nurses, as clinical experts, leaders, and change agents, to assist organizations in developing sustainable models of health care (Bryant-Lukosius et al., 2004).

There is also a growing body of high-quality research documenting the positive impact of APN roles on patient, provider, and health system outcomes for a variety of patient populations (DiCenso &

Bryant-Lukosius, 2010; Horrocks et al., 2002; Newhouse et al., 2011). These reviews indicate that the value-added component of these roles is central to the underlying purpose and characteristics of advanced nursing practice. These characteristics include the provision of coordinated, integrated, holistic, and patient-centered care focused on maximizing health, quality of life, and functional capacity (Bryant-Lukosius et al., 2004). Opportunities for innovation and improved patient and health system outcomes are more likely to occur when the introduction of APN roles represents a complementary addition to the model of care rather than a transfer or substitution of role functions between health care providers.

An initial review of the international literature identified six frequently reported barriers that were common to the effective implementation of various types of APN roles (Bryant-Lukosius et al., 2004). A subsequent study involving a review of the international literature and examination of APN role implementation in Canada reconfirmed these challenges (DiCenso & Bryant-Lukosius, 2010). Many of these barriers could be avoided through improved planning and better stakeholder understanding of the roles (Exhibit 12.2). Initial and follow-up reviews of the literature (Bryant-Lukosius et al., 2004; DiCenso et al., 2010) also indicate that the costs associated with poor APN role implementation planning are high and justify the need for more thoughtful, systematic approaches to role introduction (Exhibit 12.3).

The PEPPA Framework builds on earlier models recommending steps for introducing new health providers (Spitzer, 1978) and specifically APN roles (Dunn & Nicklin, 1995; Mitchell-DiCenso, Pinelli, & Southwell, 1996), by incorporating additional steps and strategies to

#### Exhibit 12.2  *Common Barriers to APN Role Implementation*

| |
|---|
| Stakeholder confusion about APN terminology |
| Lack of clearly defined roles and role goals or outcomes |
| Role emphasis on physician replacement or support |
| Underutilization of APN scope of practice and expertise in all role dimensions |
| Failure to address role implementation barriers |
| Limited use of evidence-based approaches to guide role development, implementation, and evaluation |

*Source*: Bryant-Lukosius, D., DiCenso, A., Browne, G., & Pinelli, J. (2004). Advanced practice nursing roles: development, implementation, and evaluation. *Journal of Advanced Nursing*, 48(5), 519–529.

**Exhibit 12.3** *The Costs of Poor APN Role Implementation Planning*

| |
|---|
| Poor stakeholder role acceptance |
| Role conflict |
| Role overload |
| Poor advanced practice nurse job satisfaction |
| Difficulty recruiting and retaining highly qualified advanced practice nurses |
| Negative impact on the quality of patient care and patient safety |
| Unrealized opportunity for innovation and to benefit from APN expertise for patients, health providers, and the health care system |
| Ineffective use of limited health care resources |
| Negative impact on long-term role sustainability |

*Source*: Bryant-Lukosius, D., DiCenso, A., Browne, G., & Pinelli, J. (2004). Advanced practice nursing roles: development, implementation, and evaluation. *Journal of Advanced Nursing*, 48(5), 519–529

address known barriers to successful APN role implementation. The aims of the framework are to:

- Use relevant data to support the need and identified goals for a clearly defined role.
- Support advanced nursing practice characterized by patient-centered, health-focused, and holistic care.
- Promote the integration of APN knowledge, skills, and expertise from all role dimensions related to clinical practice, education, research, organizational leadership, and scholarly/professional practice (Canadian Association of Nurses in Oncology [CANO], 2001).
- Create practice environments that support APN role development by engaging stakeholders from the health care team, practice setting, and health care system in the role-planning process.
- Promote ongoing role development and model of care enhancement through continuous and rigorous evaluation of progress in achieving predetermined outcome-based goals.

## CONCEPTUAL FOUNDATIONS OF THE PEPPA FRAMEWORK

The principles of participatory action research (PAR) informed the development of the framework. PAR is a democratic, systematic approach that involves individuals from organizations, education systems, and communities in promoting health and social change (Deshler & Ewert, 1995; Foote Whyte, 1991; Smith, Pyrch, & Lizardi, 1993). Key principles of PAR include active participation in cycles of reflection and action; valuing what people know and believe by building on their current understanding; collective investigation, analysis, learning, and the conscious production of new knowledge; collective decision making and action in using new knowledge to address problems; and evaluating the impact of these actions (Bowling, 1997; Deshler & Ewert, 1995; Smith, 1997).

The principles of PAR are consistent with research-based app-roaches recommended for nursing and health human resource plan-ning (Advisory Committee on Health Deliver and Human Resources, 2007; O'Brien-Pallas, Tomblin Murphy, Baumann, & Birch, 2001). First, PAR promotes the use of objective data in health care planning and deci-sions to develop, implement, and modify an APN role. Early pioneers in the development of APN roles have also emphasized the importance of valid data to support the need for new health provider roles in the same way that research evidence is used to support the introduction of new therapeutic interventions such as medications (Spitzer, 1978). Second, advanced practice nurses work collaboratively within interprofessional teams and in established relationships with other stakeholders in the health system. Stakeholder roles and relationships are influenced by their values, beliefs, experiences, and expectations. These relationships create the conditions that impact the effective delivery of health care services and can facilitate or obstruct the implementation of APN roles. Therefore, collective learning and consensus decision making in the health planning process, on the part of key stakeholders, are necessary for the effective implementation of APN roles.

The principles of PAR are consistent with research-based approaches recommended for the planning of nursing and health and human resources (Advisory Committee on Health Delivery and Human Resources, 2007; O'Brien-Pallas, Tomblin Murphy, Baumann, & Birch, 2001). These include the principles of collaborative decision making through involvement of appropriate stakeholders, ensuring that target population health care needs are foundational to any pro-cess, consideration of environmental trends and drivers (context), and a system approach to ensure comprehensiveness in planning and in the assessment of outcomes.

The PEPPA Framework also draws on Donabedian's theory for evaluating the quality of health care by proposing a structure–process–outcome evaluation of the APN role (Donabedian, 1966, 1992). This approach is consistent with other structure–process–outcome mod-els developed to evaluate APN roles (Byers & Brunell, 1998; Grimes & Garcia, 1997; Sidani & Irvine, 1999). Structures are factors that affect processes or determine how the APN role is implemented. Role structures may include characteristics of the advanced practice nurse and patient population; APN education programs; practical and financial resources; nursing and health care policies; regulatory and credentialing mechanisms; the model of care; and the physical, cultural, and organizational environment in which the advanced practice nurse works (Bryant-Lukosius et al., 2004). Process refers to what the advanced practice nurse does in the role. This includes the types of APN services and how these services are provided. To ensure maximal use of APN expertise and scope of practice, the PEPPA Framework recommends that role processes be considered across all dimensions of advanced nursing practice related to clinical practice, education, research, organizational leadership, and scholarly and professional development (CANO, 2001).

Outcomes are the results of APN role services and care and thus are affected by both structure and process factors. In the framework, outcomes may be evaluated from the perspectives of patients and families, the advanced practice nurse, other health care providers, the organization, and the broader health care system. Outcomes are determined by goals for improving the delivery of nursing and health care services established early in the APN role-planning process. A package of APN services and specific role activities for each dimension of advanced nursing practice are developed specifically to achieve these pre-established goals. Strategically linking APN role activities with pre-set goals and outcomes facilitates the selection of outcome measures that will be most sensitive to APN interventions (Burns, 2001; Minnick, 2001).

The ability to conduct meaningful evaluations of the APN role is further strengthened by linking role structures, processes, and outcomes in the early stages of role development. For example, in the PEPPA Framework, the APN role is evaluated along with the model of care in which the role is situated. This strategy aids in determining how structures within the model of care (e.g., health provider roles, role relationships, and resources), influence APN role processes and outcomes.

Finally, the PEPPA Framework posits that there is sufficient worldwide literature demonstrating that well-designed and sufficiently developed APN roles are effective in achieving positive outcomes for patients, providers, and the health care system (Brooten et al., 2002; DiCenso & Bryant-Lukosius, 2010; Fulton & Baldwin, 2004; Newhouse et al., 2011). Thus, important questions to address when evaluating APN roles are not "Are APN roles effective?" but "How are APN roles effective?" and "For which patient populations, under which conditions, and in which models of care delivery are APN roles most effective?"

## STEPS OF THE PEPPA FRAMEWORK

The PEPPA Framework involves a nine-step process (see Figure 12.1). These steps reflect the complexity of the roles and are consistent with guidelines for developing and evaluating complex health care interventions that stress the importance of (1) using the best evidence to design the intervention, (2) developing a theory or clear picture for how the different components of the intervention are expected to lead to desired outcomes, and (3) incorporating process evaluations to test and refine the intervention prior to a full scale outcome evaluation (Craig et al., 2008). Steps 1 to 6 focus on establishing role structures and processes and developing an evaluation plan. This includes health care planning and decision making about the need for an APN role and designing multi-components of the role to address identified gaps and to achieve expected outcomes. Step 7 focuses on role processes and initiating the implementation plan and introduction of the APN role. Steps 8 and 9 include the short- and long-term evaluations of the APN role and the new model of care in which it takes place to assess progress, refine the role, and promote role sustainability in achieving pre-determined goals and outcomes.

*Step 1: Define the population and describe the current model of care.*

The purpose of Step 1 is to set some parameters or limits on the health care planning process. This includes identification of a priority patient population as the central focus of the process. Second, the scope of the process is determined by focusing on relationships and interactions from a team, organizational, and/or geographic perspective. Efforts are made to describe and understand the current model of care by identifying how and when patients interact with health care providers and services.

*Step 2: Identify stakeholders and recruit participants.*

In this step, key individuals who represent important stakeholder groups that are integral to the current model of care are identified and invited to participate in the health care redesign process. Strategies are employed to ensure a breadth of input from various stakeholders, including patients and families. The selection of participants also considers their roles and responsibilities within the model of care and their importance in facilitating the implementation of the new model of care and potential APN role.

*Step 3: Determine the need for a new model of care.*

In this step, the strengths and limitations of the current model of care for meeting patient health needs are assessed from a variety of stakeholder viewpoints. This involves conducting a needs assessment

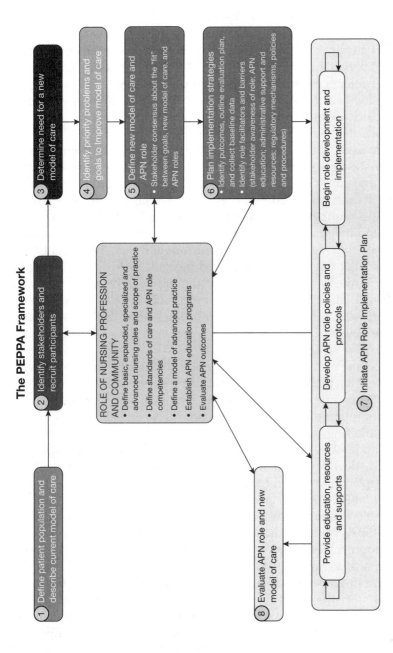

**The PEPPA Framework**

**ROLE OF NURSING PROFESSION AND COMMUNITY**
- Define basic, expanded, specialized and advanced nursing roles and scope of practice
- Define standards of care and APN role competencies
- Define a model of advanced practice
- Establish APN education programs
- Evaluate APN outcomes

1. Define patient population and describe current model of care
2. Identify stakeholders and recruit participants
3. Determine need for a new model of care
4. Identify priority problems and goals to Improve model of care
5. Define new model of care and APN role
   - Stakeholder consensus about the "fit" between goals, new model of care, and APN roles
6. Plan implementation strategies
   - Identify outcomes, outline evaluation plan, and collect baseline data
   - Identify role facilitators and barriers (stakeholder awareness of role; APN education; administrative support and resources; regulatory mechanisms, policies and procedures)
7. Initiate APN Role Implementation Plan

Provide education, resources and supports

Develop APN role policies and protocols

Begin role development and implementation

8. Evaluate APN role and new model of care

**Figure 12.1** *The PEPPA Framework: A Participatory, Evidence-Based, Patient-Focused Process for APN Role Development, Implementation, and Evaluation*

*Source:* Bryant-Lukosius, D., & DiCenso, A. (2004). A framework for the introduction and evaluation of advanced practice nursing roles. *Journal of Advanced Nursing, 48*(5), 530–540.

to collect and/or generate information about the extent, severity, and importance of unmet patient health needs and about the health care services required to meet these needs.

*Step 4: Identify priority problems and goals to improve the model of care.*

In this step, participating stakeholders come to consensus regarding unmet patient health needs that are the most important to address. Priority problems associated with unmet health needs are identified, and outcome-based goals to improve the model of care delivery and patient health are established.

*Step 5: Define the new model of care and APN role.*

This step involves identifying strategies and solutions for achieving established goals and expected outcomes. The need for new care practices and care delivery strategies is determined and the research evidence about best practices is reviewed to design the new model of care. The number, complement, and mix of health care providers required to implement the new model of care are examined. It is during this step that participants learn more about the purpose and types of various APN roles. The need for and the pros and cons of introducing an APN role rather than other nursing or health provider roles are considered. If an APN role is to be implemented, this step concludes with the development of a specific job description for an APN role within the new model of care.

*Step 6: Plan implementation strategies.*

In this step, participants develop a plan to ensure system readiness for the role. This includes obtaining funding approval (if required) and identifying potential barriers to and facilitators of role implementation. Key factors relating to advanced practice nurse and stakeholder education, marketing, recruitment and hiring, role-reporting structures, funding, and policy development are assessed. An important aspect of this stage is developing an evaluation plan and establishing timelines for role implementation and achievement of outcome-based goals.

*Step 7: Initiate APN role implementation plan.*

This step begins by initiating the role implementation plan developed in Step 6 and hiring an advanced practice nurse for the position. Full development and implementation of the APN role may take 3 to 5 years (Hamric & Taylor, 1989). During this period, efforts are made to monitor progress in role development and to modify or initiate strategies to support the implementation of the APN role. As Figure 12.1 illustrates, role implementation is a continuous process, in which the need for new organizational policies, procedures, and other supports are influenced by changes within the practice setting and the stage of APN role development.

*Step 8: Evaluate the APN role and new model of care.*

In this step, formative evaluations that systematically evaluate APN role structures, processes, and outcomes are recommended as a strategy to promote ongoing role development. Several studies have demonstrated the importance of assessing APN role structures and processes to identify role barriers and facilitators (Guest et al., 2001; Read et al., 2001). In this type of evaluation, progress in achieving outcome-based goals is monitored, and APN role structures and processes are examined to identify additional needs for supporting role development and implementation and further role enhancement.

*Step 9: Monitor APN role and model of care over the long term.*

This step emphasizes the continuous and iterative process of ensuring that the APN role and the model of care, in which it is situated, continue to be relevant, sustainable, and improved, based on new research and/or changes in the health care environment, patient needs, and treatment practices. Long-term monitoring of well-established roles is also helpful for maintaining a common vision for the role among key stakeholders (Seymour et al., 2002).

## CURRENT APPLICATIONS OF THE PEPPA FRAMEWORK

The PEPPA Framework is incorporated into the curricula of Canadian APN education programs for NPs in primary, acute, and anesthesia care (Donald, 2008; University of Toronto, Lawrence S. Bloomberg Faculty of Nursing, 2008). The APN Chair Program also used the framework as the basis for the graduate nursing course on "Research Issues in the Introduction and Evaluation of APN Roles" (McMaster University School of Nursing, Health Sciences Library, 2008). The framework has been used to inform the design of studies and systematic programs of research for APN roles in oncology (Bryant-Lukosius et al., 2007; Martelli-Reid et al., 2007; Slater, Rosenzweig, & Steele, 2009), primary health care (Martin-Misener, Reilly, & Robinson Vollman, 2010), and in long-term care (Donald, 2007; Donald et al., 2012; Kaasalainen, DiCenso, Donald, & Staples, 2007). Graduate students have used the PEPPA Framework to guide their thesis research regarding APN roles and services for patients with inflammatory bowel disease (Westin, 2009) and those requiring psychiatric mental health care (Brady, 2010).

In Canada, the framework has been recommended as a best practice for implementing APN roles (CNA, 2008) as well as nursing roles and models of care involving interprofessional teams (Virani, 2012). The framework is being used by large regional health authorities to implement new

NP roles (Sawchenko, 2007) and to develop policies to support the successful implementation of NP and CNS roles in regional health authority practice settings (Advanced Practice Nursing Steering Committee, Winnipeg Regional Health Authority, 2005; Lewthwaite et al., 2013).

Several published studies and reports document the benefits and illustrate the applicability of the PEPPA Framework for the successful implementation of APN roles in varied specialties and for other health provider roles such as advanced physiotherapist roles for patients undergoing hip and knee replacement surgery (Robarts, Kennedy, MacLeod, Findlay, & Gollish, 2008), advanced radiation therapists in cancer care (Cancer Care Ontario, 2011), and physician assistants in emergency departments (Ducharme, Buckley, Alder, & Pelletier, 2009). In a long-term care setting, the framework's emphasis on stakeholder engagement to identify role priorities, to establish a common vision, and to participate in the planning process contributed to the successful implementation of a unique NP model of care (McAiney et al., 2008). The NPs were found to improve staff confidence and reduce hospital admission rates by 39% to 43% (McAiney et al., 2008). Application of the framework's steps was found to provide the structure for guiding the process and anticipating activities for introducing a new specialized NP in cardiac surgery (McNamara, Giguere, St. Louis, & Boileau, 2009). The PEPPA Framework was found to be an effective change management tool for introducing NPs and physician assistants into the emergency department (Ducharme et al., 2009). Key framework strengths were team-building strategies to motivate and support change, and the importance of conducting a needs assessment and environmental scan to identify and address barriers to role implementation. In a project to introduce advanced physiotherapist roles, the flexibility of the framework as a planning guide enabled the redesign process to be completed over a short period of time, fostered quick wins and early buy-in to the role, and led to a new model of care that matched patients' needs with providers with the most appropriate skill set (Robarts et al., 2008).

In a recent PAR study, we examined the impact of the PEPPA Framework, a team facilitator, and a toolkit of resources specific to each step of the framework on the introduction of oncology APN roles for underserved patient populations (Bakker et al., 2009). Similar to other reports (Ducharme, et al., 2009; McAiney et al., 2008; Robarts et al., 2008), the high level of team and stakeholder engagement at each step of the framework was important for promoting their support and acceptance of the new APN role. Team function and positive group dynamics also improved over time for implementation teams involved in the role planning process. The implementation teams also noted that the framework enabled them to identify gaps in care delivery and to develop an APN role job description that was relevant to patient needs. The teams reported that a facilitator with experience in the introduction of advanced practice nurses was beneficial for moving the role-planning process along and for implementing the steps in a way that was relevant to their practice setting and patient population.

In this same study, a draft toolkit utilized and evaluated by the implementation teams was found to provide an "essential roadmap" for guiding the process and keeping the team on track. Varied resources, tools, and activities also aided in the collection of data and facilitated group decision making at each step of the framework. Real-time evaluation data and feedback collected from the implementation teams were also used to refine and augment the final toolkit that is available free of charge in an electronic format (Bryant-Lukosius, 2009). One example of a strategy and resource outlined in the toolkit is the use of a logic model that is developed in steps 4 to 6 of the framework. As Figure 12.2 illustrates, a logic model is very helpful for illustrating the complexity of the APN role and the relationship among role activities and the timing of expected outcomes. Another toolkit, based in part on the PEPPA Framework, has also been developed by the Canadian Nurse Practitioner Initiative (2006) to support health care planners and administrators with the introduction of NP roles, particularly in primary health care settings.

## APN RESEARCH DATA COLLECTION TOOLKIT

In an effort to facilitate APN-related research, the APN Research Data Collection Toolkit was developed and is fully accessible via the APN Chair Program website (http://apntoolkit.mcmaster.ca/). The objective of the toolkit is to identify instruments that could be used to facilitate data collection for monitoring and measuring a variety of variables at different stages of APN role development, implementation, and evaluation. Focused on APN, the toolkit includes instruments that have been used in research related to CNSs as well as to primary and acute care NPs. The toolkit is an ongoing initiative to create a compendium of common instruments used in APN research. It was developed with the following users in mind: APN researchers, graduate students planning APN research, and decision makers seeking to evaluate one or more dimensions of APN roles (i.e., structures, processes, and outcomes).

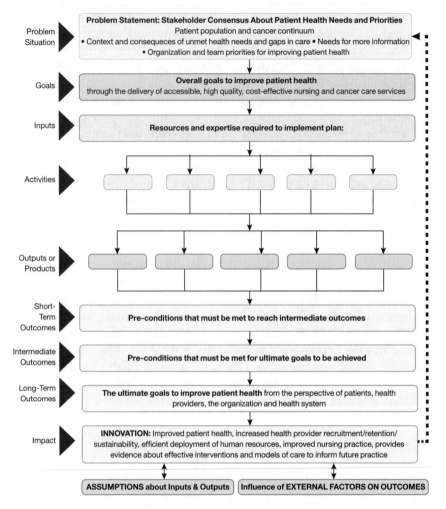

**Figure 12.2** *Logic Model for APN Role Development, Implementation, and Evaluation*

*Source:* Bryant-Lukosius, D. (2009). *Designing innovative cancer services and advanced practice nursing roles: Toolkit.* Toronto: Cancer Care Ontario. Retrieved February 5, 2013, from https://www.cancercare.on.ca/common/pages/UserFile.aspx?fileId=76090

The steps involved in producing the toolkit include (1) identifying and appraising measurement tools used in APN research, (2) compiling the results into a publicly accessible web page, and (3) promoting the website, so that those introducing and evaluating APN roles can use the resource and contribute their own instruments to it. The first step taken to identify relevant measurement tools was to review the studies included in systematic reviews of APN-focused research (e.g., Horrocks et al., 2002) and in books focused on APN-related outcome measures (e.g., Kleinpell, 2001). Second, all APN-related research conducted through the APN Chair Program was reviewed and measurement tools extracted. Third, a systematic search of the literature focused on APN practitioners was conducted. These citations were reviewed by two APN researchers to identify relevant studies. Data collection instruments identified in any relevant studies were included in the toolkit.

Once a relevant measurement tool is identified, the primary author is contacted and asked to provide any additional information regarding the measurement instrument, an electronic copy of the instrument itself, and permission to post the tool on the APN Toolkit website. Exhibit 12.4 illustrates the type of information compiled for each instrument. The instruments are organized according to the steps of the PEPPA Framework, so that users of the website can link the instruments with the distinct steps described in this framework (e.g., needs assessment, describing the model of care, defining the APN role, role implementation and practice patterns, barriers to and facilitators of APN integration, and outcomes evaluation). The summary developed for each instrument is sent to the instrument developer, who is asked to review it for accuracy.

The APN Toolkit website is housed on a secure server in the McMaster University domain area. Navigation of the web page is available through a sidebar menu, as well as through the table of contents. To further facilitate ease of information retrieval, there is a keyword search function where users can enter a keyword to see if it is contained anywhere in the APN Toolkit website. Links to a PDF copy of the instrument are available to users, where permission has been granted by authors. Users are invited to submit references for instruments, updates, and corrections via a web form. Users are also invited to submit any tools they have created that are not yet in the toolkit.

The APN Toolkit is an ever-growing resource that currently houses summaries of over 100 instruments. This toolkit will be an important resource for those introducing and evaluating APN roles by making available existing instruments that have been used, for example, to conduct needs assessments, measure practice patterns, identify barriers and facilitators, and evaluate provider and patient outcomes related to APN.

In summary, the establishment of a nationally funded research chair has facilitated the training of the next generation of Canadian nurse researchers who will continue to expand our knowledge about the effective development and deployment of APN roles for improving

**Exhibit 12.4** *An Example of an APN-Related Data Collection Tool as Summarized in the APN Data Collection Toolkit.*

---

### *Misener Nurse Practitioner Job Satisfaction Scale (MNPJSS)*

Original Citation—Misener TR, Cox DL. Development of the Misener Nurse Practitioner Job Satisfaction Scale. *Journal of Nursing Measurement.* 2001; 9(1):91–108.

Contact Information De Anna L. Cox College of Nursing University of South Carolina, Columbia, SC 29208, USA. Phone: 803–777-4390 dlcox@gwm.sc.edu

Price and Availability—Published in original citation. Contact author for permission to use.

Brief Description of Instrument—Assessment of job satisfaction of primary care NPs. Scale Format—44 items each measured using a 6-point Likert scale. Response options: "Very Satisfied" 6, "Satisfied" 5, "Minimally Satisfied" 4, "Minimally Dissatisfied" 3, "Dissatisfied" 2, and "Very Dissatisfied" 1 point. One item for global satisfaction measured on a 10-point scale, 10 being the highest level of job satisfaction. Administration Technique—Self-administered questionnaire. Scoring and Interpretation—Total score is obtained by summing all 44 items. Subscale score is obtained by summing the subscale items. Factors and Norms—6 factors determined by factor analysis: (1) Intrapractice Partnership/Collegiality, (2) Challenge/Autonomy, (3) Professional, Social, and Community Interaction, (4) Professional Growth, (5) Time, and (6) Benefits. Item mean (SD) reported in original citation. Internal Consistency—Cronbach's alpha on entire scale: 0.96; Cronbach's alphas on subscales range from 0.79 to 0.94. Content and Face Validity—Instrument development based on literature review, review of existing instruments, and input from numerous NP experts. Strengths—Easy to administer and score, covers a wide variety of previously published factors associated with job satisfaction. Limitations—Relies heavily on factor analysis results to justify subscale, lacking theoretical rationale. Published APN studies using instrument—See original citation. PEPPA Framework Category—8 patient, provider, and health system outcomes. Initially, through the CHSRF/CIHR Chair in APN and now CCAPNR, APN researchers, educators, health providers, and decision makers have access to critically appraised tools for conducting APN-related research. As a relatively new resource, the PEPPA Framework has demonstrated wide applicability for the introduction of advanced nursing and other health provider roles. The framework is suitable for designing and evaluating the complex nature of APN roles and can be employed to inform APN curricula and health care policies in support of APN, to establish systematic approaches for role evaluation, and to develop APN-focused programs of research.

## Answers to Chapter Discussion Questions

1. Like APN roles, complex health care interventions are those that have a number of interacting components, address difficult health care problems or behaviors, target a number of groups or organizations, aim to improve several and/or variable outcomes, and are flexible or tailored to specific health care contexts (Craig et al., 2008).

2. Common barriers to conducting APN role evaluations that provide meaningful results about role outcomes include lack of advanced practice nurse research expertise, failure to utilize relevant theoretical frameworks and rigorous research methods in designing the role and role evaluation plan, lack of clearly defined roles with pre-determined outcomes that are linked with APN role activities, lack of baseline data to permit future comparative evaluations, and the use of outcome measures not sensitive to APN role activities (Bryant-Lukosius et al., 2004; DiCenso et al., 2010).

3. Key principles of PAR include active participation in cycles of reflection and action; valuing what people know and believe by building on their current understanding; collective investigation, analysis, learning, and the conscious production of new knowledge; collective decision making and action in using new knowledge to address problems; and evaluating the impact of these actions (Bowling, 1997; Deshler & Ewert, 1995; Smith, 1997). These principles promote the generation and use of objective data critical for health care planning and introduction of new roles. Advanced practice nurses work collaboratively within interprofessional teams and in established relationships with other stakeholders in the health system. These rela-

tionships create the conditions that influence the effective delivery of health care services and can facilitate or obstruct the implementation of APN roles. Therefore, collective learning and consensus decision making in the health-planning process are necessary for the effective implementation of APN roles.

4. Structures are factors that affect processes or determine how the APN role is implemented (i.e., advanced practice nurse education, patient population, nursing and health care policies). Process refers to what the advanced practice nurse does in the role (i.e., types of APN services and how these services are provided). Outcomes are the results of APN role services and care and thus are affected by both structure and process factors (i.e., improved patient quality of life, improved health care provider satisfaction, and reduction in wait times). The PEPPA Framework proposes that the role structures, processes, and outcomes and their relationships within the context of the model of care and organizational environment should be determined during the early stages of role development and evaluated throughout the role implementation journey.

## REFERENCES

Advanced Practice Nursing Steering Committee, Winnipeg Regional Health Authority. (2005). *A guide to the implementation of the nurse practitioner role in your health care setting.* Retrieved February 5, 2013, from http://www.wrha.mb.ca/professionals/nursing/files/NP-Toolkit.pdf

Advisory Committee on Health Delivery and Human Resources. (2007). *A framework for collaborative pan-Canadian health human resources planning.* Ottawa, ON: Author.

Bakker, D., Bryant-Lukosius, D., Wiernikowski, J., Conlon, M., Baxter, P., Green, E., . . . DiCenso, A. (2009). Enhancing knowledge, promoting quality: Evaluating the implementation of oncology APN roles. Oral presentation. *International Conference on Cancer Nursing*, Atlanta, Georgia.

Bowling, A. (1997). *Research methods in health: Investigating health and health services.* Philadelphia, PA: Open University Press.

Brady, R. L. (2010). *Introducing a new psychiatric mental health nurse practitioner role in a mental health agency* (Master's thesis). Available from ProQuest Dissertations and Theses Database. (UMI No. 1475129)

Brooten, D., Naylor, M. D., York, R., Brown, L. P., Hazard Munro, B., Hollingsworth, A. O., et al. (2002). Lessons learned from testing the quality cost model of advanced practice nursing (APN) transitional care. *Journal of Nursing Scholarship, 34*, 369–375.

Bryant-Lukosius, D. (2009). *Designing innovative cancer services and advanced practice nursing roles: Toolkit.* Toronto: Cancer Care Ontario. Retrieved

February 5, 2013, from https://www.cancercare.on.ca/common/pages/UserFile.aspx?fileId=76090

Bryant-Lukosius, D., & DiCenso, A. (2004). A framework for the introduction and evaluation of advanced practice nursing roles. *Journal of Advanced Nursing, 48,* 530–540.

Bryant-Lukosius, D., DiCenso, A., Browne, G., & Pinelli, J. (2004). Advanced practice nursing roles: Issues affecting role development, implementation, and evaluation. *Journal of Advanced Nursing, 48,* 519–529.

Bryant-Lukosius, D., Green, E., Fitch, M., Macartney, G., Robb-Blenderman, L., McFarlane, S.,...Milne, H. (2007). A survey of oncology advanced practice nurses in Ontario: Profile and predictors of job satisfaction. *Canadian Journal of Nursing Leadership, 20*(2), 50–68.

Burns, S. M. (2001). Selecting advanced practice nurse outcome measures. In R. M. Kleinpell (Ed.), *Outcome assessment in advanced practice nursing* (1st ed., pp. 73–90). New York, NY: Springer Publishing.

Byers, J., & Brunell, M. (1998). Demonstrating the value of the advanced practice nurse: An evaluation model. *AACN Clinical Issues, 9,* 296–305.

Canadian Association of Nurses in Oncology. (2001). *Standards of care, roles in oncology nursing, role competencies.* Kanata, ON: Author.

Canadian Nurse Practitioner Initiative. (2006). *Implementation and evaluation toolkit for nurse practitioners in Canada.* Retrieved February 4, 2013, from http://23072.vws.magma.ca/cna/documents/pdf/publications/Toolkit_Implementation_Evaluation_NP_e.pdf

Canadian Nurses Association. (2008). *Advanced nursing practice—A national framework.* Ottawa, ON: Author.

Cancer Care Ontario. (2011). *Clinical specialist radiation therapist implementation sustainability project: Toolkit.* Toronto: Cancer Care Ontario. Retrieved February 5, 2013, from https://www.cancercare.on.ca/common/pages/UserFile.aspx?fileId=119464

Craig, P., Dieppe, P., Macintyre, S., Michie, S., Nazareth, I., & Petticrew, M. (2008). Developing and evaluating complex interventions: The new Medical Research Council guidance. *British Medical Journal, 337.* doi:10.1136/bmj.a1655.

Davies, B., & Hughes, A. M. (2002). Clarification of advanced nursing practice: Characteristics and competencies. *Clinical Nurse Specialist, 16,* 147–152.

Deshler, D., & Ewert, M. (1995). *Participatory action research: Traditions and major assumptions.* Retrieved November 19, 2001, from www.oac.uoguelph.ca/~pi/pdrc/articles/article.1

DiCenso, A., & Bryant-Lukosius, D. (2010). *Clinical nurse specialists and nurse practitioners in Canada: A decision support synthesis.* Ottawa, ON: Canadian Health Services Research Foundation. Retrieved February 5, 2013, from http://www.chsrf.ca/PublicationsAndResources/ResearchReports/CommissionedResearch/10–06-01/b9cb9576–6140-4954-aa57–2b81c1350936.aspx

DiCenso, A., Bryant-Lukosius, D., Martin-Misener, R., Donald, F., Carter, N., Bourgeault, I.,...Kioke, S. (2010). Factors enabling advanced practice nursing role integration. *Canadian Journal of Nursing Leadership, 23*(special issue), 211–238.

Donabedian, A. (1966). Evaluating the quality of medical care. *Milbank Memorial Quarterly, 44,* 166–203.

Donabedian, A. (1992, November). Commentary: The role of outcomes in quality assessment and assurance. *Quality Review Bulletin, 18*(11), 356–360.

Donald, F. (2007). *Collaborative practice by nurse practitioners and physicians in long-term care homes: A mixed method study.* Unpublished doctoral thesis, McMaster University.

Donald, F. (2008). *The Ontario Primary Health Care Nurse Practitioner Program.* (Integrative practicum, provincial course professor; personal communication).

Donald, F., Martin-Misener, R., Carter, N., McAiney, C., Kaasalainen, S., Ploeg, J.,...Dobbins, M. (2012). *The nurse practitioner role in Canadian long-term care settings: A mixed-methods study.* In 7th International Council of Nurses International Nurse Practitioner/Advanced Practice Nursing Network (INP/APNN) Conference, London, UK. Oral presentation, Accepted for August 20–22.

Ducharme, J., Buckley, J., Alder, R., & Pelletier, C. (2009). The application of change management principles to facilitate the introduction of nurse practitioners and physician assistants into six Ontario Emergency Departments. *Healthcare Quarterly, 12*(2), 70–77.

Dunn, K., & Nicklin, W. (1995, January–February). The status of advanced nursing roles in Canadian teaching hospitals. *Canadian Journal of Nursing Administration, 8*(1), 111–135.

Foote Whyte, W. (1991). *Participatory action research.* London, England: Sage.

Fulton, J. S., & Baldwin, K. (2004). An annotated bibliography reflecting CNS practice and outcomes. *Clinical Nurse Specialist, 18,* 21–39.

Grimes, D. E., & Garcia, M. K. (1997). Advanced practice nursing and work site primary care: Challenges for outcomes evaluation. *Advanced Practice Nurse Quarterly, 3,* 19–28.

Guest, D., Peccei, R., Rosenthal, P., Montgomery, J., Redfern, S., Young, C., Wilson-Barnett, J., et al. (2001). *Preliminary evaluation of the establishment of nurse, midwife and health visitor consultants. Report to the Department of Health.* University of London, Kings College.

Hamric, A. (2000). A definition of advanced nursing practice. In A. B. Hamric, J. A. Spross, & C. M. Hanson (Eds.), *Advanced nursing practice: An integrative approach* (pp. 53–73). Philadelphia, PA: W. B. Saunders.

Hamric, A. B., & Taylor, J. W. (1989). Role development of the CNS. In A. B. Hamric & J. Spross (Eds.), *The clinical nurse specialist in theory and practice* (2nd ed., pp. 41–82). Philadelphia, PA: W. B. Saunders.

Horrocks, S., Anderson, E., & Salisbury, C. (2002). Systematic review of whether nurse practitioners working in primary care can provide equivalent care to doctors. *British Medical Journal, 324,* 819–823.

Kaasalainen, S., DiCenso, A., Donald, F., & Staples, E. (2007). Optimizing the role of the nurse practitioner to improve pain management in long-term care. *Canadian Journal of Nursing Research, 39*(2), 14–31.

Kleinpell, R. (Ed.). (2001). *Outcome assessment in advanced practice nursing* (1st ed.). New York, NY: Springer Publishing.

Lewthwaite, B., Hearson, B., Cusack, C., Sawatzky-Dickson, D., Robertson, J., Doerksen, K., Yasinski, L., Streeter, L., Avery, L., & Boitson, S. (2012). A guide for successful integration of a clinical nurse specialist. Winnipeg Regional Health Authority. Retrieved February 5, 2013, from http://www.wrha.mb.ca/professionals/nursing/files/CNS-Toolkit.pdf

Martelli-Reid, L., Bryant-Lukosius, D., Arnold, A., Ellis, P., Goffin, J., Okawara, G.,...Hapke, S. (2007). *A model of interprofessional research to support the development of an advanced practice nursing role in cancer care.* Poster presentation at the Canadian Association of Nurses in Oncology Conference, Vancouver, BC.

Martin-Misener, R., Reilly, S. M, & Vollman, A. R. (2010). Defining the role of primary health care nurse practitioners in rural Nova Scotia. *Canadian Journal of Nursing Research, 42*(2), 30–47.

McAiney, C. A., Haughton, D., Jennings, J., Farr, D., Hillier, L., & Morden, P. (2008). A unique practice model for nurse practitioners in long-term care homes. *Journal of Advanced Nursing, 62*, 562–571.

McGee, P., & Castledine, G. (2003). A definition of advanced practice for the UK. In P. McGee & G. Castledine (Eds.), *Advanced nursing practice* (2nd ed., pp. 17–30). Oxford, England: Blackwell.

McMaster University School of Nursing, Health Sciences Library. (2008). *Finding resources for Nursing 706: Research issues in the introduction and evaluation of advanced practice nursing roles.* Retrieved February 5, 2013, from http://www.apnnursingchair.mcmaster.ca/education_researchissues.html

McNamara, S., Giguere, V., St. Louis, L., & Boileau, J. (2009). Development and implementation of the specialized nurse practitioner role: Use of the PEPPA framework to achieve success. *Nursing and Health Sciences, 11*, 318–325.

Minnick, A. (2001). General design and implementation challenges in outcomes assessment. In R. M. Kleinpell (Ed.), *Outcome assessment in advanced practice nursing* (1st ed., pp. 91–102). New York, NY: Springer Publishing.

Mitchell-DiCenso, A., Pinelli, J., & Southwell, D. (1996). Introduction and evaluation of an advanced nursing practice role in neonatal intensive care. In K. Kelly (Ed.). *Outcomes of effective management practice* (pp 171–186). Thousand Oaks, CA: Sage.

Newhouse, R. P., Stanik-Hutt, J., White, K. M., Johantgen, M., Bass, E. B., Zangaro, G.,...Weiner, J. P. (2011). Advanced practice nurse outcomes 1990–2008: A systematic review. *Nursing Economics, 29*(5), 230–250.

O'Brien-Pallas, L., Tomblin Murphy, G., Baumann, A., & Birch, S. (2001). Framework for analyzing health human resources. In *Canadian Institute for Health Information. Future Development of Information to Support the*

*Management of Nursing Resources: Recommendations.* Ottawa, ON: Canadian Institute for Health Information.

Read, S., Jones, M. L., Collins, K., McDonnell, A., Jones, R., Doyal, L., . . . Scholes, J. (2001). *Exploring new roles in practice (ENRIP) final report.* Sheffield: University of Sheffield. Retrieved February 5, 2013, from http://www.shef.ac.uk/content/1/c6/01/33/98/enrip.pdf

Robarts, S., Kennedy, D., MacLeod, A. M., Findlay, H., & Gollish, J. (2008). A framework for the development and implementation of an advanced practice role for physiotherapists that improves access and quality care for patients. *Healthcare Quarterly, 11*(2), 67–75.

Sawchenko, L. (2007). An evidence-informed approach to the introduction of nurse practitioners in British Columbia's Interior Health Authority. *Links, 10*(3), 4. Retrieved February 5, 2013, from http://www.cfhi-fcass.ca/Migrated/PDF/Links/links_v10n3_e.pdf

Seymour, J., Clark, D., Hughes, P., Bath, P., Beech, N., Corner, J., . . . Webb, T. (2002). Clinical nurse specialists in palliative care. Part 3. Issues for the Macmillan Nurse role. *Palliative Medicine, 16,* 386–394.

Sidani, S., & Irvine, D. (1999). A conceptual framework for evaluating the nurse practitioner role in acute care settings. *Journal of Advanced Nursing, 30*(1), 58–66.

Slater, A., Rosenzweig, M., & Steele, C. (2009). Workflow analysis in one community oncology outpatient setting: Advanced practice nurse versus physicians. *Oncology Nursing Forum, 36*(3), 33.

Smith, S. E. (1997). Deepening participatory action-research. In S. E. Smith & D. G. Willms (Eds.), *Nurtured by knowledge: Learning to do participatory action-research* (pp. 173–264). New York, NY: Apex Press.

Smith, S. E., Pyrch, T., & Lizardi, A. (1993). Participatory action-research for health. *World Health Forum, 14,* 319–324.

Spitzer, W. O. (1978). Evidence that justifies the introduction of new health professionals. In P. Slayton & M. J. Trebilcock (Eds.), *The professions and public policy* (pp. 211–236). Toronto: University of Toronto Press.

University of Toronto, Lawrence S. Bloomberg Faculty of Nursing. (2008). *Nurse Practitioner in Anesthesia Care Program. Course outlines.* Retrieved February 5, 2013, from http://bloomberg.nursing.utoronto.ca/academic/programs/graduate-diploma/post-master-of-nursing-np-field-diploma-in-anaesthesia-care

Virani, T. (2012). *Interprofessional collaborative teams.* A commissioned report for the Canadian Nurses Association and published by the Canadian Health Services Research Foundation. Retrieved February 5, 2013, from http://www.chsrf.ca/Libraries/Commissioned_Research_Reports/Virani-Interprofessional-EN.sflb.ashx

Westin, L. (2009). *Advanced nursing practice in nurse-led inflammatory bowel disease support service* (Master's thesis). Retrieved February 5, 2013, from https://dspace.library.uvic.ca:8443//handle/1828/4120

# Index